Clinics in Developmental Medicine

# Medical Care of Newborn Babies

PAMELA A. DAVIES

R. J. ROBINSON

J. W. SCOPES

J. P. M. TIZARD

J. S. WIGGLESWORTH

1972

Spastics International Medical Publications

LONDON : William Heinemann Medical Books Ltd.

PHILADELPHIA : J. B. Lippincott Co.

First Published 1972

Reprinted 1978


ISBN 0 433 32375 2

Pamela A. Davies, M.D., F.R.C.P.,
Senior Lecturer in Paediatrics.

R. J. Robinson, B.M., D. Phil., M.R.C.P.,
Senior Lecturer in Paediatrics.*

J. W. Scopes, M.B., Ph.D., F.R.C.P.,
Reader in Paediatrics.

J. P. M. Tizard, B.M., F.R.C.P.,
Professor of Paediatrics.†

J. S. Wigglesworth, M.D., M.R.C.Path.,
Senior Lecturer in Paediatric Pathology.

Neonatal Department of the Institute of
Child Health, University of London;
Neonatal Research Unit, Hammersmith Hospital,
London W.12.

*Now Consultant Paediatrician and Paediatric
Neurologist, Guy's Hospital, London S.E.1.

†Now Professor of Paediatrics, University of Oxford,
John Radcliffe Hospital, Headington, Oxford.

Printed in England at THE LAVENHAM PRESS LTD., Lavenham, Suffolk.

# Contents

*See introductory page to each Section for page numbers of each sub-section listed below.*

# Introduction

For some years we have prepared duplicated sheets of instructions* for the neonatal residents at Hammersmith Hospital. These sheets are revised when too heavily amended by entries in the departmental diary or when superseded by departmental folklore handed down from resident to resident. This book is an attempt to prepare our instructions in a form suitable for publication. We have omitted from the text matters which are only pertinent to Hammersmith Hospital but we have not altered the primary purpose of the handbook, which is to provide detailed instructions for resident paediatricians working in a maternity department with an intensive care nursery as well staffed and equipped as our own. Thus, some of our instructions—for instance those relating to respiratory failure—may be too involved and impracticable for the paediatrician working in the conventional special care nursery. Nevertheless, we hope that the book will contain much information of value to all paediatricians who care for newborn babies.

This is not a textbook of neonatal paediatrics. We have largely omitted descriptions of aetiology and pathogenesis, although we admit we have not been entirely consistent in this respect. The book aims to tell the paediatric resident what to do when faced with common problems of illness in the newborn and also with rare disorders in which recognition and correct handling are matters of immediate importance. Events move quickly in the neonatal period and we hope that this book will help the resident who has no time to consult a senior or a library. On the other hand, we do not expect even our own residents to follow its instructions slavishly; we would much rather they did their own thinking and retained a properly critical attitude to the printed word. Moreover, since there is no branch of medicine in which new knowledge is being more rapidly accumulated, we realize that some sections of our book may need early revision.

A glance at the Table of Contents will show that the book is problem, rather than disease, orientated. This has necessarily resulted in our having to make numerous cross-references as an alternative to being repetitious. We hope the reader will not find this too irritating and will find the index useful.

In preparing this book, we found that our instructional sheets did not cover anything approaching all the information that the paediatrician caring for newborn babies needs to have readily available. We also discovered that there was a good deal of relevant information which none of the five of us had at our finger-tips. Thus we have had to do much 'looking-up', but we hope we have made obvious what information is derived from personal experience and what has been acquired from others, without in every instance making reference to original sources. Some references are

---

*Many of these instructional sheets were first prepared when Dr. John Davis (now Professor of Child Health and Paediatrics at Manchester University) worked at Hammersmith Hospital. He will probably recognise his own ideas and even his own phraseology in many parts of this book, which would have been vastly improved had he had a hand in its production.

inserted because we have little or no personal experience of the matter under discussion, others because the matter is one of very recent knowledge or because the original source supplies fuller technical details of practical importance.

### Sex

Faced with the choice of referring pronomically to the newborn baby as 'he or she', 'he', 'she' or 'it', we have unanimously decided in favour of 'he'. In actual practice we usually know the baby's sex (see p. 41 and p. 60), not only because we think it polite to do so but also because sex often has a bearing on the nature or severity of illness in the newborn.

### 'Consultant', 'Resident' and 'General Practitioner'

We realize that a few words of explanation concerning the designation of doctors may be necessary for foreign readers. 'Consultant' is the term applied to the trained paediatrician in a permanent hospital post; he is a specialist who usually only sees patients on referral from general practitioners and other doctors. 'Resident', in British hospital terminology, means resident—at least for most of the week! Our neonatal residents are trainee paediatricians who have usually completed two or more years hospital work since qualification and who have had at least six months' previous experience of hospital paediatrics. With the help of research fellows who have had clinical neonatal experience, our three neonatal residents run a rota which ensures that there are always two on duty in the hospital day and night.

The 'General Practitioner' (G.P.) is the family doctor providing primary medical care.

### Intensive Care Nurseries

In an intensive care nursery, at present, the saving of life and health is perhaps only marginally better than in the conventional special care unit. Nevertheless, we are sure that an intensive care nursery does provide the best chances of saving life and of lessening the risks of permanent handicap in survivors of serious perinatal illness. However, we believe that more could be done nationally were more vigorous attempts made to ensure that babies at special risk of perinatal disaster were delivered in selected maternity units—those not only particularly well staffed and equipped from an obstetric standpoint, but also possessing an intensive care nursery. Much of our 'trade' is in newborn babies born elsewhere, where facilities for intensive care do not exist and where it is unrealistic to suppose they will exist in the forseeable future. But transfer is a second-rate procedure from the baby's (and mother's) point of view.

At present women with certain types of abnormal pregnancy (*e.g.* severe Rhesus isoimmunisation) are confined in selected maternity hospitals. We are aware, of course, that some obstetric difficulties and disasters cannot be anticipated, but we have come across very many instances where mothers whose pregnancies caused obvious risks to the fetus or newborn were confined in hospitals or nursing homes in which there was insufficient provision for the treatment of a sick newborn baby. The choice of place of confinement should lie not so much between home, G.P.

obstetric unit and hospital, but between all these three and selected maternity units in general hospitals with adequate paediatric services. Even when there have been no ill-omens, the life of the fetus or newborn may suddenly be threatened and it is our view that a mother who unexpectedly goes into premature labour should be transferred to a selected maternity unit, rather than be admitted to the unit at which she has been booked, although we fully recognize the psychological disadvantages to the mother of entering a hospital as a complete stranger.

## Acknowledgments

There is still so much to learn about the ill—and indeed the healthy—newborn baby that research and clinical care go hand in hand, perhaps more so than in any other branch of medicine. We believe that we have high standards of clinical care at Hammersmith and that these standards are in no small measure due to our research activities.

The Neonatal Research Unit was founded in 1961 by the Nuffield Foundation, which continued to support it until 1967. Since then the Unit has been supported by the Wellcome Trust and we have also received important benefactions from the National Fund for Research into Crippling Diseases, The Sir William Coxen Trust, the Worshipful Company of Clothworkers, the Variety Club of Great Britain, the Children's Research Fund, Liverpool, and the British Epilepsy Association. We are thus greatly indebted to all these charitable foundations for the initiation and maintenance of our work.

Of the individuals who have helped us, we must particularly mention Sister Margaret Castle, the Sister in charge of our intensive care nursery. She has a fund of knowledge, great technical skill, energy and determination. Thus the Unit has a special reputation for postgraduate training of nurses, such that we are always very well staffed in terms of quality and quantity. This book is written from the standpoint of the doctor, but we are well aware that nursing care is at least as important as medical care in the treatment of the ill newborn baby.

Next, we must thank our residents and ex-residents, in whom we have been exceptionally lucky. Dr. David Harvey (Consultant Paediatrician at Queen Charlotte's Maternity Hospital), Drs. David Baum, Richard Robinson and Juan Beca have all read the MS of this book and we are grateful to them for some helpful and practical suggestions*. The work of the department has depended on the excellence of our technical staff and we particularly wish to mention our former chief technician Mr. John Stevens, M. PHIL. M.I. BIOL., FIMLT, (now Principal Biochemist, The Courtauld Institute, The Middlesex Hospital) and his successor Mrs. Dorothy Harris, FIMLT. Others of our colleagues are acknowledged in the text.

We gratefully acknowledge our indebtedness to our obstetric colleagues. There have always been good obstetric/paediatric relationships at Hammersmith, thanks to the foundations of collaboration laid by the late Sir Alan Moncrieff and the late Professor James Young. These good relationships have been maintained by the

---

*We are particularly grateful to Dr. N. R. C. Roberton for valuable suggestions made in the proof stage of this book.

goodwill and co-operation of Professor J. C. McClure Browne and his colleagues, amongst whom we especially wish to mention Mr. Harry Gordon. Professor McClure Browne has also read the MS of this book, and we are most grateful to him for his helpful advice.

The reader of this book will find that there are numerous occasions when the only advice we can give the resident is to call in one of our expert colleagues, and we acknowledge our indebtness to all of them—clinicians and pathologists too numerous to mention individually. It is very seldom that the Hammersmith Hospital and Royal Postgraduate Medical School cannot provide the appropriate expert adviser. Finally we are most appreciative of the expert advice given us and the friendly forbearance shown us by Dr. Martin Bax and Mr. Bernard Hayes.

# Section 1: Problems Predicted in Pregnancy

*NOTES*

# Introduction

The term 'prenatal paediatrics' expresses two obvious facts—that life does not begin at birth, and that the paediatrician should be keenly interested in the health of the fetus, while recognising that ultimate responsibility for its care must lie with the obstetrician.

Optimum fetal and neonatal care obviously depends on close and willing collaboration between obstetrician and paediatrician: we make joint rounds of the antenatal ward and special care nursery, and have a weekly meeting at which problem pregnancies and neonatal progress are discussed. When the obstetricians have decided that early induction of labour is essential, they warn us; when the decision is difficult they discuss with us the relative risks of prolongation of intra-uterine existence versus premature birth.

The neonatal and obstetric residents exchange information, and it is particularly important for the former to keep the latter up to date about the progress of an ill newborn baby so that the obstetrician knows what is happening when he sees the mother or father.

The paediatrician should have expert knowledge on the risk of recurrence of both inherited and intra-uterine environmentally determined disease, and of the rapidly expanding possibilities for the prenatal diagnosis of structural and biochemical deformities in the embryo or fetus.

This section outlines the principal methods used in the prenatal diagnosis of fetal abnormality and other fetal problems, and then gives some practical instruction for the paediatrician.

# Prenatal Diagnosis

The purposes of prenatal diagnosis are:

(1) to diagnose abnormalities of the fetus at a stage when the pregnancy can be terminated;

(2) to assess fetal growth or well-being in late pregnancy, to aid in planning the place, time and mode of delivery, to perform treatment (in Rh haemolytic disease), and to organise facilities for neonatal care.

Many of the techniques involved in the diagnosis of fetal disorders or in the assessment of fetal well-being are still under evaluation, while others require highly specialised laboratory facilities. In any one obstetric department it is likely that only some of these methods will be on trial or in routine use, and the neonatal paediatrician should acquaint himself with their uses and limitations.

### Diagnosis of Fetal Abnormalities in Early Pregnancy

The diagnosis of fetal abnormalities may be made by amnioscopy, chemical examination of the amniotic fluid, or amniotic cell culture. Only the last is in practical use at present, and it is only of value if it can be carried out sufficiently early to allow termination of pregnancy, and if the risk of abnormality is high enough to outweigh the small risk of damage or abortion to the normal fetus and to the mother.

The three following types of examination may be performed on cells from amniotic fluid.

(1) Staining cells for chromatin to identify male fetuses in the case of x-linked recessive disease, *e.g.* haemophilia, muscular dystrophy. Fluorescent staining may be used to identify the Y chromosome.

(2) Cell culture for karyotype, to confirm sex and to identify chromosomal abnormalities, *e.g.* Down's syndrome.

(3) Cell culture for enzyme assay to identify inherited metabolic disease, *e.g.* galactosaemia.

This is a rapidly expanding field, but the application of these techniques is limited at present by the difficulty of obtaining amniotic fluid samples in early pregnancy, and difficulties in culture of amniotic cells.

### Fetal Diagnosis and Assessment in Late Pregnancy

The main indications for fetal investigation in late pregnancy are:

(1) rhesus iso-immunisation;

(2) uncertainty about gestational age;

(3) suspected fetal growth retardation; and

(4) risk of fetal distress.

4

**Types of Investigation**

*Intra-uterine*

(1) Examination of amniotic fluid:

(*a*) bilirubin, for assessment of severity of Rh haemolytic disease (see p. 7);

(*b*) pregnanetriol, for diagnosis of congenital adrenal hyperplasia;

(*c*) lipid (Nile blue sulphate) staining of epithelial squames from amniotic fluid, to assess gestational age (particularly in suspected fetal growth retardation);

(*d*) creatinine content, also to assess gestational age;

(*e*) lecithin/sphingomyelin ratio, to assess maturity of surfactant synthesis.

(2) Examination of fetal scalp blood, for the assessment during labour of acidosis in fetal distress and of anaemia in haemolytic disease and feto-maternal haemorrhage.

(3) Fetal electrocardiography by means of scalp electrodes, to diagnose fetal distress.

*Observation of the Fetus by Extra-uterine Means*

(1) Measurement of rate of placental transfer of labelled amino-acids (seleno-methionine) across the placenta, to assess fetal growth-rate.

(2) Ultrasonic measurement of fetal dimensions, especially biparietal diameter of the head, to assess gestational age before 30 weeks gestation, and growth-rate thereafter.

(3) Fetal electrocardiography by external abdominal electrodes to diagnose fetal distress.

(4) Assay of maternal hormone excretion (24-hour urinary output of pregnanediol and oestriol), to assess the efficiency of placental function and the health of the feto-placental unit.

(5) X-rays may help in the diagnosis of congenital malformations, but there are pitfalls in their use for assessment of gestational age.

# Maternal Conditions Which May or May Not Affect the Fetus

The remainder of this section deals with maternal conditions about which the paediatrician may be informed in the antenatal period, and gives brief instructions on what action the neonatal resident should take, and what he should expect, when the baby is born.

When any of the problems listed below has been present during pregnancy, the paediatric resident should attend the birth of the baby. The baby need not necessarily be transferred to the special care nursery, unless this is specifically stated below, or unless one of the indications for transfer listed on p. 45 is present.

**Previous Abnormal Infant or Perinatal Death**

Find out what was wrong with the previous baby, if possible the exact diagnosis. Obtain the case notes or request a summary from the hospital where the baby was born.

In the case of genetically-determined disease, find out the inheritance and the risks of recurrence (see Blyth and Carter 1969, McKusick 1968)*.

Remember that certain disorders not genetically determined may recur, *e.g.* smallness for dates, haemolytic disease of the newborn, and some cases of premature birth such as those associated with cervical incompetence.

**Complications of Pregnancy**

*Hypertension or Toxaemia*

These may lead to obstetrical intervention, and are sometimes associated with retarded fetal growth (*q.v.*). Find out what drugs the mother has been given: they may cause depression of the baby's activity, especially sucking, or functional intestinal obstruction. (See p. 15 *et seq.*)

*Retarded Fetal Growth* (*Smallness for Dates*)

When the obstetrician diagnoses intra-uterine growth failure, he may decide to induce labour or to do a caesarean section. The paediatric resident should be present at delivery and be prepared to deal with the immediate problems of the small-for-dates baby (*i.e.* birth asphyxia) or, if the estimate of length of pregnancy was wrong, a pre-term baby.

*Rhesus Incompatibility*

The obstetrician will try to assess the presence and severity of haemolytic disease

---

*Blyth, H., Carter, C.O. (1969) 'A guide to genetic prognosis in paediatrics.' *Developmental Medicine and Child Neurology*, Suppl. 18.
McKusick, V. A. (1968) *Mendelian Inheritance in Man.* 2nd edn. Baltimore: Williams & Wilkins.

in the fetus from about mid-pregnancy onwards, for the following three reasons:
(1) the very severely affected fetus may require intra-peritonal transfusion;
(2) early induction of labour may be necessary; and
(3) the paediatrician needs to know what to expect at birth.

The obstetrician bases his assessment on the following four factors.
(1) The history of previous pregnancies and the severity of disease in previously affected children.
(2) The zygosity of the father. All infants of a homozygous father will be Rh positive, but there is a fifty-fifty chance that the infant of a heterozygous father will be Rh negative and thus unaffected. In individuals with a Rh-positive (D) phenotype, it is only possible to obtain incomplete information about the genotype. Statements about zygosity for the Rh(D) factor in the Rh-positive father can therefore only be expressed in terms of probability, based on the known distribution in the population of the different combinations of genes for the three pairs of Rh factors. (One should not necessarily take a cynical view concerning the birth of an Rh-negative baby to a mother whose husband is said to be homozygous Rh positive.)
(3) The titres of indirect Coombs antibody in maternal serum. In general, rising titres or very high titres (greater than 1:128) suggest an affected baby, though there are exceptions, especially with second and subsequent affected babies.
(4) Optical density difference (O.D.D.) at 450nm between the base-line optical density of amniotic fluid and the peak which occurs in affected babies. The O.D.D. tends to become less with advancing pregnancy, so interpretation is not simple. See Liley's Chart (Fig. 1, next page). In general, a high O.D.D. (greater than 0.1) or a rising O.D.D. suggests a severely affected infant.

None of these methods of estimating severity of the haemolytic process before birth is entirely reliable, and mistakes can be made in either direction.

The obstetricians usually decide to deliver severely affected babies early, so the paediatrician should be prepared for a baby who has problems of pre-term delivery *and* haemolytic disease of the newborn.

We have a formal arrangement whereby the obstetricians inform us whenever an Rh-negative mother's delivery is imminent, and in any case the duty neonatal resident keeps in touch with activities in the labour rooms.

When an affected infant is to be born, the resident should arrange that fresh Group O, Rh-negative blood is available. The action to be taken at birth is described on pp. 65 and 66.

The resident should visit the mother before the baby is born, either in the ante-natal ward or in the labour room, so that she is acquainted with the doctor who will be caring for her baby and knows what has been planned.

*Abnormal Quantity of Liquor*
*Polyhydramnios*. In an appreciable proportion of cases in which this diagnosis is made there is no fetal abnormality. However, neurological or alimentary tract disorders which cause difficulty in swallowing, and anencephaly, are associated with a high incidence of hydramnios. Exclude oesophageal atresia by passing a tube into

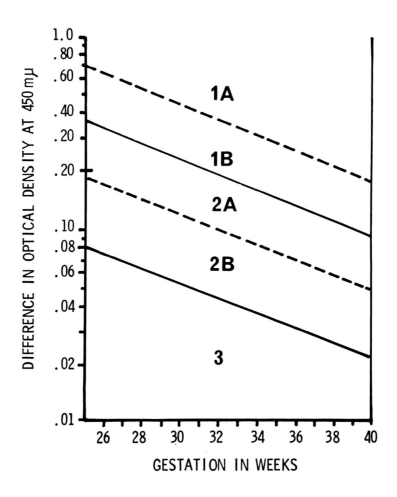

**Fig. 1.** Modification of Liley's chart for prediction of the severity of fetal disease in Rhesus isoimmunisation. When the optical density difference (O.D.D.) of amniotic fluid is related to gestational age, the zone into which the point falls gives a prediction of the severity to be expected. In general, within zone 3 the baby will be unaffected or very mildly affected. In zones 2B and 2A the baby will show increasing severity of disease and premature delivery is likely to be indicated. In zones 1B and 1A the baby will be severely affected; the obstetrician will probably give an intra-uterine transfusion or effect immediate delivery. Points falling in zone 1 will frequently be associated with babies who are already hydropic. We are grateful to Professor A. W. Liley for permission to use this simplified table.

the stomach (p. 50).*

*Oligohydramnios.* This may be caused by abnormalities interfering with the passage of fetal urine (renal agenesis or hypoplasia), or obstructive lesions in the renal tract. Renal agenesis is associated with pulmonary hypoplasia and therefore with extreme difficulties in resuscitation. Oligohydramnios leads to certain distortions of the fetus (*e.g.* Potter face, or limb deformities) and it is probably responsible for some cases of talipes equinovarus. It is also associated with placental insufficiency and, therefore, intrapartum asphyxia.

### Multiple Pregnancy

The babies are likely to be delivered before term. The paediatric resident should anticipate trouble to the extent of ensuring that there are enough trained persons and pieces of equipment to deal with resuscitation in each baby—especially the second and subsequent ones. For the determination of zygosity, see pp. 69 and 70.

### Antepartum Haemorrhage

Be prepared for premature delivery, severe birth asphyxia, respiratory distress and anaemia.

### Malpresentation

The baby may be malformed or may suffer from birth asphyxia or birth injury. Nasal obstruction or laryngeal oedema may complicate face presentation.

### Prolonged Rupture of Membranes

If the membranes have been ruptured more than 48 hours, find out the results of the vaginal swabs and what antibiotics have been given to the mother. Take nose, throat and umbilical swabs from the newborn baby. Watch for signs of infection. Do not give prophylactic antibiotics (but see p. 167).

## Maternal Conditions Incidental to Pregnancy
### Diabetes Mellitus

If the mother's diabetes is well controlled with insulin there are likely to be no problems in the baby except transient hypoglycaemia. In babies born to mothers whose diabetes is less well controlled, the following problems may occur.

(1) The obstetrician may deliver the baby by caesarean section, sometimes before term.

(2) The baby may be large for dates and liable to mechanical difficulties during delivery, especially of the shoulders.

---

*Minority Report.* We have had some splendid arguments in writing this book; this one can only be resolved by a minority report. Polyhydramnios is diagnosed in about four per thousand pregnancies at Hammersmith Hospital, whereas the incidence of oesophageal atresia is about 0.3 per thousand. To pass a tube down a newborn baby's gullet when the only indication for doing so is polyhydramnios in his mother seems to me to be an act of impertinence comparable to doing a lumbar puncture in *every* older child who is brought to hospital having had a fit. If a baby born to a mother with poly-hydramnios were drooling saliva I would certainly pass an oesophageal catheter at once. Otherwise I would have the baby kept under observation for about six hours and only fed when it was clear that he showed no signs of drooling or choking.

J.P.M.T.

(3) The baby may develop hypoglycaemia (see p. 147). In our experience, hypoglycaemia in the first few hours of life is almost inevitable in all babies of diabetic mothers, but does not cause symptoms and does not need treatment. Hypoglycaemia may be rather more severe and prolonged when maternal diabetic control is less satisfactory. Very severe and prolonged hypoglycaemia sometimes occurs in babies whose mothers have been treated with sulphonylurea drugs such as chlorpropamide.

(4) The baby may develop hyaline membrane disease.

Congenital malformations (especially in the sacral region) are slightly commoner in babies born to diabetic mothers.

If there has been moderate or severe birth asphyxia, or if the baby develops respiratory difficulties, he must be transferred to the special care nursery. In general, we feel it wise to do so anyway for the first 48 hours. Early feeding is recommended. Blood glucose should be checked by 'Dextrostix' (Ames) at 6, 12 and 24 hours. For management of hypoglycaemia, see p. 148 *et seq.*

*Thyrotoxicosis*

Find out what treatment the mother has had in the past and is having now, and whether her long-acting thyroid stimulator (LATS) has been estimated. This substance, passed across the placenta in the IgG fraction of antibodies, appears to be responsible for congenital thyrotoxicosis in the infant, which is therefore a self-limiting condition. However, not all infants of affected mothers have clinical symptoms; and further, a euthyroid mother who has previously had a thyroidectomy may give birth to an affected baby, as LATS will persist in her blood.

In many affected infants there may be a deceptive period of well-being for a few days after birth, presumably due to the controlling effect of maternal antithyroid drugs before they are completely excreted by the infant.

The syndrome of very marked thyroid enlargement present at birth (sometimes responsible for dystocia) and accompanied by symptoms of hypothyroidism, is now rarely if ever seen, and was presumably due to maternal overdosage with antithyroid drugs.

It is not necessary to transfer the baby routinely to the special care nursery, but he should not be discharged from hospital before the eighth day of life since symptoms have sometimes first appeared as late as this.

Save cord blood for estimation of LATS (this is undertaken by very few laboratories at present, and is time-consuming and expensive).

Signs of thyrotoxicosis in the infant include:
    tachycardia;
    congestive cardiac failure which may occur with alarming rapidity;
    diffuse swelling of the thyroid, usually not marked;
    exophthalmos—usually only if present in the mother;
    overactivity and jitteriness;
    ravenous appetite—often with static weight or even weight loss;
    diarrhoea.

10

TREATMENT

Treat cardiac failure if present (see p. 215).

*Antithyroid drugs:* potassium iodide (5mg, 8-hourly, orally). Carbimazole may also be necessary (2.5mg, 8-hourly, orally). Reduce gradually once symptoms are controlled.

Length of treatment will depend on the severity of the initial symptoms to some extent, but is rarely necessary beyond a few weeks of age.

## Cushing's Disease

The possible fetal problems when a mother has Cushing's disease are the same as those when a mother is on steroids (see p. 18). The baby may be small for dates, and symptoms of steroid withdrawal should be watched for after birth, though they are unlikely to occur.

## Addison's Disease

If the Addison's disease is caused by tuberculosis, find out if the mother has active pulmonary tuberculosis.

We have had one case of a baby born to a mother with auto-immune Addison's disease in which antibodies were transferred to the fetus, and an apparent Addisonian crisis took place a few days after birth.

The mother will be on replacement steroids but these should not affect the fetus (see p. 18).

## Simmond's Disease

First reconsider the diagnosis of (a) Simmond's disease or (b) pregnancy! However, there certainly are cases of women with hypopituitarism in whom pregnancy has been induced with gonadotrophic drugs. In the two cases we have seen there have been no neonatal problems directly referable to the hypopituitarism. The mother is likely to be on replacement steroids but these should not affect the fetus.

## Hyperparathyroidism

The baby may develop hypocalcaemic fits. Feed on breast-milk if possible, and if not possible see that the baby is not overfed with cow's milk.

## Cyanotic Heart Disease

The baby will almost certainly be severely growth-retarded (see p. 90, and 'Birth asphyxia' p. 32).

## Malignant Disease

*Malignant disease diagnosed and treated prior to pregnancy.* This will seldom present any problem to the baby. Radiotherapy or chemotherapy with antimitotic drugs or folic acid antagonists in early pregnancy (given before it was realized that the patient was pregnant) is likely to cause abortion or fetal malformation, in particular microcephaly following radiotherapy. If the mother has a lymphoma or Hodgkin's disease she may be on treatment with steroids (see p. 18). If a tumour of the maternal

11

genital tract has been excised, planned delivery by caesarean section may be necessary.

*Malignant disease diagnosed in pregnancy.* The necessity for treatment by surgery or radiotherapy may dictate the mode and timing of delivery.

*Spread to placenta and baby.* Metastatic deposits in the placenta occur rarely in a variety of forms of malignant disease, including carcinoma of breast and lung; however, spread to the baby has only been described on a few occasions in association with malignant melanoma. In several cases the infant has had metastases at birth but these have sometimes undergone later regression. Chorionepithelioma arising in the placenta rarely spreads to both mother and infant. The condition usually presents in the infant with haemoptysis, anaemia and hepatomegaly before it is diagnosed in the mother, but the symptoms have not been recorded earlier than two weeks of age.

### Sickle Cell Anaemia and Sickle Cell Trait

There is an increased perinatal mortality in infants of mothers with this condition, largely explained by perinatal asphyxia. Be prepared for an asphyxiated baby at birth. There is no point in testing the baby for sickle cell anaemia at birth, but this should be done at the age of, say, four months.

### Thrombocytopenic Purpura (*Idiopathic or Drug Induced*)

The presumed autoimmune antibody, formed against a platelet antigen which is responsible for the maternal disease, is transferred to the infant and may cause the same condition in him temporarily. A number of thrombocytopenic mothers do, however, produce unaffected infants, while some who appear to be in clinical remission at delivery, and even those who have been cured by splenectomy, occasionally have thrombocytopenic babies.

In affected infants the liver and spleen are not usually enlarged.

The risk of haemorrhage is greatest at or shortly after delivery, and when the platelet count is below about $15,000/mm^3$. Petechiae or larger purpuric spots occur most commonly and may be widespread—unlike those of 'traumatic' asphyxia (see p. 47). Bleeding may occur from the nose or umbilicus, the gut or genito-urinary tract, or from injection sites. Intracranial haemorrhage can prove lethal. The indications for replacement of blood-loss are those of other haemorrhagic neonatal disorders (see p. 209); use fresh whole blood. There is no justification for splenectomy, and little, on available evidence, for the use of steroids.

Keep the infant in hospital until the cord has separated. After discharge from hospital, arrange follow-up until his platelet count has risen to normal. For other causes of neonatal thrombocytopenic purpura, see p. 208.

### Ulcerative Colitis

If the mother's illness is severe and she is on steroid therapy, the infant may be small for dates and/or born before term. There is also the theoretical, but improbable, risk of adrenal crisis in the infant following steroid withdrawal (see p. 18).

### Disseminated Lupus Erythematosus

The infant may be affected by (*a*) disease itself or (*b*) maternal drug therapy (steroids or cyclophosphamide). The majority of the liveborn infants appear to escape unscathed, though there is an increased risk of abortion, premature delivery, stillbirth and low birthweight for gestation.

Save a specimen of cord blood—both LE cells and anti-nuclear factor may be demonstrated, and can persist for several weeks after birth. Transient anaemia, thrombocytopenia and leucopenia have been noted. In the rare event of bleeding accompanying the thrombocytopenia, see p. 209 for treatment.

Examine the infant carefully. Lesions resembling discoid lupus erythematosus may be present on the face and scalp at birth and persist for several weeks, leaving atrophic scars. Endocardial fibro-elastosis with widespread fibrosis of other organs has been reported, proving rapidly fatal. *These complications are rare.*

### *Myasthenia Gravis*

About one-quarter of the babies born to mothers with myasthenia gravis will have temporary myasthenia themselves. This may manifest itself by respiratory difficulties, feeding difficulties and floppiness. Signs may be present at or within a few hours of birth, and usually consist of respiratory insufficiency—rapid, shallow breathing and intermittent cyanosis—or difficulty in sucking and swallowing. The normal newborn baby usually keeps its mouth and eyes shut except when crying or feeding. Reduced mobility of the face, with eyes and mouth open, should suggest the diagnosis, which is supported by the finding of generalised hypotonia.

A test dose of 0.05mg prostigmine, 0.3mg pyridostigmine bromide or edrophonium chloride 1mg (0.1ml 'Tensilon') by intramuscular injection will confirm the diagnosis. Maintenance therapy consists of 1 to 5mg of prostigmine or 4 to 20mg of pyridostigmine bromide orally with feeds. The size and frequency of the dose will have to be adjusted according to the degree and duration of relief of symptoms, and must be reduced as spontaneous recovery takes place.

It is probably wise to transfer the baby to the special care nursery for the first 24 hours.

### *Psychiatric Illness and Social Problems*

These may clearly have all sorts of repercussions on the infant. The subject is too large to be discussed here, but it is as important for the paediatrician to know if a mother has mental illness or difficult home circumstances as it is for him to know about the physical complications of her pregnancy. The reader is referred to Tylden (1969)* for a fuller discussion of this subject.

### Maternal Drugs Which May Affect the Embryo, Fetus and/or Newborn

Drugs taken by the mother reach the fetal blood-stream and, in some cases, the amniotic fluid, via the placenta. Very rarely, they may be directly administered; sometimes intentionally, as during intra-uterine peritoneal transfusion, and some-

Tylden, E. (1969) 'Psychiatry in childbearing.' *In* Holmes, J. M. (Ed.) *Obstetrics.* Concise Medical Textbooks. London: Baillière.

times accidentally, when local anaesthetic intended for the mother is injected into the fetus.

All drugs taken by a mother in the first trimester of pregnancy, particularly the first eight weeks, have to be considered as possible teratogens. There is need for great caution, however, before incriminating any one drug; it is usually only when the introduction of a new preparation coincides with a steep increase in incidence of a previously rare anomaly that it can be done with near certainty, as with thalidomide for example. This drug, the antimitotic and immunosuppressant drugs, and the androgens are the only ones which can be listed as having teratogenic potential. Others such as anticonvulsants, particularly barbiturates, aspirin, and dextroamphetamine are under suspicion, but the evidence is only equivocal as yet.

You should always question the mother of a congenitally malformed infant about drugs taken in pregnancy (and about illness), but try to convey at the same time that any association between the abnormality and pregnancy happenings is extremely unlikely. All parents with malformed babies probably have some feelings of guilt, and these should not be intensified by the nature of your questioning. You should also ask the general practitioner if he would consult his records, for few mothers remember with accuracy that they took a particular drug at a particular time. However, many women take drugs during pregnancy without medical supervision or awareness.

Some of the maternal drugs which may have undesirable effects on the fetus and newborn are listed in Table I under the pharmacological classification of the British National Formulary (1971). In the majority, and except where indicated by an asterisk in the Table, maternal medication has to be given at the end of pregnancy or in labour to produce these effects.

We have tried to compile as complete a list as possible of drugs which may affect the fetus or newborn. Some of the effects recorded have only been reported very rarely, or even in single cases. Some of the drugs listed would not normally be given to a patient known to be pregnant, and some are now rarely used. We have *not* listed drugs which may disturb differential growth in the embryo, *e.g.* thalidomide.

### Excretion of Drugs by the Breast

Precise knowledge about excretion of drugs in breast-milk is often lacking, but the evidence available suggests that practically all products taken by the mother will be excreted in her milk in some form. The amounts are usually small, however, and in general are no contra-indication to breast-feeding. The definite exception is a mother who has been given radioactive iodine, and possible exceptions are mothers who have been given other drugs which may affect thyroid function. Purgatives, other than liquid paraffin or bulk purgatives, should be avoided by the breast-feeding mother, as they may cause diarrhoea in the baby.

A useful article is that by Knowles (1965)* on the excretion of drugs in milk.

### Maternal Drug Addiction
See p. 222.

*Knowles, J. A. (1965) 'Excretion of drugs in milk.' *Journal of Pediatrics*, **66**, 1068.

## TABLE I
### Maternal drugs which may affect the fetus and/or newborn

| Maternal drug | Possible effect on fetus and/or newborn | Action which may be required |
|---|---|---|
| **ANAESTHETIC**<br>General | Respiratory depression. Halogenated hydrocarbons, *e.g.* halothane, trichlorethylene, reach fetus more easily than nitrous oxide because of high lipid solubility. | Treatment of birth asphyxia. |
| Local | Fetal bradychardia and fall in pH, neonatal bradycardia, apnoea and convulsions following use in paracervical block—probably due to faulty technique with accidental injection into the fetal presenting part. | As above. If marked depression, consider exchange transfusion, and aspirate stomach (drug present in gastric secretions). |
| Spinal, epidural, caudal | Intra-uterine hypoxia will occur if there is sudden maternal hypotension. | Treatment of birth asphyxia. |
| **ANALGESIC**<br>Aspirin | Prolonged prothrombin time leading to neonatal haemorrhage; decreased serum albumen binding capacity. | Give phytomenadione injection B.P. 1mg I.M. (vitamin K$_1$) after birth; watch for haemorrhage. |
| Aspirin, phenacetin and codeine | Heinz bodies in peripheral blood (in presence of maternal Heinz body anaemia). | |
| Diamorphine, morphine, pethidine; used in labour. | Respiratory depression. | Treatment of birth asphyxia. Give nalorphine injection B.P. 0.25 to 1.0mg (depending on gestational age) slowly I.V. or I.M. |
| in drug addicts | *Withdrawal symptoms (usually towards end of first 24 hours, occasionally later), *e.g.* hyperirritability, increased tone, myoclonus, shrill cry, vomiting and diarrhoea, dehydration. | In presence of symptoms treat with either pheno-barbitone or chlorpro-mazine; intravenous fluids may be necessary in presence of watery stools. (See also p. 222.)<br>*(continued)* |

*In general, these drugs have to be given throughout pregnancy to produce harmful effects.

Table I (cont.)

| Maternal drug | Possible effect on fetus and/or newborn | Action which may be required |
|---|---|---|
| **ANTIBACTERIAL** | | |
| Nitrofurantoin | Haemolytic anaemia in G6PD-deficient infants. | |
| Streptomycin (and dihydrostreptomycin) | *Occasional VIIIth nerve damage, vestibular and auditory; slight hearing loss, sometimes unilateral. | |
| Sulphonamides | Haemolytic anaemia in G6PD deficiency. | |
| long-acting | Hyperbilirubinaemia and displacement of bilirubin from protein-binding sites. | |
| Tetracyclines | Chelates with calcium, and is therefore deposited in tissues undergoing mineralisation, e.g. bone, tooth buds. Milk teeth may be stained. | |
| **ANTICOAGULANT** | | |
| Coumarins | Fetal and neonatal haemorrhage due to prolonged prothrombin time. (In practice, these anticoagulants are usually withdrawn one week before labour is anticipated, when heparin, which does not cross the placenta, is given instead. Thus this problem is only likely to occur in unexpectedly early delivery.) | Obtain cord blood for coagulation studies and give the baby phytomenadione injection B.P. 1mg I.M. If prothrombin time is greatly prolonged or if you have to wait more than say two hours to find out, it is safer to give 10ml/kg of fresh frozen plasma I.V. or, if available, concentrate of factors II, VII, IX and X. Alert the nursing staff to the possibility of the baby bleeding. |
| **ANTICONVULSANT** | | |
| Phenobarbitone, phenytoin | *Neonatal haemorrhage due to deficiency of vitamin K dependent factors. | As above. |

(continued)

*In general these drugs have to be given throughout pregnancy to produce harmful effects.

TABLE I (cont.)

| Maternal drug | Possible effect on fetus and/or newborn | Action which may be required |
|---|---|---|
| **ANTIDIABETIC** Oral hypoglycaemic agents, sulphonylureas | Insulin release from pancreatic cells; hypoglycaemia, sometimes prolonged. | Check blood sugar levels and be prepared to treat hypoglycaemia. |
| **ANTIHYPERTENSIVE** Reserpine | Stuffy nose, nasal discharge, lethargy and respiratory depression. | Cautious use of ephedrine nasal drops B.P.C. one drop in each nostril, if nasal symptoms severe enough to interfere with feeding. Do not use more than once or twice a day, and stop as soon as possible. |
| Ganglion blockers | Paralytic ileus. | Intravenous feeding may have to be substituted for oral during first days of life. |
| **ANTIMALARIAL** Quinine | Thrombocytopenia purpura. *Deafness. | Watch for haemorrhage. |
| Chloroquine | *Deafness and abnormal retinal pigmentation. | |
| **ANTITHYROID** Carbimazole, methylthiouracil, propylthiouracil, sodium iodide | *Goitre, hypothyroidism when dosage poorly controlled. (Drugs more usually mask symptoms of neonatal thyro-toxicosis in first days of life; see p. 10.) | Relief of airways obstruct-ion if goitre sufficiently large. Thyroid replace-ment therapy (thyroxine 0.025mg daily may be necessary initially). |
| Sodium iodide ($^{131}$I) solution | Hypothyroidism. | Thyroid replacement therapy as above. |
| **CHOLINERGIC** Edrophonium chloride, neostigmine, physo-stigmine, pyridostig-mine bromide | About $\frac{1}{4}$ of infants of myasthenic mothers have transient muscular weakness which might represent drug withdrawal rather than the effects of a transplacentally acquired endogenous factor. | Watch for respiratory and feeding difficulties and floppiness, and be prepared to treat with neostigmine etc. (See p. 13.) |

*(continued)*

*In general, these drugs have to be given throughout pregnancy to produce harmful effects.

TABLE I (cont.)

| Maternal drug | Possible effect on fetus and/or newborn | Action which may be required |
|---|---|---|
| **CORTICOSTEROID** | | |
| Cortisol and analogues | Theoretical risk of adrenal crisis after birth, but few well-documented reports. ? Increased risk prematurity and/or intra-uterine growth retardation—probably due in part to underlying maternal disease. | Careful watchfulness first few days of life. |
| **DIURETIC** | | |
| Thiadiazine group | Possible thrombocytopenic purpura. (Direct effect on platelet count following neonatal administration not confirmed.) | Watch for haemorrhage. |
| **EXPECTORANTS AND COUGH SUPPRESSANTS** | | |
| Iodine-containing proprietary mixtures, not in B.N.F., available without prescription, used for asthma, bronchitis, etc. | *Goitre, hypothyroidism. | Relief of airways obstruction if goitre sufficiently large. Thyroid replacement therapy may be necessary initially. |
| **HORMONE** | | |
| Androgens (e.g. testosterone), oestrogens (stilboestrol) and progestogens (ethisterone and norethisterone) | *Virilisation of female fetus; clitoral enlargement sometimes with varying degrees of fusion of labio-scrotal folds. | Establish that sex is female as soon as possible (see p. 60); reconstructive surgery may be necessary later. Re-assure parents that menstruation and ovulation will be normal. |
| **INTRAVENOUS DEXTROSE AND WATER SOLUTION** | | |
| (Causing maternal hyponatraemia) | Hyponatraemia–hypotonia, lethargy, convulsions. | Intravenous saline usually not necessary if oral feeding started early. |
| **NEUROMUSCULAR BLOCKING** | | |
| d–tubocurarine | *Arthrogryposis. | |
| **SEDATIVE AND TRANQUILISER** | | |
| Barbiturates | Diminished responsiveness to breastfeeding; less forceful and effective sucking; diminished visual attentiveness. Enzyme induction. | |
| Lithium carbonate | Respiratory depression and hypotonia. | |

(continued)

*In general, these drugs have to be given throughout pregnancy to produce harmful effects.

**Table I (cont.)**

| Maternal drug | Possible effect on fetus and/or newborn | Action which may be required |
|---|---|---|
| Phenothiazines | Extra-pyramidal dysfunction—generalised tremors, increased muscle tone, opisthotonus; symptoms persisting weeks or months after birth. | These are *not* drug withdrawal symptoms, so do not prescribe more! |
| Promazine (in combination with pethidine, and causing profound maternal hypotension) | Intra-uterine hypoxia. | Treatment for birth asphyxia. |
| *VITAMIN* | | |
| Water-soluble analogues of vitamin K | Haemolytic anaemia, hyper-bilirubinaemia, kernicterus. | |
| Vitamin D | Infantile hypercalcaemia—evidence for definite association controversial. | |
| *MISCELLANEOUS* | | |
| Bromethol ('Avertin'), resulting in profound maternal hypotension | Intra-uterine hypoxia. | Treatment for birth asphyxia. |
| Magnesium sulphate (used in treatment of eclampsia) | Peripheral neuromuscular block and central depression. | In severe cases, assisted ventilation and exchange transfusion may be necessary. |
| Naphthalene (pregnancy craving for mothballs) | Haemolytic anaemia in G6PD-deficient infants. | |
| Propanolol (adrenergic blocking agent used in premedication for obstetric anaesthesia) | Birth asphyxia. | Treatment for birth asphyxia. |
| Tobacco | *Retardation fetal growth. | |

*In general, these drugs have to be given throughout pregnancy to produce harmful effects.

### Known Infectious Disease in the Mother

In general, the fetus seems to be well protected against infectious disease acquired by the mother during pregnancy. However, certain infections appear to be readily transmitted to the fetus via the placenta, and the baby may also be infected during parturition, especially from cervical lesions.

When the obstetrician knows of a definite infective illness in the mother, certain steps may be necessary to rule out, or confirm and possibly treat, infection in the baby. Proof of involvement will lie in the isolation and identification of the infecting organisms. Confirmatory evidence may be provided in certain cases from specific IgM fluorescent antibody tests. The interpretation and usefulness of these and of antibody titres and immunoglobulin levels are discussed in the section 'Infection' (see p. 162 and p. 166), along with the clinical features of the various infections.

Table II (pp. 21-26) indicates action necessary at birth. Note that a specimen of cord blood is necessary in many cases, and that the placenta should be saved. Also note that some of these infections will seldom, if ever, be diagnosed in a pregnant woman; we include them for completeness.

**TABLE II**

**Investigation of newborn in cases of known maternal infection**

| Maternal infection | Possible clinical involvement of fetus and/or newborn (see also p. 164) | Source for isolation of infecting organism | Additional tests | Further action |
|---|---|---|---|---|
| **BACTERIAL*** | | | | |
| Bowel pathogens (acute illness, or carrier state), usually:- Enteropathogenic Esch. coli Salmonellae Shigellae | Enteritis. | Faeces (send several specimens). | | Keep infant with mother, making sure the latter is instructed in strict personal hygiene. Isolate from other infants. If infant remains well in first days and stool cultures negative, send both home as soon as possible, informing G. P. first. If infant becomes ill with positive stool cultures, start antibiotic treatment (see p. 201) in view of possibility of blood-stream invasion at this age. Transfer out of Maternity Department if acceptable alternative possible. |
| Listeria monocytogenes | See footnote.† Pneumonia, septicaemia, meningitis. | CSF, blood, faeces. | Placental histology. | Start antibiotic treatment (see p. 168) after taking specimens if infant appears ill at or shortly after birth. |
| Mycobacterium tuberculosis | Respiratory and/or abdominal tuberculosis. | Gastric washings, faeces. | Chest x-ray. | Separate healthy infant from sputum-positive mother. Arrange for BCG vaccination. Try to find substitute mother (within family or with help of Medical Social |

(*continued*)

*Only unusual bacteria have been listed here; any others may be involved.
†The effect on the newborn may be inapparent, mild or severe. The spectrum of involvement ranges from nothing obvious on complete examination to widespread system involvement, the central nervous system frequently taking the brunt.

**TABLE II (cont.)**

| Maternal infection | Possible clinical involvement of fetus and/or newborn (see also p. 164) | Source for isolation of infecting organism | Additional tests | Further action |
|---|---|---|---|---|
| | | | | Worker) for 2-3 months. Sputum-negative mother and healthy infant can stay together, but arrange for BCG vaccination before discharge. If the infant appears to be healthy, no investigations are needed on him. If he becomes ill after birth and congenital tuberculosis (*very* rare and onset not immediate) seems a possibility, start anti-tuberculosis treatment, first obtaining specimens. |
| *Neisseria gonorrhoeae* | Ophthalmia. | Eye swabs. | | Prevention: instil 1% $AgNO_3$ into eyes shortly after birth. Treatment: see p. 169. |
| *Vibrio fetus* | See footnote.† Meningoencephalitis. | CSF. | Placental histology. | Start antibiotic treatment (see p. 168) after taking specimen if infant appears to be ill at or shortly after birth. |
| *FUNGAL* *Candida albicans* | Oral and perineal moniliasis (relatively common). Pulmonary, generalized skin infection (rare). Yellowish-white pinpoint necrotic nodules on umbilical cord. | Mouth swab, faeces. Skin swab (diagnosis of lung infection usually only made at autopsy). | | Oral lesions usually develop towards end of the first week. See p. 171 for treatment. |

22

| | | | | |
|---|---|---|---|---|
| **PROTOZOAL** | | | | |
| *Plasmodium* (*malaria*) | Congenital malaria. | Blood smear. | Baby's serum for specific IgM fluorescent antibody. Placental histology. | Start antimalarial treatment (see p. 171) if diagnosis established. |
| *Toxoplasma gondii* | See footnote†. Meningoencephalitis, choroidoretinitis, hepatitis, thrombocytopenia. | Organism may be seen on Wright stained CSF sediment. | Baby's serum for specific IgM fluorescent antibody. Paired maternal and cord sera for complement fixation and dye tests; repeat at 3-4 months of age. Placental histology. | Start antitoxoplasma treatment (see p. 172) if infection apparent. If inapparent but fluorescent antibody test positive, arrange for careful follow-up, to include eye examination. |
| **SPIROCHAETAL** | | | | |
| *Treponema pallidum* (syphilis) | See footnote†. Rashes, hepatitis, periostitis. | | Baby's serum for specific IgM fluorescent antibody. Paired maternal and cord sera for cardiolipin W.R., V.D.R.L., slide test and Reiter protein CFT; repeat at 3-4 months of age. Placental histology. | Start antisyphilitic treatment (see p. 172) if infection apparent, and if inapparent but fluorescent antibody test positive. Arrange for follow-up. |
| **VIRAL** | | | | |
| *Arbovirus* | | | | |
| Western equine encephalitis | Encephalitis. | CSF, throat swab. | Cord serum for IgM. | Arrange for follow-up. |
| *Herpesvirus* | | | | |
| Cytomegalovirus (CMV) | See footnote†. Small for dates, meningoencephalitis, choroidoretinitis, hepatitis, thrombocytopenia. | Freshly voided urine, throat swab. | Baby's serum for specific IgM fluorescent antibody. | If involvement severe, no treatment, as CNS will have been seriously damaged; if |

*(continued)*

†The effect on the newborn may be inapparent, mild or severe. The spectrum of involvement ranges from nothing obvious on complete examination to widespread system involvement, the central nervous system frequently taking the brunt.

**TABLE II (cont.)**

| Maternal infection | Possible clinical involvement of fetus and/or newborn (see also p. 164) | Source for isolation of infecting organism | Additional tests | Further action |
|---|---|---|---|---|
| | | | Cord IgM. Paired maternal and cord sera for complement fixing antibody titre; repeat at 3-4 months of age. | inapparent or mild, consider treatment with idoxuridine (see p. 172). Arrange for follow-up, and remember that viral excretion by infant (often prolonged) is potential hazard for pregnant women. |
| *Herpesvirus hominis* (simplex) majority type 2 | See footnote†. As for cytomegalovirus; also skin vesicles. | Fresh vesicular lesions, CSF, throat swab. | | As for cytomegalovirus. |
| *Varicella-zoster* (chicken pox, herpes zoster) | Congenital varicella. Congenital herpes-zoster. | Fresh vesicular lesion. | | Separate temporarily from mother only if no evidence of disease in the baby and if the mother is still infectious; keep apart from other infants. |
| *Myxo- or paramyxo- viruses* Influenza | (Abortion.) | | | Separation of healthy infant from his mother is only necessary if she is still infectious at delivery (*i.e.* for 5 days after appearance of rash in measles, for 1 week after disappearance of swelling in mumps). Infant should be isolated from other infants, as he may contract the infection. |
| Measles | (Abortion), congenital measles. | Throat swab. | | |
| Mumps | (Abortion.) | | | |
| *Picornaviruses* Coxsackie | See footnote†. Meningitis, enteritis. | Faeces, throat swab. | Cord serum for IgM. Paired sera for complement fixing, neutralizing and | Isolate from other infants. Arrange follow-up. |
| ECHO | See footnote†. Meningitis, enteritis. | Faeces, throat swab. | | As above. |

| | | | | |
|---|---|---|---|---|
| Poliovirus | (Abortion), congenital polioencephalitis or carditis. | Faeces, throat swab. | haemagglutination inhibition titres; repeat at 3-4 months of age. | As above. Be prepared for respiratory failure. |
| *Poxvirus* | | | | |
| Vaccinia (smallpox vaccination) | (Abortion), congenital vaccinia. | Fresh vesicular lesions. | | If infant is involved, fetal or very early neonatal death is likely. |
| Variola (smallpox) | (Abortion), congenital variola. | Fresh vesicular lesions. | | You should never be involved if the mother is correctly diagnosed for she will be in an isolation hospital. If she is not, and you make the diagnosis, send the mother and infant there at once and inform the Medical Superintendent, M.O.H., etc. |
| *Other* | | | | |
| Hepatitis (SH/Au Ag) | Hepatitis. | Blood. | Cord serum for IgM. | Instruct mother in strict personal hygiene. Avoid breast-feeding if nipples cracked. ? immunoglobulins. Arrange follow-up. |
| Rubella | See footnote†. Malformations if mother affected in first trimester: cardiac defects, cataract, deafness. Also small for dates, hepatitis, thrombocytopenia, defects in metaphyses. | Throat swab, urine. | Baby's serum for specific IgM fluorescent antibody. Cord serum for IgM. Paired maternal and cord sera for complement fixing, neutralizing and haemagglutination inhibition titres; repeat at 3-4 months of age. | Arrange for follow-up, with particular reference to detection of hearing and visual impairment. Remember that viral excretion by infant (often prolonged) is a potential hazard for pregnant women. |

(continued)

†The effect on the newborn may be inapparent, mild or severe. The spectrum of involvement ranges from nothing obvious on complete examination to widespread system involvement, the central nervous system frequently taking the brunt.

**TABLE II (cont.)**

| Maternal infection | Possible clinical involvement of fetus and/or newborn (see also p. 164) | Source for isolation of infecting organism | Additional tests | Further action |
|---|---|---|---|---|
| *OTHER*<br>*Mycoplasma hominis* | Ophthalmia. Pneumonia, (superficial abscesses reported, but probably rare). | Eye swabs, warn laboratory that special media may be necessary. | | For treatment, see p. 169. |
| *TRIC agent* | Ophthalmia. | Anaesthetise conjunctiva with 1 % amethocaine and 1/10,000 adrenalin, and when blanched, evert lids and scrape tarsal surface firmly with spatula. Spread material onto slide, dry in air, and ask laboratory to examine for special type cytoplasmic inclusion bodies. | | For treatment, see p. 171. Arrange for follow-up. |

# Section 2: Problems at Birth

The neonatal resident should be present at the birth of the baby if any of the conditions described in the previous section—Problems Predicted in Pregnancy—was present, or if there is fetal distress, or if the delivery is instrumental or otherwise abnormal.

*NOTES*

# Abnormal Amniotic Fluid

**Blood-stained Liquor**

The source of blood is usually maternal. If swallowed by the fetus, melaena may occur soon after birth, often with the first meconium, and so is distinguishable from the melaena of haemorrhagic disease of the newborn which usually does not occur until the second or third day.

If the source of blood is fetal (from a placental vessel for instance) the infant may be shocked and anaemic at birth (see p. 37 and p. 206).

**Meconium-stained Liquor**

Breech presentation apart, meconium in the liquor is usually taken to be a sign of fetal distress, although many infants who pass meconium *in utero* are perfectly normal at birth. However, birth asphyxia and respiratory obstruction due to meconium at laryngeal level should be anticipated. If the liquor has been aspirated into the lungs *in utero*, respiratory distress may occur after birth; pneumothorax should always be considered as a further complication in the case of sudden collapse (see p. 140). The skin, umbilical cord and nails may be meconium stained. The passage of meconium *in utero* is very rare in an asphyxiated *pre-term* infant, but this sign has been reported as occurring frequently in cases of listeriosis.

**Foul-smelling Liquor**

This is usually associated with bacterial infection and chorioamnionitis. For management see p. 167.

**Abnormal Quantities of Liquor**

See p. 7.

# The Umbilical Cord and Placental Transfusion

In uncomplicated deliveries, the care of the cord will normally be the responsibility of the midwife, but the paediatric resident should know the usual procedure.

**Cutting the Cord**

About one-third of the blood volume of the conceptus is in the placenta. After birth, part of the blood is transferred to the baby as the placental transfusion. The amount involved is from 30-100ml. Factors which facilitate this transfer of blood are (a) gravity—if the baby is lower than the placenta; (b) the first breaths—which open the pulmonary circulation: and (c) a uterine contraction—which squeezes blood from the placenta to the baby. In most cases the major part of the placental transfusion occurs within the first 30 seconds after birth. Immediate clamping of the cord will deprive the baby of the transfusion. Delayed clamping of the cord is associated with fewer signs of respiratory distress syndrome (RDS) in the first 24 hours though it is not clear whether this means a lower incidence of RDS, or less severe RDS in those cases which are affected. The placental transfusion provides iron stores for the baby, but a very large placental transfusion may lead to an excessively high haematocrit with viscous blood and problems therefrom (see p. 228).

Allow the baby to be just below the level of the placenta and do not clamp the cord immediately, *i.e.* wait at least 20-30 seconds, preferably after the first gasps. Do not 'milk' the cord.

In seriously asphyxiated babies do not delay resuscitation: it may be necessary to clamp at once in order to get on with laryngoscopy and intubation.

**Tying the Cord**

After any immediate problems of birth have been dealt with, spray the base and first two centimetres of cord with Polybactrin (polymyxin, bacitracin, neomycin) spray. Apply a plastic clip 1 to 2cm from the umbilicus and cut the cord cleanly. Spray the cut end with Polybactrin.

Various cord clips are available; and a sterilized elastic band will serve well. Any system used must continue to give compression as the Wharton's jelly under the clip is squeezed away. Tying with a string or tape has the disadvantage that compression is lost when the jelly exudes, and bleeding may ensue. If, for some reason, tape must be used, a second tie should be put in place and the ties inspected and retied if necessary after an hour or two.

*CAUTION.* Very rarely, the cord contains a hernia with a viscus or omentum in it. If the proximal part of the cord is very thick, place the clip distally, beyond the distended part, and ask the surgeon to have a look. Remember also the possibility of Beckwith's syndrome (omphalocele or enlarged cord, combined with high birthweight, enlarged tongue, large liver and kidneys, mild microcephaly and neonatal hypoglycaemia).

30

**Obtaining Cord Blood**

(1) Blood can be obtained freely by inserting a needle into the umbilical vein after the cord is clamped and while the placenta is still *in utero*.

(2) During the third stage of labour, after the cord has been clamped and cut, blood will usually flow freely if the clamp on the placental end is released. Such blood may be contaminated by Wharton's jelly, and this may cause a false positive direct Coombs Test.

(3) After the placenta has separated, the fetal veins are usually sufficiently distended for it to be easy to enter one with a needle and extract up to 10ml. Sometimes only a drop or two can be obtained.

(4) Hanging the placenta in a large funnel, with the cord through the stem, will usually distend the veins so that a maximal amount of blood can be obtained either by releasing the clamp or entering the vein with a needle.


**Umbilical Arteries**

The cord vessels should be counted on the cut end of the cord; there are usually two arteries and one vein. In cases where a single umbilical artery is found, look especially carefully for other congenital abnormalities. About 20 to 40 per cent of babies with a single umbilical artery have other congenital malformations which are detectable in the neonatal period—especially oesophageal atresia and imperforate anus. There may be hidden malformations involving, for example, the kidneys or heart.

# Birth Asphyxia and Resuscitation

## Causes of Asphyxia

Birth asphyxia may take the form of failure to breathe, failure to expand the lungs, or both. In practice, initial failure to breathe is much commoner than initial failure to expand the lungs, although it is obvious that one will lead to the other.

When a baby does not gasp or cry at birth it is because the respiratory centre is depressed and cannot respond to the inevitable sensory bombardment that occurs at birth. There are three main reasons for this: (a) prolonged intra-partum asphyxia; (b) recent intra-partum asphyxia, combined with the effects of narcotic drugs which have crossed the placenta from the mother; and (c)—least common under conditions of modern obstetric practice—actual brain-stem injury in the form of haemorrhage or herniation.

Failure of adequate expansion of the lungs in response to a normal respiratory effort may result from extreme prematurity, from congenital malformation of the respiratory tract, or from airway obstruction. Obstruction is usually caused by thick mucus (occasionally meconium) at the level of the larynx.

## Immediate Effects of Asphyxia

In experimental asphyxia of fetal or newborn mammals the following sequence of events consistently occurs (Dawes 1968)*. There is a short period of dyspnoea which ends abruptly and is followed by a longer period of apnoea ('primary apnoea'): this is followed by a period of repeated single gasps which become somewhat more frequent and weaker before ceasing altogether: the animal is then apnoeic again ('terminal apnoea') and, unless revived by artificial oxygenation, its heart rate and blood pressure continue to fall until it is dead. There are good reasons for thinking that this sequence of events occurs in the human baby, although the situation may be complicated by partial or intermittent intra-partum asphyxia. It must also be remembered that part or all of this sequence of events may have occurred *in utero* or in the birth canal before the baby is seen.

### Primary Apnoea

A baby in primary apnoea will usually appear blue rather than white, show small spontaneous movements (especially of the eye-lids and lips), lie with normal flexural tone, show some reflex responses to manipulation and, on auscultation, will often, but not invariably, be found to have a relatively rapid or an accelerating heart-rate.

Even if one does nothing, the first gasp will usually occur spontaneously, but it may be expedited by a number of different physical and chemical stimuli. (It is this period of primary apnoea that is extended by anaesthetics or narcotics such as morphine or pethidine.)

*Dawes, G. S. (1968) *Fetal and Neonatal Physiology*. Chicago: Year Book Medical Publishers Inc. Chapter 12.

*Gasping*

The gasping movements which eventually ensue are powerful and lead to expansion of the lungs and initiation of normal respiration, provided the airway is clear. Thus in most cases of birth asphyxia, respiration will be established spontaneously and without the need for artificial respiration after a period of 'primary' apnoea—a fact which needs to be taken into account in evaluating old and new methods of resuscitation.

*Terminal Apnoea*

Uncommonly, the infant is in 'terminal' apnoea, having already passed his last gasp at the time of birth, and in this case resuscitation is a matter of urgency and is genuinely lifesaving. The baby in terminal apnoea will appear white rather than blue, show no spontaneous movements or reaction to stimulation, will lie outstretched and limp and will always have a slow, and sometimes a slowing, heart-rate.

There is no response to physical or chemical stimuli and there is evidence that brain damage may occur in this period, rather than in primary apnoea. Resuscitation can only be achieved by raising arterial oxygen tension by means of artificial ventilation and, when successful, an improvement in heart rate and colour will precede the first gasp.

Our instructions for resuscitation are based on these facts. However, primary and terminal apnoea are not always clearly distinguishable. We therefore intubate most apnoeic babies as if they were in terminal apnoea, with the realization in retrospect that artificial respiration has probably been unnecessary, when gasping has preceded an improvement in colour.

**Assessment of the Baby at One Minute after Birth**

We employ a modification of the Apgar system, but do not routinely apply a score, although the now traditional Apgar score can be derived from the information we collect on the form reproduced on p. 34.

The information is collected on all babies born at the Hammersmith Hospital, observations being made as far as possible at one minute after birth (regardless of whether the cord has been tied or cut). The heart rate is counted by placing a stethoscope over the chest; while this is being done the baby's colour, respirations, tone and posture are noted. Pharyngeal suction will usually have been carried out before one minute and the response should also be noted.

**Instructions for Resuscitation**

New residents should read these instructions and learn them as soon as possible after taking up their appointments. They should familiarize themselves with the equipment and should practice intubating first on the model, then on dead babies, and then under supervision on ill babies needing intubation in the special care nursery.

Most cases of birth asphyxia (*i.e.* apnoea at one minute following delivery) are anticipated at Hammersmith and the resident should be in the delivery room prepared to cope with the situation. The remaining unexpected cases of birth asphyxia are also, by-and-large, the least serious.

CONDITION OF BABY AT _____ MINUTE(S) AFTER BIRTH
(at 1 minute whenever possible)

*Please tick appropriate square*

| | | | |
|---|---|---|---|
| Apex beat by auscultation | Inaudible | Rate if present: | /min. |
| Respiration | Absent | Gasping or irregular | Regular or rhythmical |

Did the baby gasp or cry before the age of 1 minute? YES/NO

| | | | |
|---|---|---|---|
| Muscle tone and movement | Limp | Normal muscle tone: no movement | Spontaneous movement of the limbs |
| Response to nasal or pharyngeal catheter within first minute | None | Grimace | Cough |
| Colour of trunk | Grey or white | Blue | Pink |

*In cases of asphyxia:*

| | | | |
|---|---|---|---|
| Heart-rate at 1 minute | Slowing | Steady | Quickening |
| Response to resuscitation | Pink before gasp | | Gasp before pink |

On being called to the delivery room in cases of anticipated birth asphyxia:
(1) check the equipment on the trolley;
(2) turn on the heater over the trolley;
(3) ensure that the incubator is heated.

When the baby is born:
(1) start (or have an assistant start) the clock on the trolley and the tape-recorder to which you may dictate notes;
(2) suck out the airways when the head is delivered (note the baby's response to this stimulus);
(3) as soon as the cord is clamped and cut, transfer the baby to the resuscitation trolley and, if you have an assistant, have him attach the ECG leads;
(4) assess the baby's state (see above). This is usually done one minute after complete delivery, but should be done at once if the baby is obviously asphyxiated.

*Presumed 'Primary' Apnoea*
If the baby has not gasped by one minute after delivery, the pharynx and nose should again be aspirated with the mucus catheter. In practice, this will be quite ineffective in removing a plug of mucus at laryngeal level and it is doubtful if aspiration

of amniotic fluid is of great importance. However, the posterior pharyngeal wall is a sensitive reflexogenic zone and application of the mucus catheter may well initiate the first gasp.

If the baby still remains apnoeic but shows all the favourable signs of primary apnoea (blue rather than white, small spontaneous movements, good muscle tone, heart rate over 100 or rising) it is theoretically not unreasonable to await events. However, in practice, we usually try to expedite the first gasp by flicking the baby's feet, by aspirating the pharynx again, or by applying intermittent positive pressure to the airways with a bag and mask (which may cause a gasp by eliciting Head's paradoxical reflex).

If you are uncertain whether the baby is in primary or terminal apnoea; if there is any deterioration in the baby's state; or if spontaneous gasping is not quickly followed by regular respiration, intubate at once.

*Presumed 'Terminal' Apnoea*
(1) Inspect the cords with a laryngoscope, aspirate mucus, meconium, etc. under direct vision, and intubate*, using an oro-tracheal tube with a shoulder on it, having attached the Y-piece adaptor.
(2) Attach the side limb of the adaptor to a supply of 40% oxygen, which should be flowing at two litres per minute. Set the pressure-valve release to 30-35cm $H_2O$. Occlude the other limb of the Y-adaptor with your thumb until the pressure reaches 30cm, then remove your thumb for two seconds to allow elastic recoil of the lungs. Watch chest movement and auscultate on either side to check that both lungs are being inflated. Repeat this rhythmically. The rate should be about 30 per minute, *i.e.* not too rapid. The flow rate of oxygen will limit the time it takes to achieve the desired pressure and may have to be adjusted slightly. Occasionally, higher pressures will be necessary for the initial inflation (up to 60cm$H_2O$), but the intention is to inflate the lungs by *repeated* pressures rather than by one massive blow. (If intubation proves impossible, bag-and-mask or mouth-to-mouth ventilation are the best alternatives.) Artificial respiration must be carried on until regular respiration is established or until the baby is dead.

Do not be in too great a hurry to remove the endotracheal tube after respiration is established following serious asphyxia. Wait until adequate ventilation has been established for 5 to 10 minutes; if it is decided to transfer the baby to the special care nursery immediately, leave the endotracheal tube *in situ* until he has arrived there and settled down.
(3) In any baby thought to have been in terminal apnoea, alkali should be administered as soon as spontaneous respiration or adequate artificial ventilation has been established. Insert an umbilical venous catheter and inject 10ml of 7% THAM or 8.4% bicarbonate, followed by 5ml of 20% dextrose. This injection should not be

---

*During suction and/or intubation, make sure that all connecting links between tubes and metal are firm. We have seen a small suction catheter disappear down the oesophagus because of a loose connection. Others have reported similar accidents with endotracheal tubes. If this happens ask a surgeon skilled in infant oesophagoscopy to see the child without delay, for there is a risk that the tube may cause oesphageal rupture. Removal under anaesthesia usually presents no difficulties, but prevention is better than cure.

too rapid, *i.e.* take two minutes or more. Nalorphine may also be given if the mother has been given morphia or pethidine within 12 hours of the baby's birth. It also should be administered intravenously (see below).

(4) All babies thought to have been in terminal apnoea should be left in the incubator on the labour ward and observed frequently for two or three hours. If any doubt then remains about the baby's condition, transfer him to the special care nursery. (*N.B.* The use of analeptics, unnecessary in primary apnoea, is useless and positively harmful in terminal apnoea.)

*Cardiac Arrest or Severe Bradycardia (HR < 30/min) in Terminal Apnoea*

Proceed as follows if the baby is pale, motionless, limp, and has a very low or absent heart-rate. (If the fetal heart has been heard until shortly before the delivery of an apparently dead baby, we believe that attempts at revival should be carried out. In our small experience of long-term survivors, brain damage has been frequent, but by no means invariable.)

If you are single-handed, give 5 to 10 beats of external cardiac massage before intubating. (Even with unventilated lungs, this has been shown to aid resuscitation in animals.) Place two fingers on the sternum (above 2nd costal cartilage) and press the upper sternum sharply back towards the spine at the rate of about one per second. There is a danger of rupturing the liver if the pressure is exerted too far down (*i.e.* caudally) on the sternum. (An alternative method of applying cardiac massage to the newborn is to put your hands around the baby's chest and compress the upper sternum with both thumbs.) Then proceed as for terminal apnoea (see above).

In the case of the 'stillborn' baby, cardiac massage should be continued at the same time as artificial ventilation until heart action is restored—or the baby is clearly dead. If you have any difficulty in intubating it is best to continue cardiac massage while attempting to inflate the lungs by bag and mask, or mouth-to-mouth ventilation, say four times a minute.

*Delayed Apnoea*

A number of babies, usually those born to mothers who have had general anaesthesia, cry at once but then quickly become apnoeic. Such babies should be treated as for primary apnoea, with aspiration under direct vision, intubation and IPPV if the heart rate slows or the general condition deteriorates. They start to breathe again, but sometimes only after several minutes. If the mother has had morphine or pethidine, consider using nalorphine (see p. 38).

**Other Emergencies at Birth**

*Respiratory Obstruction*

If a baby makes respiratory efforts at birth, but these are accompanied by sucking of the chest wall and no improvement in the baby's colour, there is probably obstruction by a plug of mucus or meconium at the laryngeal level. Pharyngeal aspiration is useless and laryngoscopy is called for urgently so that any obstruction may be aspirated under direct vision: after even brief delays, the obstructing material is sucked down into the bronchi.

When a baby born covered with meconium develops these signs, the nasopharynx should be aspirated, then the cords under direct vision, followed by intubation. This is the exceptional situation when suction may be applied directly to the endotracheal tube and the suction maintained while the tube is pulled out. The procedure may have to be repeated.

Babies with respiratory obstruction at birth will need to be watched particularly carefully for signs of respiratory distress over the next few hours. They may develop a tension cyst or spontaneous pneumothorax (see p. 140). Take a lateral chest film to demonstrate the presence or absence of mediastinal emphysema. Rarely, obstruction is due to an anatomical defect (webs, cysts, stenosis). The only hope is to get an endotracheal tube beyond it.

*Fetal Haemorrhage*

If a baby at birth is very pale, with air hunger and tachycardia (particularly in cases of twinning, ante-partum haemorrhage or incision of the placenta at caesarean section), fetal haemorrhage may have occurred. The cord blood should be 'milked' into the baby before the cord is tied and an immediate transfusion of up to about 30 ml blood per kg should be given.

*Surgical Emergencies*

There are several reparable conditions which may present as respiratory difficulties shortly after birth: the operator should keep them in mind. The more important ones are:
(1) oesophageal atresia with tracheo-oesophageal fistula (p. 49);
(2) choanal atresia (p. 53);
(3) Pierre Robin syndrome (p. 51);
(4) diaphragmatic hernia (p. 50);
(5) pneumothorax (p. 140);
(6) gross ascites (p. 67).

## Notes on Various Resuscitative Procedures

*Laryngoscopy and Endotracheal Intubation*

The larynx must first be inspected. The baby is laid flat, with the neck slightly flexed and the head extended on the neck. The endotracheal tube is held in the right hand. The laryngoscope and jaw are held in the left hand between the thumb, index and middle fingers, and the blade is held along the tongue with the tip anterior to the epiglottis. The cricoid cartilage is then pressed towards the spine using the fourth and little fingers, thus obliterating the oesophagus and bringing the larynx into view. Any obstructing mucus or meconium should be aspirated under direct vision. The endotracheal tube is now inserted, care being taken not to insert it so far that it enters one main bronchus, thus occluding the other. A guide is to insert the tube not farther from the mouth than the distance between the acromion process and the elbow. If there is any doubt as to whether the tube is correctly placed, apply your lips to the tube and puff once or twice while listening to the lungs (the contents of your mouth—20-50ml; *not* the contents, of your lungs—3-5 litres!).

In desperate circumstances, if the laryngoscope light fails at the crucial moment or you cannot get the endotracheal tube in place by the conventional method, insert your right index finger into the baby's throat until you feel the epiglottis and, about 1cm further on, a depression where the cords are. Keeping this finger in place, guide the endotracheal tube along the finger till it enters the larynx. We have succeeded in intubating the oedematous larynx of a hydropic baby this way, when the usual method had failed.

*Mouth-to-mouth or Bag-and-mask Ventilation*

If intubation proves impossible, either of these methods is a second best alternative. For mouth-to-mouth ventilation, the baby's head should be extended and the mouth of the operator should cover the baby's mouth and nose. The operator should blow out his cheeks to inflate the baby's lungs, which should not be subjected to the full volume of expiration. The baby's lungs should be allowed to recoil spontaneously before the next inflation, 12 breaths a minute being satisfactory. To make this manoeuvre safe and efficient, the larynx should be pushed back gently against the spine to occlude the oesophagus. For bag-and-mask ventilation see that the mask fits closely around the baby's nose and mouth, and that the blow-off valve is set to $30cmH_2O$.

**Drugs**

IN THE APNOEIC BABY, ARTIFICIAL VENTILATION MUST PRECEDE THE ADMINISTRATION OF DRUGS.

*Alkali*

THAM or bicarbonate is given intravenously in a dose of about 3ml/kg (of 7% THAM or 8.4% $HCO_3$). A polyvinyl umbilical catheter is filled with sterile normal saline and the end is left attached to the synringe as a precaution against air embolism. The cord is cleaned with 70% isopropyl alcohol, a ligature is tied loosely near the umbilicus, and the cord is cut off with sterile scissors about 2cm from the umbilicus. The cut end is gripped with Spencer Wells forceps and the catheter is inserted 5-7cm into the umbilical vein which appears on the cut surface of the cord. Blood can usually be freely aspirated by gentle suction, and a specimen should be taken under anaerobic conditions (for later estimation of pH and base deficit), the syringe being put in the refrigerator on the resuscitation trolley. Alkali is then given slowly, taking about two minutes over the injection.

*Nalorphine*

If the baby is thought to have been affected by pethidine or morphine given to the mother (*i.e.* when spontaneous respiration does not begin after successful artificial respiration or when spontaneous respiration is shallow) give 1mg of nalorphine, if possible intravenously, injecting 1ml of normal saline before giving the nalorphine to exclude a nonspecific effect and 1ml afterwards to wash the nalorphine in. (We would like to know if the baby was morphinized, and when nalorphine is given intramuscularly it is never possible to be certain that an improvement of respiration is not coincidental.)

*Analeptics*

We do not use any analeptics (*e.g.* nikethamide, ethamivan) and consider them undesirable and dangerous for a number of reasons.

## Warmth

An asphyxiated baby can get very cold during resuscitation.
(1) Turn on the heater over the trolley before his birth.
(2) Quickly dab him dry.
(3) Transfer him to the preheated incubator as soon as possible.
(4) When resuscitating in places other than where the trolley is situated, wrap as much of the child in a silver swaddler* as is consistent with an adequate view of the chest.

The labour wards should be as warm as is consistent with the mother's well-being. The incubator in the labour ward should be kept at 36°C.

## Gastric Aspiration

This is *not* done as a routine (even for infants of diabetic mothers or for babies born after caesarean section). There is a danger of mucus carried up from the stomach obstructing the glottis as one withdraws the tube. However, if the baby is thought to have swallowed a large quantity of blood, liquor or meconium, there is a case for emptying the stomach. Use a polyvinyl feeding tube and aspirate with a syringe. Before withdrawing the tube, inject 2 or 3ml of sterile water rapidly to wash away any mucus from the end of the tube.

## Notes

During resuscitation, jot down notes whenever possible (and use the ECG and the tape-recorder).

Following the recovery or death of the baby, careful notes should be written indicating the exact times at which various procedures were carried out and when the onset of gasps and of regular respirations took place. Try to make a retrospective assessment of the degree of asphyxia, based principally on the response to resuscitation (gasp before pink = primary apnoea; pink before gasp = probable terminal apnoea). The baby should be re-assessed for the record at about five minutes and ten minutes after birth.

*Lewis Griptight Ltd.

# Routine Examination at Birth

(At Hammersmith, this examination is done by the obstetric resident).

All apparently healthy newborn babies should be examined within an hour or two of birth.

(1) Assess whether the baby is pre-term or small for dates from his gestational age and weight, and measure the head-circumference in case this is not done later. (It is better to measure head-circumference after 24 hours. See charts on p. 326 and p. 327).

(2) Look for jaundice (which should not be present at this age), central cyanosis and anaemia.

(3) Look for birth trauma.

(4) Look for those congenital malformations which are not immediately obvious, but which are serious and yet treatable. Look in particular for the following.

(*a*) Excessive salivation or frothiness at the mouth, which might suggest oesophageal atresia (see p. 49).

(*b*) Evidence of respiratory difficulty or obstruction. (Apart from 'medical' causes of respiratory distress, consider choanal atresia (p. 53), diaphragmatic hernia (p. 50), Pierre Robin syndrome (p. 51), oesophageal atresia (p. 49) and congenital lobar emphysema (p. 122).

(*c*) Cleft palate (see p. 51 and p. 59).

(*d*) Viscera protruding into the umbilical cord (see p. 30 and p. 54).

(*e*) Abdominal tumours (see p. 199).

(*f*) Imperforate anus (see p. 60).

(*g*) Abnormal genitalia (see 'Ambiguous sex' p. 60, 'Hooded prepuce' p. 64, and 'Genitalia' p. 246).

(*h*) Midline lesions over the spine which may have a track connecting with the subarachnoid space.

(*i*) Single umbilical artery and single transverse palmar crease. Though neither of the anomalies is important in itself, other congenital anomalies may co-exist and should be especially looked for.

This very quick examination is far from being a complete one, but other possible congenital abnormalities will either be too obvious to miss, or can safely be left until the final discharge examination (p. 81) or until the symptoms are reported.

# General Approach to the Parents of Deformed or Ill Babies

Talking to parents is, of course, an everyday part of the paediatrician's life, but it does sometimes present particular difficulties when the child is a newborn baby, because the parents will probably not know the paediatrician and neither they nor the paediatrician will know the child. Furthermore, the mother, who will be the first parent involved—and sometimes the only one—is herself a patient who has just been through the physically and emotionally exhausting experience of labour. If there is a member of the paediatric staff who has looked after other children in the family, he will find it much easier to talk to the parents and will be the best person to do so. Our joint rounds of the antenatal wards allow us to meet some mothers before labour begins, but still only a minority of those likely to have babies with neonatal problems. Usually the obstetrician will be the member of the hospital staff who knows the mother best, and it is often very helpful for him to speak to the mother first and introduce the paediatrician to her.

Nevertheless, there will often be situations where the paediatrician simply has to arrive on the scene as a total stranger, and announce that the baby has some serious illness or abnormality. He then must be aware of the difficulties and do his best in spite of them.

Before talking to the parents, be sure to find out (and remember) the baby's sex. Failure to do so means you will either have to commit the solecism of calling the baby 'it', or engage in impossible circumlocutions to avoid using 'he' or 'she', or confess that you do not know, so that (except in cases of ambiguous sex) the mother may, not unreasonably, have little faith in your assessment of her baby's problems.

## Deformed Babies

Today more and more babies are, so to speak, 'ordered' by their parents and childbirth can less and less be looked upon as an act of God, a bit of good luck or of bad luck. And, as Dr. Alfred White Franklin has pointed out, when parents order a baby, they order a perfect one. Thus the shock, grief and bewilderment of having produced a congenitally malformed baby and the sense of personal responsibility for it are perhaps greater today than they have ever been in the past.

When the mother has seen her *obviously* deformed baby, the resident paediatrician should see her at once to give her a brief explanation, to tell her what has to be done and to assure her that he will let her husband know as soon as possible. He should aim to tell the truth and nothing but the truth, but not necessarily the whole truth all at once. He should then inform the consultant paediatrician, the child's father and the general practitioner.

If the baby has a malformation which will be obvious to the mother on detailed inspection but which she has not yet seen, it may be best to try to get hold of the father to tell him first, and ask him whether he wants you to tell his wife or to do so himself.

41

However, this should not be done if it will involve a delay of more than, say, an hour before the mother is told; if she is specifically asking about the baby's normality, she must not be fobbed off with evasions or falsehoods.

When a malformation is obvious to the doctor or midwife but not to the parents, the paediatrician faces a difficult decision. This situation most commonly arises in the case of a baby with Down's syndrome. A majority of mothers will recognize that there is something wrong, either from the baby's or from the midwife's appearance and expression. Such a mother deserves an immediate, full and truthful explanation. We prefer that the consultant paediatrician should give this, but if this will involve delay in answering the mother's questions, any member of the midwifery or medical staff should be authorised to give a sympathetic, factual but brief explanation, leaving the consultant paediatrician to have further discussion with both parents.

Even when the mother is apparently perfectly happy about her baby, it is commonly accepted today that she should be told at once about abnormality. We have no departmental policy, and there are considerable disagreements between ourselves as to what should be done. Furthermore, no single one of us always does the same. Many mothers who were not told at once have subsequently said they were glad—'it gave me time to get fond of him, doctor'. The decision about when to tell will depend on numerous but sometimes imponderable considerations. The general practitioner must always be consulted. Of course, one may make the wrong decision (or the right one) and subsequently be blamed by the parents. But this is one of many situations in which a doctor should be prepared to shoulder the blame in the best interests of his patients.

Talking to the parents of a congenitally malformed baby is involved and difficult, and is one situation in which age and experience really do help. It is as important to listen as to talk. What does the malformation mean to the parents? They may have wild misconceptions about its causation and implications for the child's future. Cleft lip and palate, especially if bilateral, is a hideous deformity; many parents have no idea that today the plastic surgeons will usually make it scarcely detectable. 'Before' and 'after' photographs are kept in the paediatric department and should be shown to the parents. A baby with Down's syndrome may be thought of as having to lead a vegetative and helpless existence for the whole of his lifetime; in fact children with Down's syndrome walk and feed themselves by about $2\frac{1}{2}$ years and talk at about $4\frac{1}{2}$ years. Hypospadias may be regarded as a cause of infertility; it is not.

The parents will also want to know how it has happened—'Is it our fault, doctor?' At least the answer to that question is simple enough, but one can seldom tell the parents the exact causation of a congenital deformity. They should be told that we are all carriers of disease processes—indeed, it appears to be a condition of healthy survival—and that malformations may be caused by chance co-incidence of many factors, none of which is in itself decisive or controllable.

Parents will also want to know what are the chances of a future child being affected. If you don't know, consult the authorities referred to on p. 6.

If the young paediatrician has the task of 'breaking the news' he may not always realize that, however sympathetic and well thought-out his explanation, the parents will never listen. They cannot do so, since their minds are whirling with considerations of immediate practical importance: 'What shall I say to my mother-in-law? What shall I say to the neighbours?', and so on. Thus it will be necessary to see them again and repeat this explanation. Remember to assure the parents that they will get continued support from the medical services and not be left in doubt as to how they should care for their baby.

Sometimes it will greatly help the parents to meet other parents of a child with a similar abnormality, but such introductions should only be arranged with considerable thought and care. In general, it is important for the parents to belong to the same social class. Joining parents' societies and reading literature designed for parents may often be helpful: consult the medical social worker about what literature and organisations are available in relation to the child's particular problems.

### Ill and Low-birthweight Babies

Illness and low birthweight do not have the same emotionally charged connotations as congenital malformations, but what has been said above about one's first approach to the parents is largely applicable to these slightly different situations. Both parents must be informed as soon and as fully as possible about the baby's condition, and must be kept informed of his progress or of any important changes. It is particularly important for the paediatrician to keep closely in touch with the mother and visit her at least once a day. A mother of a seriously ill child would normally want to be with him most of the time. This is usually impossible for the recently delivered mother, but she should at least feel that she knows what is happening.

In the early days, it is sometimes best to talk to the mother in rather general terms about the baby's progress, reserving more detailed and technical explanations for the father to pass on to her as he sees fit. Clearly, however, mothers vary greatly in what information they can assimilate and cope with in the puerperium.

On first seeing the mother, discuss with her how she intended to feed the baby, and point out the advantages of breast milk, particularly the high-protein milk of the first week, for the ill or low-birthweight baby. Explain that she can express her milk and that there is a sporting chance that she will eventually be able to breast-feed her baby, however immature. If she wants to do so, make sure her lactation is not suppressed. It is also kind and helpful to give the mother some idea of how long the baby will be in the special care nursery before being ready to go home. This can only be a guess (and you should say so), but it should be a better informed guess than the mother's own. For a low-birthweight baby, reckon that he will regain his birthweight in about 2 weeks, then gain about 200g per week, and that he will be ready to go home when he weighs about 2250g. Small-for-dates babies may be quicker; babies below 1200g birthweight slower.

### Mothers and Their Low-birthweight Babies

The mother of a low-birthweight baby should be encouraged to visit him as much as possible, as soon as she is fit enough. Even if he is in an incubator and receiving intensive care, she should be allowed to touch and handle him (provided he is well enough to be handled) and to feel that he belongs to her and not to the hospital.

The only exception we would make is in the case of a very ill baby, who seems virtually certain to die; we would not, of course, discourage her from visiting her baby and seeing and touching him as much as she wanted, but we would not put pressure on her to form an attachment which would increase her sense of bereavement when he died.

When the low-birthweight baby is well enough to come out of the incubator, his mother should if possible handle him regularly, feed him, change him and talk to ·him. We are not certain how important this is from the baby's point of view at the time, but we are certain it is important for the mother, and hence in the long run for the baby.

**Fathers**

Remember that in the case of a baby born in wedlock the father is the legal guardian and any serious problem concerning the baby should be discussed fully with him. If the natural father of an illegitimate baby visits and shows an interest (and they usually do today) he should, with the mother's approval, also be consulted and involved in any decision concerning the baby's health.

# Indications for Transfer to the Special Care Nursery

Babies need to be transferred to the special care nursery if they require observation or treatment which are not available on the ordinary postnatal wards. This is clearly a matter for individual judgement, but transfer will almost invariably be necessary in the following situations.

(1) *Birthweight less than about* 2000g. Apart from any specific problems of prematurity or smallness for dates, these babies need extra warmth and observation, and are unlikely to be ready to go home when their mother goes. However, some of these babies may be able to breast-feed, and their mothers should be encouraged to do this if it is possible.

(2) *Gestational age less than 35 weeks*. Apart from any other problems, the baby will probably require some tube feeds.

(3) *Illness*. The great majority of illnesses occurring immediately after birth are respiratory, and present with signs of respiratory distress—whatever the cause. Persisting respiratory distress is an indication for transfer, but when signs are mild it is reasonable to observe the baby in the labour ward incubator up to the age of four hours. If the signs resolve during this time and the baby is well, he may go to the postnatal ward.

Most other illnesses and most of the *serious* congenital malformations are indications for transfer.

Transfer from the postnatal ward to the special care nursery is indicated for babies who develop fits, significant vomiting, evidence of intestinal obstruction, haemorrhage, or other dangerous illness.

The decision as to whether a baby with serious infection should go to the special care nursery or elsewhere may be difficult. A baby with diarrhoea of presumed enteral infective origin should be transferred to a children's ward rather than to the special care nursery. On the other hand, a baby with a presumed gram-negative septicaemia could reasonably go to the isolation cubicle of the special care nursery. The facilities for neonatal intensive care would certainly be valuable to him, and he would be much less likely to constitute a real danger to the other babies. No set rules can be laid down: each case must be dealt with on its merits. Similar considerations apply to the admission of babies from other hospitals to the special care nursery: we no longer routinely apply the rule that such babies cannot be admitted after the age of 48 hours.

(4) *Anxiety*. In some cases where the doctors, midwives, or parents are particularly anxious about a baby, it may be sensible to transfer him temporarily to the special care nursery for observation—even in the absence of indications (1), (2) or (3) above. Examples are maternal illnesses which it is feared may lead to sudden and serious trouble to the baby in the early neonatal period (*e.g.* thyrotoxicosis, myasthenia gravis, thrombocytopenia) and previous unexplained neonatal deaths. The consultant should decide about transfer in these cases.

45

(5) *Contra-indications to transfer.* The main disadvantage of transfer to the special care nursery is that it partially separates the mother and baby. This is very undesirable in situations where the mother may find it difficult to form an attachment to the baby. Examples are Down's syndrome and disfiguring malformations such as cleft lip and severe talipes. In these cases, transfer should be avoided unless there are over-riding medical reasons for it.

We do not routinely transfer to the special care nursery babies who have had abnormal deliveries, *e.g.* caesarean section or forceps, unless there is some other indication for transfer. The policy about such babies must depend on how reliably they can be observed in the maternity department.

**Keeping the Mother Informed**

At the best, it is very disappointing to the mother for the baby to be taken away from her and transferred to the special care nursery. At the worst, she may fear that something is being hidden from her or that the baby will die. The neonatal resident should visit the mother at least once a day for the first few days that the baby is in the special care nursery, and certainly as long as the baby's condition is causing anxiety. See also p. 43.

# Birth Trauma

Serious obstetric trauma at birth is now fortunately uncommon. Minor injury in newborn babies usually heals well but it must be remembered that any injury may represent a portal of entry of infection. A baby's skin is easily lacerated or bruised.

## Superficial Abrasions

These may occur after the use of forceps or the ventouse extractor, and by minor accidental incisions at caesarean section. If an incision is gaping widely, ask the obstetrician (politely) to put in a suture while he is still scrubbed up, and has needles and sutures available. In general, leave abrasions clean and dry, but at any sign of purulence take a swab and treat appropriately. (see 'Infection', p. 167).

## Petechiae and Bruising

'Traumatic cyanosis'—that is cyanosis and petechiae *confined* to the head and neck—is not in our experience associated with obvious birth trauma. (Make quite certain that petechiae or cyanosis do not occur elsewhere on the body). The prognosis is good and no action is necessary other than to explain the situation to the mother (for the baby may look spuriously ill).

Petechiae of the conjunctivae or subconjunctival haemorrhages are commoner in Negro babies than in Causasian babies. They may alarm mothers, but they do not affect vision and disappear spontaneously.

Bruising may be extensive in short-gestation babies, especially when delivered by the breech. No action is necessary at birth, but remember that jaundice may be aggravated at 3 to 4 days.

## Fractures

Obvious skull fractures are rare, although it is probable that many cephal-haematomata—not present at birth—are associated with small skull fractures. These latter are not of any clinical significance and we do not routinely x-ray the skull in cases of cephalhaematoma. Even depressed fractures will usually disappear spontaneously and surgical elevation is rarely necessary. The fracture to the cranium, *per se*, therefore requires no treatment other than gentle handling. Associated intracranial damage may present as birth asphyxia at this stage (see p. 32).

Fractures of the clavicle or humerus may occur after breech extraction or shoulder impaction. They may first become apparent because the baby cries when handled, or does not move the affected upper limb and has an asymmetrical Moro reflex. These fractures heal quickly and, even if badly aligned, moulding takes place spontaneously and the end result is good unless an epiphysis has been damaged, in which case there may be permanent shortening of the limb. Confirm the fracture by x-ray and inform the orthopaedic consultant. Probably no action other than gentle handling is necessary, but some prefer to bandage with a crêpe bandage (the clavicle by a figure-of-8 across the back of the shoulders, and the humerus, *gently*, to the side of the chest). Remember that there may be an associated brachial plexus palsy.

Fractured femur is rare, but we have seen an occasional case. Seek orthopaedic advice. The leg may be left to heal, or bandaged over the abdomen. Gallows traction is not necessary. All bandages incorporating the chest or abdomen must be sufficiently loose not to obstruct respiration.

Fractures of the cervical spine or avulsions of the cervical cord may occur, especially during difficult breech extractions, but these injuries are now very rare indeed. Sometimes a crack may be heard during delivery. The child usually lies with arms abducted and is completely flaccid below the lesion. Later the bladder enlarges and becomes palpable because of an inability to pass urine spontaneously.

Always consider the possibility of osteogenesis imperfecta, especially if there is more than one fracture. Feel the skull for defects in the membrane bones and the ribs for irregularities.

### Nerve Injury

Facial palsy may occur whether or not forceps have been used. Facial palsy due to trauma usually recovers well, sometimes in a day or two, sometimes after weeks, but may be difficult to differentiate from the rarer prenatal facial palsy in which the prognosis is not so good. Bilateral facial palsy suggests a central lesion such as agenesis of the seventh nerve nucleus. If the child cannot close his eye, methylcellulose drops should be instilled.

Brachial plexus palsy may occur after breech extraction or shoulder impaction. The paresis may escape unnoticed for a day or two. When the upper roots are affected (Erb's palsy) the arm hangs limply and internally rotated with the elbow extended. Rarely, the diaphragm may also be paralysed. Klumpke's paralysis (lower roots) appears as wrist-drop and flaccid paresis of the hand, and is similar to radial nerve paresis—in which there may be signs of bruising over the anterolateral aspect of the upper arm. Inform the orthopaedic surgeon and apply a clove-hitch of crêpe bandage to the child's wrist, pinning the bandage to the cot above the shoulders in such a way as to prevent undue stretching of paralysed muscles. For wrist-drop, make a light padded cock-up splint from a wooden spatula or of plaster of paris. In general, one may expect recovery, but the course may be anything from days to months.

### Visceral Trauma

Visceral trauma and liver or adrenal haemorrhage may present as unexpected collapse, usually not at birth (see p. 218).

### Intracranial Injury

Modern obstetric practice has greatly reduced the incidence of serious intra-cranial injury. When it does occur, the presenting signs may be birth asphyxia, with delay in establishing spontaneous regular respirations even after resuscitation (see p. 32), or 'abnormal behaviour following perinatal hazard'—especially cerebral irritation or cerebral depression (see p. 181).

# Congenital Malformations Needing Urgent Treatment

The malformations described under this heading all require immediate action to be taken. The first five (oesophageal atresia, congenital diaphragmatic hernia, Pierre Robin syndrome, choanal atresia, omphalocele) are life-threatening, and are likely to lead to death if not treated promptly. Though none of them is met very frequently in an average-sized maternity department, it is essential that the neonatal paediatrician should know how to recognize them, and what to do when they are diagnosed.

Myelomeningocele is included in this section because a decision about early surgical treatment must be made immediately after birth, and talipes equinovarus is included because prompt treatment is important if permanent deformity is to be avoided.

**Oesophageal Atresia and Tracheo-oesophageal Fistula**

These two anomalies are generally associated, by far the commonest combination being the one in which the fistula connects the lower trachea with the lower oesophageal pouch, *i.e.* the oesophagus below the atretic portion. Though the condition is generally referred to as 'tracheo-oesophageal fistula' or simply 'T.O.F.', the oesophageal atresia is the more lethal anomaly, for it leads to direct aspiration into the lungs of accumulated pharyngeal mucus and of any feeds which may disastrously be given if the diagnosis is missed.

*Grounds for Suspicion of Oesophageal Atresia*

The condition should be suspected before or during labour if there is poly-hydramnios (see p. 7). At birth the baby will generally have a short period of undistressed breathing, with or without prior resuscitation. Within minutes or hours, excessive saliva will accumulate in the mouth, and the baby will develop signs of respiratory distress or obstruction accompanied by cyanosis. These symptoms will be temporarily relieved by pharyngeal suction but this will be required frequently. The diagnosis should be made before a feed is given: if it is not, feeding will cause serious choking, respiratory difficulty and cyanosis.

The grounds for suspicion are therefore:
(1) polyhydramnios;
(2) the infant being 'mucusy';
(3) respiratory distress, choking and/or cyanosis temporarily relieved by pharyngeal suction; or
(4) respiratory distress, choking or cyanosis precipitated by feeding (but it is a failure of care if the diagnosis has to be arrived at in this way).

49

*Diagnosis*

When any of the above grounds for suspicion is present, an attempt should be made to pass a stomach tube via the oesophagus. Failure to reach the stomach establishes the diagnosis; success rules it out. The only diagnostic snag is that a flexible stomach-tube may curl up in the upper oesophageal pouch and appear to have passed further than it has. To avoid this error, use a fairly stiff and preferably radio-opaque catheter, *e.g.* a No. 5 Jacques. If it appears to have reached the stomach, aspirate some contents and test with blue litmus (stomach contents are acid at birth). If the catheter fails to pass, take an x-ray of the chest and upper abdomen with it in position. This will show the level of the obstruction and also the outline of the air-containing upper oesophageal pouch.

Oesophageal atresia is commonly associated with other congenital anomalies (apart from tracheo-oesophageal fistula). Look especially for evidence of imperforate anus and congenital heart disease.

*Management*

(1) See that no feeds or fluids are given by mouth.

(2) Alert the paediatric surgeon and arrange operating theatre, anaesthetist and blood.

(3) Follow the surgeon's instructions as to pre-operative management. This will always include frequent pharyngeal aspiration, followed by laryngoscopy and tracheal suction if pharyngeal suction does not relieve the respiratory symptoms. A drip will usually be required (see 'Intravenous fluids', p. 99), but give as little fluid as possible pre-operatively.

*Post-operative Management*

Intensive care will be required for at least a week. The resident must be prepared to sleep on the spot, or not at all. Pulmonary complications are common and account for a high proportion of deaths; they may occur insidiously or with alarming rapidity. If the child 'goes off' suddenly, ensure the upper airways are clear, look for clinical signs of pneumothorax and make sure that the chest tube connected to the underwater seal drain is patent. Frequently the cause of sudden deterioration, which may present as either respiratory distress or apnoea, is mucus on the larynx or in the bronchi. If none of the above problems is identified, use a laryngoscope *early*—for suction and, if necessary, endotracheal intubation and tracheo-bronchial suction. In more insidious deterioration, get a chest x-ray (?pneumothorax, ?collapse) and consider infection.

The pharynx will, in any case, need frequent suction. Immediate post-operative feeding will be intravenous, and the surgeon will advise on milk feeds by gastrostomy or nasogastric tube, depending on the procedure. Feeding by mouth must wait at least until the child has been shown to be able to swallow his oral secretions.

## Congenital Diaphragmatic Hernia

Persistence of the pleuro-peritoneal canal, with massive herniation of abdominal contents into the thorax (generally on the left side), displacement of the mediastinum, and hypoplasia or compression of the lungs, may present at birth. The baby will either fail to become pink or to establish spontaneous respiration at resuscitation (and it may be obvious that lung compliance is grossly diminished so that the lungs do not inflate properly with the usual positive pressure of $30 cmH_2O$), or will establish spontaneous respirations which clearly do not ventilate the lungs adequately. In this case the baby will have poor chest movement, gross recession and persisting cyanosis. Respirations will often be slow and gasping.

Rarely, a lesser degree of herniation may present in the neonatal period, or even later, with signs of respiratory distress or of intestinal obstruction or a combination of the two. The diagnosis would immediately be made from the chest or abdominal x-rays which are mandatory when such symptoms are present.

*Grounds for Suspicions of Diagnosis*

(1) Failure of resuscitation; spontaneous respirations established inadequately or not at all.

(2) Evidence of grossly diminished lung compliance; lungs will not inflate with normal pressure.

(3) Displacement of heart to the right; apex beat palpable or audible on this side.

*Confirmation of Diagnosis*

If all the above signs are present the diagnosis is virtually certain. It may be confirmed by chest x-ray which shows bowel loops on the left side of the thorax. The only pitfall is that bowel does not look like bowel on an x-ray until it contains air, so a very early x-ray may be difficult to interpret. Make sure the radiographer puts the right or left marker on the film correctly, so that it is clear on which side the heart lies.

*Management*

The principles of management are to maintain ventilation as adequately as possible, if necessary using positive pressure ventilation, via an endotracheal tube, by hand or machine (but *not* using a bag-and-mask since this will cause gaseous distention of the stomach and bowel and further compression of the lungs), and to operate as soon as possible to reduce the hernia. Pass a stomach-tube, and aspirate stomach contents, including air, frequently, to reduce bowel distension. When there is serious respiratory difficulty, the resident should try to arrange for the baby to go straight from the labour ward to theatre, and remain with him to attend to his ventilation.

These babies generally have extreme respiratory difficulties post-operatively, for they often have too little pulmonary tissue to achieve adequate ventilation even when compression is relieved. Treat as for any other case of respiratory failure and watch for bronchial obstruction with thick secretions and for pneumothorax.

**Pierre Robin Syndrome**

The essential features of this syndrome are a small lower jaw (micrognathia) and a tendency to backward displacement of the tongue (glossoptosis), leading to respiratory obstruction. A central cleft palate is a very common association, though

51

not an essential feature of the syndrome. Babies with Pierre Robin syndrome present two major problems: respiratory distress or obstruction presenting at or soon after birth and caused by glossoptosis; and feeding difficulties which often last for several months and which are probably caused by neuromuscular weakness or inco-ordination affecting the tongue and pharynx.

*Grounds for Suspicion of Diagnosis*

(1) Obstructed respiration (gross recession, cyanosis, gasping) at or soon after birth. If this is seen, examine the jaw and palate.

(2) Small lower jaw. If this is noticed, see if the palate is cleft.

(3) Cleft palate. When this is found, look carefully at the baby's profile to assess the lower jaw.

If (1) and (2) are present the diagnosis is established and the management described below should be started. If (2) and (3) are present without (1) nurse the baby prone, and see that he is observed carefully for any signs of respiratory difficulty. For management of cleft palate without glossoptosis, see p. 59.

*Management*

*Respiratory obstruction.* Respiratory obstruction due to glossoptosis is an acute medical emergency. The immediate management is to place the baby prone to allow the tongue to fall forward. If this does not relieve the obstruction, try the effect of inserting an infant oral airway. If this also fails, insert an endotracheal tube to ensure the airway while further plans are made. Various methods have been suggested for relieving the respiratory obstruction; all depend on holding the tongue forward. We have found the method of Dennison (1964)* to be simple and highly effective in all of the small number of cases where we have used it. The baby is nursed prone. The head is lifted off the mattress by a length of tube-gauze suspended from a drip stand and attached to the head with adhesive plaster. The tongue is thus held forward by gravity. The baby may be successfully spoon or bottle-fed in this position, or may require tube-feeding. If this method failed to relieve obstruction, we would arrange a joint consultation with the plastic surgeon and orthodontist, and accept their advice on the best method of holding the tongue forward surgically or mechanically.

The respiratory difficulties commonly settle in the first few weeks of life, after which the baby may be nursed in a normal position.

*Feeding difficulties.* These babies have much more severe feeding difficulties than those with cleft palate alone; sucking and swallowing are often weak and unco-ordinated. There is no panacea for these difficulties, which may last for months. It is generally best to allow the nursing staff to find the best method of feeding—spoon-feeding, or feeding with an ordinary wide-bore teat or a flanged teat, may prove best. In some cases feeds will have to be given by tube, at least in part, for many weeks. However difficult feeding proves, we believe it is important (*a*) to involve the mother in it as soon as possible—she will probably manage much better than people expect—and (*b*) to give the baby some experience of sucking, if only on a dummy, as there may be a critical period for learning to suck.

*Dennison, W. M. (1964) 'Surgery in the newborn.' *British Medical Journal*, ii, 1443.

Watch for aspiration pneumonia, for otitis media, and also for glaucoma (see p. 244) which is sometimes seen in association with Pierre Robin syndrome.

*Repair of palate.* Whether or not the plastic surgeon or orthodontist have been called as an emergency because of respiratory obstruction, a joint consultation with these two specialists should be arranged as soon as possible to formulate a long-term policy.

## Choanal Atresia

The normal newborn baby breathes entirely through his nose, and is unable to breathe through the mouth except when crying. In choanal atresia, the posterior nasal air passage is blocked by a bony or membranous septum, and the baby has severe respiratory difficulties dating from birth.

*Grounds for Suspicions of Diagnosis*

(1) Respiratory difficulty, obstruction or cyanosis dating from birth, relieved by crying or worsened by feeding.

(2) Respiratory difficulty only on feeding.

(3) The presence of mucus casts in the nostrils, or nasal discharge.

Mucus casts aspirated from the nostrils have sometimes first drawn attention to the condition at birth. A characteristic glairy nasal discharge may occur; it is not usually seen in the immediate neonatal period, but may be the first sign in the unilateral cases which are not emergencies.

*Diagnosis*

(1) Listen over the nostrils with a stethoscope: in the normal baby, air can readily be heard going in and out.

(2) Hold a cold bright surface, *e.g.* a metal spatula, beneath the nostrils. In the normal baby, it will mist in a pattern corresponding with the nostrils.

(3) The definitive test is to attempt to pass a catheter through each nostril. It will not pass if there is choanal atresia.

*Management*

The alternatives are either operation to relieve the choanal obstruction, or establishment of a satisfactory oral airway. We prefer the latter method, believing that operation is best deferred until the nasal passages are bigger. However, some experienced paediatric surgeons prefer immediate operation.

For immediate treatment, insert an infant oral airway. Subsequently a simpler airway may be made from a teat, with the hole greatly enlarged, tied in position. If these methods do not work, consult the orthodontist who may construct an oral plate incorporating an airway.

Tube-feeding may be required at first. Within the first few days or weeks the baby will generally learn to breathe through the mouth without mechanical aids. Operation will be done electively later.

**Exomphalos (Omphalocele) and Gastroschisis**

In these conditions, abdominal contents protrude through a defect in the belly wall.

In exomphalos, the abdominal contents protrude where the umbilical cord should be inserted. They are covered with a transparent membrane (peritoneum and amnion), and the umbilical cord joins the hernial sac at some point. Occasionally, the sac may be ruptured before birth. In gastroschisis, there is a defect in the abdominal wall away from the umbilicus, usually on the right side. Through this protrude stomach and intestine, not covered by membrane. The coils of intestine are greatly thickened and covered by gelatinous green exudate.

Views on the treatment of these conditions are still controversial, but the following facts have to be taken into account.

(1) The size of the sac, or protruberant contents if there is no sac.

(2) Whether there is an intact sac or, if there is no intact sac, whether the bowel looks clean and healthy (suggesting recent rupture of the sac) or is thickened and covered in exudate (suggesting that there was no sac—as in gastroschisis—or that the sac was ruptured prenatally).

(3) Whether there are other important congenital anomalies present—there often are. (If the baby has a large tongue, consider the possibility of Beckwith's syndrome (see p. 30) and watch for hypoglycaemia.)

*Immediate Management*

(1) Cover the lesion with moist saline packs or, as Mr. R. B. Zachary suggests, with a plastic bag strapped to the abdominal wall.

(2) Pass a stomach tube and suck out air and gastric contents every 10 minutes to prevent intestinal distension.

(3) Ascertain the facts as to (1), (2) and (3) above, then consult the surgeon and follow his advice.

The surgeon may choose to operate and close the defect, possibly using a prosthesis or to treat it conservatively, applying scarifying agents such as 1% mercurochrome to the sac and allowing it to epithelialize.

**Myelomeningocele**

There are no difficulties in recognition or diagnosis: the difficulty is to know what to do. This involves non-medical considerations which we cannot discuss here. Some authorities believe that a radical surgical approach is right in all cases of myelomeningocele. Our own view has been for many years that radical treatment is not appropriate in the most severe cases. We recognize that this view would not be acceptable to everyone and we would not disagree strongly with those who follow a different policy. Our only strong disagreement would be with those who are certain about what they and everyone else should do for these children.

*Management*

*Assessment at birth.* As soon as possible after birth, make an assessment of the following features.

SITE, NATURE AND EXTENT OF THE MYELOMENINGOCELE

What is the level of the lesion? Usually it is thoraco-lumbar, but it may be higher or lower. What are its dimensions? What does it look like? Do not waste time on unprofitable speculation as to whether it is a myelocele, myelomeningocele, meningocele, etc.: these distinctions are of doubtful theoretical value and of no practical value. The only important distinction concerns whether the lesion is fully covered by skin or not. Very rarely it is: in such cases no urgent treatment is required and the immediate prognosis is good. Far more commonly, the lesion is not covered by skin; there is a central yellowish-red area consisting of exposed deformed neural tissue, surrounded by bluish membranes, merging into bluish skin. There may be some oozing of the CSF.

DEGREE OF HYDROCEPHALUS

Practically all cases of myelomeningocele have an associated Arnold-Chiari malformation, and most either have or develop hydrocephalus. Measure the head-circumference, the size of the fontanelles and the width of separation (if any) of the sutures. If possible, transilluminate the head in the dark; translucency of the head suggests that the cerebral mantle is thinned to less than 1cm.

STRUCTURE AND FUNCTION OF THE LOWER LIMBS

In the severest cases, where there has been marked prenatal paralysis of the lower limbs, these will be deformed. Congenital dislocations of the hips or knees, mis-shapen bones, talipes, or contractures—or any combination of these features—may be present, and the limbs may look like those seen in arthrogryposis. Look for these structural abnormalities. Then assess motor and sensory function, trying to establish the spinal level of any defect. Observe (1) spontaneous movement of lower limbs, and (2) reflexes.

(1) Spontaneous movement of lower limbs, particularly hip extension, which is often defective since it involves segments below L4, and which is important in walking.
(2) Reflexes. A reasonable selection is:

(a) withdrawal response on stimulation of sole of foot: observe hip flexion (L1-4), knee (L4-S3) and dorsiflexion of ankle (L4-S1);
(b) crossed-extension response: observe hip extension (L5-S2), knee extension (L2-4) and planter flexion of the foot (S1-2);
(c) plantar grasp response (L4-S1);
(d) adductor jerk (L2-4);
(e) knee jerk (L2-4);
(f) ankle jerk (S1-2).

Note that the presence of functions which depend on a particular spinal level does not necessarily mean that the spinal cord is intact down to that level. There may be an 'isolated' cord segment above which the long tracts are interrupted. Look especially for paradoxical responses to tendon taps, which may indicate isolated cord function.

There is a particularly helpful article by Dr. Gordon Stark (1971)* on assessment of lower-limb function at birth in these babies.

SPHINCTER FUNCTION

Is the anus patulous? Is the anal reflex present? Is there dribbling incontinence of urine, and is the bladder palpably distended?

OTHER CONGENITAL ANOMALIES

Look quickly for other important malformations.

*Decision on Strategy*

When the initial assessment has been made, it must be decided whether treatment is to be radical or conservative, and this decision must be made by the consultant paediatrician, in consultation with the general practitioner if possible. It will be based on all the information collected in the initial assessment, together with a knowledge of the child's family. We try to assess the parents' feelings and capabilities without actually asking them to make the decision about treatment. In general, our policy is to begin radical treatment unless there is severe hydrocephalus or severe involvement of the lower limbs (and/or sphincters). Read Dr. John Lorber's article†.

Conservative treatment consists of general nursing care, feeding, and circumspect symptomatic treatment.

*Radical Treatment*

Radical treatment means embarking on a highly complicated programme of medical and surgical care which will continue for very many years and probably for a lifetime. It is clearly impossible to cover all the details here. In the first few weeks there will be five main considerations.

(1) *Closure of defect.* This should be done as soon as possible, preferably within hours of birth, to prevent infection. A primary skin closure is generally possible. While awaiting surgery, cover the lesion with moist saline-packs. After closure, the baby should be nursed prone. A sling attached to two pieces of adhesive plaster, one on each side of the anterior abdominal wall, may relieve the tension on the suture line. Watch for anaemia post-operatively, since the baby may lose an appreciable amount of blood during closure.

(2) *Treatment of hydrocephalus.* Hydrocephalus usually progresses rapidly after closure of the myelomeningocele. The neurosurgeon should be informed about the case as soon as radical treatment is started, and his advice taken about subsequent treatment of the hydrocephalus. Measure the head-circumference daily. Usually the shunt operation for hydrocephalus is deferred till the back is healed. However, a rapid build-up of CSF pressure may interfere with healing and ventricular taps may be necessary to relieve pressure (see p. 281). They have the disadvantage that they may create intracerebral cysts.

*Stark, G. (1971) 'Neonatal assessment of the child with myelomeningocele.' *Archives of Disease in Childhood*, **46**, 539.

†Lorber, J. (1971) 'Results of treatment of myelomeningocele. An analysis of 524 selected cases, with special reference to possible selection for treatment.' *Developmental Medicine and Child Neurology*, **13**, 279.

(3) *Bladder function.* The baby may have retention of urine and/or dribbling incontinence. Retention can generally be dealt with by manual expression, but sometimes the bladder needs to be drained. In this case we prefer suprapubic bladder puncture to catheterization. In all babies, but especially those with dribbling incontinence, check the urine every 3 to 7 days for evidence of infection.

(4) *Infection.* If the baby becomes ill, consider especially urinary infection (examine urine), ventriculitis or meningitis (do a ventricular tap if these seem at all likely), and septicaemia (do a blood culture). For treatment of infection, see p. 167.

(5) *Orthopaedic problems.* Orthopaedic treatment takes a relatively low priority at this stage, but it is sensible to consult the orthopaedic surgeon early so that he can formulate a plan of management.

### Talipes Equinovarus

A 'club-foot' is a deformity obvious to parents and doctor alike. It constitutes an emergency in that, if the lesion is untreated, a life-long crippling results, whereas if the bones are artifically placed in a normal position in the first days of life and subsequent management is thorough, there is a good chance that a normal foot and ankle will develop.

*Findings*

There are varus (inversion) and equinus (plantar flexion) deformities of the ankle, and the foot cannot be placed in the normal position, let alone over-corrected. (In minor, apparent abnormalities of the foot, the ability to over-correct slightly is the distinguishing sign that the foot is essentially normal.)

*Action*

Tell the parents about the abnormality (see p. 41) and explain the prognosis. Arrange for the orthopaedic surgeon to see the child, but if it will be a day or two before he comes, strap the foot as follows.

(1) Paint the toes, foot and entire leg to mid thigh with compound Benzoin tincture.

(2) Cut two 1cm squares of 'elephant felt' (felt that is 3-4cm thick and adhesive on one surface) and apply over each malleolus of the ankle.

(3) Use 2.5cm zinc oxide non-stretchable tape. Hold the foot by the toes so that the knee and ankle are each at a right-angle (Fig. 2). Apply a pre-cut strip of strapping downwards along the medial aspect of the calf, over the medial malleolus (which is protected by felt) and, pressing the ankle to correct the varus deformity, carry the plaster up the lateral aspect of the calf and over the superior surface of the thigh, where the knee is bent (Fig. 3).

(4) Start another pre-cut strip of plaster on the dorsum of the foot, carry it around the medial side of and under the foot, then up the lateral side of the calf (pressing to correct the varus deformity) and over the bent knee to the superior surface of the thigh as before (Fig. 4).

(5) Tidy the strapping on the calf by two *loose* circumferential pieces of strapping around the calf.

There are two consequences of such strappings: (*a*) the varus deformity, but not the equinus, is partially corrected; and (*b*) each time the baby attempts to straighten his knee the varus deformity is moved into a slightly better (*i.e.* more corrected) position: there is thus a mild manipulation whenever the baby kicks his legs.

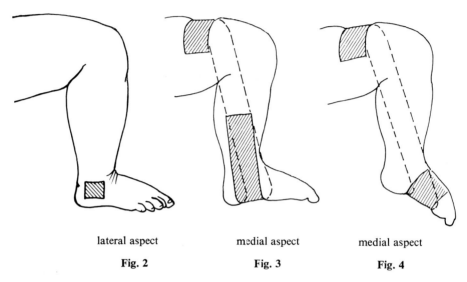

lateral aspect        medial aspect        medial aspect

**Fig. 2**        **Fig. 3**        **Fig. 4**

**Figs. 2-4.** Diagrams of strapping for talipes equinovarus. Details of the procedure are described in the text. Fig. 2 shows the correct position of the leg and ankle, with both knee and ankle at a right-angle. A small square of adhesive felt protects the malleolus. Fig. 3 shows the first length of strapping in place (viewed from the medial aspect). Fig. 4 shows the second length of strapping in place. This second length is applied on top of the piece illustrated in Fig. 3, which has not been drawn into Fig. 4 in order that the details of the position of the latter strapping can be more clearly illustrated.

# Other Malformations Requiring Early Action

The malformations described under this heading are not immediately life-threatening, but it is important that their implications should be understood, and that they should be discussed with the parents soon after birth.

**Cleft Lip and Cleft Palate** (see also Pierre Robin syndrome, p. 51.)

These malformations may occur separately or together*. Cleft lip is a very disfiguring deformity in the newborn, especially if it is bilateral; the most urgent matter is therefore to explain the present situation and future prospects to the parents. Cleft palate alone is not disfiguring, but is also likely to cause great anxiety to the parents concerning the development of speech. In the case of either deformity, therefore, one doctor (preferably the consultant) should see the parents as soon as possible to discuss the problems (see p. 41). In the case of cleft lip, it is particularly helpful to show the parents photographs of children who have had this malformation repaired.

*Plan for Management*

A consultation with the plastic surgeon should be held as soon as possible to make a plan for management. It is very helpful in counselling the parents to be able to tell them what to expect. The timing of operation must be left largely to the surgeon, but from the point of view of the parents—and of their attitude to, and handling of, the child—there is much to be said for repairing the cleft lip before the child leaves hospital.

The programme for management of cleft palate will be more complicated than that for cleft lip and will ultimately involve the plastic surgeon, orthodontist, speech therapist and, probably, ENT specialist. The repair of the palate will probably be deferred till the age of about a year, but before the child leaves hospital it should be clear—and the parents should know—which consultant is primarily responsible for his general care and for co-ordinating the activities of the other specialists involved. Remember that otitis media is an almost universal complication of cleft palate; see that this is watched for carefully and treated promptly, by drainage if necessary.

*Feeding Problems*

Cleft lip rarely causes important feeding problems, and breast-feeding will probably succeed if the mother wishes. Cleft palate is more troublesome from this point of view and breast-feeding is not usually successful but, except in the case of Pierre Robin syndrome (p. 51), feeding problems are rarely major and long-lasting.

When the baby with a cleft palate does have initial difficulty in feeding, several different methods can be tried. A flanged teat is often recommended but usually

---

*Central cleft palate is genetically distinct from the commoner lateral cleft palate; it is not accompanied by cleft lip, but is more likely to be associated with other malformations.

does not help. Frequently the baby will soon be able to feed from an ordinary teat with a large hole. Spoon-feeding will almost invariably succeed, but it is perhaps better first to try a method by which the baby learns to suck. Tube-feeding will very rarely be required.

**Imperforate Anus and Other Anorectal Anomalies**

Anorectal anomalies are complex and variable. Their management is a matter for specialist surgical advice. If an anomaly is detected in this region at birth, call the surgeon and do nothing further till his advice has been obtained. There is no point in taking x-rays in the first 24 hours of life with the baby held upside down to establish the level of atresia, for air may not have yet reached the rectum. Imperforate anus is usually combined with a fistula from the rectum. In the male, this fistula may be recto-vesical or recto-urethral, and meconium staining of the urine should be looked for. Urinary infection is probable if there is a recto-vesical fistula. In the female, there may be a recto-vaginal or recto-cloacal fistula. Meconium is therefore passed from the vagina, and the diagnosis of anorectal anomaly may be missed if the perineum is not carefully inspected.

Remember that there may be associated congenital anomalies in other regions, *e.g.* oesophageal atresia.

**Ambiguous External Genitalia**

This problem is uncommon, but failure to recognize its importance, or incorrect management can lead to much subsequent unhappiness for both parents and child.

The external genitalia of the virilized female, imperfectly masculinized male and hermaphrodite may be very similar, and usually consist of an inappropriately sized phallus, an opening along its ventral surface or in the perineum, and rugose skin representing scrotum or fused labia. An uninformed guess about the sex of such an infant must be avoided, and the parents told at once that doubt exists. At the same time they should be sympathetically and firmly assured that the appropriate sex of rearing can be decided once certain necessary investigations are complete. This should always be possible by the time registration of the birth is necessary at six weeks of age, and usually well before.

Uncertainty as to how and what to tell close relatives and near neighbours often means considerable additional anxiety for the parents, and they should announce the birth to as few people as possible. An offer to give simple explanations for them, to the child's grandparents for instance, may be welcomed; and the suggestion that they give the baby one of those names applicable to either sex (*e.g.* Frances(is), Hilary, Evelyn, Jo(e), Pat, Robin), may also be helpful.

Until the diagnosis is established, remember that the child may have congenital adrenal hyperplasia, and may become seriously ill from adrenal insufficiency. Check the serum electrolytes and measure the blood-pressure twice weekly until a firm diagnosis is made.

*Diagnosis*

*Any* ambiguity of the external genitalia merits investigation.

Enquiry should be made of the family history, with special note of unexplained deaths in infancy, of short adults who were tall children with sexual precocity, or of sterility in adults of either sex. At the same time, any evidence of virilization in the mother herself or of a history of virilizing drugs in the pregnancy can be noted. The flow-sheet shown on the next page sets out the main steps necessary for diagnosis. (We thank Dr. R. W. H. Edwards for help in its preparation.)

The essential first investigation is to establish the sex chromosome complement, either by chromosome counting or by sex chromatin determination. The latter may be unreliable in the first few days of life. Consult the laboratory first: they may wish to take the buccal smear themselves. If not, scrape the inside of the infant's cheek with the edge of a wooden spatula and smear the deposit on to a clean glass slide which must then be put immediately into 1 : 1 ether-alcohol to fix for 30 minutes before staining.

(1) *Chromatin-negative* (*or X Y karyotype*) *infants.* See flow-sheet for possible causes. A full description of all of them is not possible, and the references cited below* will be found helpful.

Once the rare form of congenital adrenal hyperplasia (CAH) due to 3β-hydroxy-steroid dehydrogenase deficiency and associated with incomplete masculinization in the male is ruled out by urinary steroid estimation (see below), the final diagnosis will depend on the chromosomal karyotype and on an urethrogram or other contrast radiography of the lower genito-urinary tract, and possibly laparatomy and gonadal biopsy.

In the chromatin-negative cases, the decision as to the appropriate sex for rearing will depend on the size of the phallus rather than on the karyotype. If the phallus is small, the female sex should be chosen, and the appropriate surgery undertaken later, with removal of testicular tissue.

*Note.* Complete forms of the testicular feminizing syndrome may have *normal female genitalia* at birth, but the diagnosis should be suspected if inguinal or labial testes are palpable, usually in association with a hernia.

(2) *Chromatin-positive* (*or female karyotype*) *infants.* See flow-sheet for possible causes. Congenital adrenal hyperplasia is the most likely, and it is important to establish the diagnosis without delay, for treatment prevents the progressive virilization which otherwise occurs, and salt-losing leading to adrenal crisis can be anticipated and treated.

Chromosomal females with virilisation from congenital adrenal hyperplasia or maternal drugs should be reared as female. In 'hermaphrodites', the sex of rearing depends on the size of the phallus.

**Congenital Adrenal Hyperplasia**

This is an automosal recessive inborn error of metabolism characterised by an inability to synthesise cortisol from cholesterol, and a compensatory rise in pituitary ACTH, which leads to adrenal cortical enlargement and excess androgen production. For a description of the metabolic pathways and enzymes concerned in the production

*Dewhurst, C. J., Gordon, R. R. (1969) *The Intersexual Disorders.* London: Ballière.
Schlegel, R. J., Gardner, L. I. (1969) 'Ambiguous and abnormal genitalia in infants: differential diagnosis and clinical management.' *In* Gardner, L. I. (Ed.) *Endocrine and Genetic Disease of Childhood.* Philadelphia and London: W. B. Saunders.

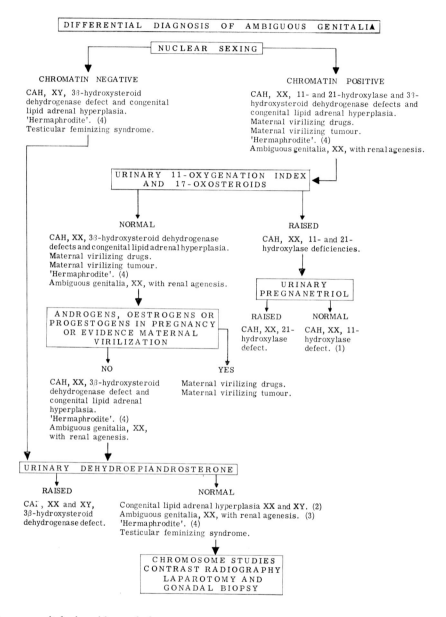

DIFFERENTIAL DIAGNOSIS OF AMBIGUOUS GENITALIA

NUCLEAR SEXING

CHROMATIN NEGATIVE

CAH, XY, 3β-hydroxysteroid dehydrogenase defect and congenital lipid adrenal hyperplasia.
'Hermaphrodite'. (4)
Testicular feminizing syndrome.

CHROMATIN POSITIVE

CAH, XX, 11- and 21-hydroxylase and 3β-hydroxysteroid dehydrogenase defects and congenital lipid adrenal hyperplasia.
Maternal virilizing drugs.
Maternal virilizing tumour.
'Hermaphrodite'. (4)
Ambiguous genitalia, XX, with renal agenesis.

URINARY 11-OXYGENATION INDEX AND 17-OXOSTEROIDS

NORMAL

CAH, XX, 3β-hydroxysteroid dehydrogenase defects and congenital lipid adrenal hyperplasia.
Maternal virilizing drugs.
Maternal virilizing tumour.
'Hermaphrodite'. (4)
Ambiguous genitalia, XX, with renal agenesis.

RAISED

CAH, XX, 11- and 21-hydroxylase deficiencies.

URINARY PREGNANETRIOL

RAISED

CAH, XX, 21-hydroxylase defect.

NORMAL

CAH, XX, 11-hydroxylase defect. (1)

ANDROGENS, OESTROGENS OR PROGESTOGENS IN PREGNANCY OR EVIDENCE MATERNAL VIRILIZATION

NO

CAH, XX, 3β-hydroxysteroid dehydrogenase defect and congenital lipid adrenal hyperplasia.
'Hermaphrodite'. (4)
Ambiguous genitalia, XX, with renal agenesis.

YES

Maternal virilizing drugs.
Maternal virilizing tumour.

URINARY DEHYDROEPIANDROSTERONE

RAISED

CAH, XX and XY, 3β-hydroxysteroid dehydrogenase defect.

NORMAL

Congenital lipid adrenal hyperplasia XX and XY. (2)
Ambiguous genitalia, XX, with renal agenesis. (3)
'Hermaphrodite'. (4)
Testicular feminizing syndrome.

CHROMOSOME STUDIES
CONTRAST RADIOGRAPHY
LAPAROTOMY AND
GONADAL BIOPSY

CAH = congenital adrenal hyperplasia.
(1) Pregnanetriol may be slightly raised in the severe condition, with very high 11-oxygenation index (*e.g.* 4 - 8).
(2) Steroid output listed as normal for convenience, but characterised by complete *lack* of steroid synthesis with severe salt-losing.
(3) Death will have occurred shortly after birth.
(4) This term is misused without apology as a veil for every permutation of sex chromosome mosaicism, including Klinefelter and Turner variants.
NOTE: Some very rare syndromes of multiple congenital anomalies, some with associated autosomal chromosomal abnormality, have not been included, and the references on p. 61 should be consulted for these.

of cortisol from cholesterol, see Visser (1966) and Cathro (1969)*. Of the several enzyme defects described so far as responsible for this condition, 21-hydroxylase deficiency occurs most commonly. A salt-losing syndrome, presumed to be due to defective aldosterone production, is present in about one-third of such children, in the majority of those with 3β-hydroxysteroid dehydrogenase deficiency, and in the rare congenital lipoid adrenal hyperplasia (presumptively due to a 20,22 desmolase defect). Hypertension is frequently present in the 11-hydroxylase defect, and the blood pressure should always be recorded.

*Note.* In CAH due to 17-hydroxylase deficiency, both genetic females *and* genetic males have *normal* female external genitalia. Hypertension will develop later. Together with those genetic males who have CAH due to 11- and 21-hydroxylase defects, the condition is likely to go undiagnosed in the neonatal period, though a salt-losing crisis may supervene in the latter, usually at any time from the second week of life onwards. Occasionally there might be slight pigmentation of scrotum and nipples.

*Establishment of Diagnosis*

This must be undertaken by a laboratory experienced in steroid chemistry, and the investigations are most reliably interpreted from the second or third week of life rather than earlier; in doubtful cases they may need to be repeated later still. Chromatographic methods may be required for clarification of the various defects.

(1) *Abnormal urinary steroid excretion.* (*a*) RANDOM SAMPLE (20ml) for 11-oxygenation index: this gives the ratio of cortisol precursors to cortisol, cortisone and metabolites and is normally below 0.7. An index of greater than unity is diagnostic of CAH.

(*b*) 24-HOUR SAMPLE—17-oxosteroids (17-ketosteroids): diagnostic levels greater than 1mg/24 hours (11-and 21-hydroxylase defects).

—pregnanetriol: excretion raised above 0.2mg/24 hours in 21-hydroxylase defects; occasionally, and to a lesser extent, in 11-hydroxylase defect.

—tetrahydro-compound S (THS): excretion negligible in normal newborn, increased in 11-hydroxylase defect. (This determination is technically difficult.)

—dehydroepiandrosterone (DHA): excretion negligible in the normal newborn, increased in 3β-hydroxysteroid dehydrogenase defect.

(2) *Plasma 17-hydroxyprogesterone*—may be helpful if there is difficulty in obtaining 24-hour urine specimens. Diagnostic levels (11- and 21-hydroxylase defects) will be above 0.5μg/100ml.

(3) *Electrolytes*—in the salt-losing variety, blood urea and serum potassium are raised, standard bicarbonate and serum sodium lowered. Hyperkalaemia (serum potassium more than 7mEq/litre) or tall T waves on the EEG may be the earliest signs of the salt-losing syndrome.

*Visser, H. K. A. (1966) 'The adrenal cortex in childhood. Part I: physiological aspects. Part II: pathological aspects.' *Archives of Disease in Childhood*, **41**, 2 and 113.
Cathro, D. M. (1969) 'Adrenal cortex and medulla.' *In* Hubble, D. (Ed.) *Paediatric Endocrinology*. Oxford: Blackwell.

*Treatment*

(1) *Maintenance.* All cases of congenital virilizing hyperplasia should be treated with corticosteroids for life. Dosage has to be adjusted to allow normal growth to occur and urinary steroids to return to normal levels, and will vary with individuals.

(*a*) Cortisone tablets, B.P. (5 and 25mg tablets, crushed), 25mg/day orally, divided into 2 doses, one-third of the total daily dose in the morning and two-thirds in the evening. (Stabilisation may be managed on as little as 15mg daily, or as much as 37.5mg daily in some cases.) If vomiting, substitute cortisone injection B.P. (25 mg/ml).

(*b*) In salt-losing variety (i) fludrocortisone tablets, B.P. (0.1mg tablets, crushed), 0.05-0.2mg/day orally, divided into 3 or 4 doses. If vomiting, substitute aldosterone (see below). DOCA is no longer available. (ii) Sodium chloride, orally 2-6g/day, in divided doses. This may only be necessary for a limited initial period.

(2) *Salt-losing crisis.*

(*a*) Cortisone injection B.P. (25mg/ml)—25mg I.M. or I.V. b.d.

(*b*) Aldosterone injection (0.5mg/ml)—1mg I.M. or I.V. once; repeat if necessary during first 24 hours.

(*c*) 0·9% NaCl in 5 or 10% glucose solution, intravenously, at a rate of 120ml/kg bodyweight/day.

(*d*) Substitute sodium chloride by mouth when possible, 4-8g daily (available as 0.5-1g capsules; can be put in feed).

NOTE. When the infant is stabilised and ready for discharge, it is important to make sure that the parents understand the absolute necessity of regular medication. They must also realise that maintenance doses of steroids will need to be doubled or trebled at the onset of any infection and that, if vomiting occurs, intramuscular drugs will have to be substituted. They must therefore seek advice at the beginning of any illness. Thus it is also essential that the infant's general practitioner be informed in advance of discharge, so that he can ensure he has a stock of the necessary drugs for emergency treatment.

(3) *Surgery.* In females, early operative reduction in size of the phallus is increasingly favoured for psychological reasons from both the parents' and the infant's viewpoints. Vaginal reconstruction should be carried out later.

## Hooded Prepuce

Occasionally the penis of a newborn baby appears to have been prenatally and untidily circumcised. Inspection shows that the prepuce covers only the dorsal and lateral aspects of the glans penis and on closer inspection a hypospadias—usually glandular—will be detected. Circumcision is absolutely *contra-indicated* since the prepuce will later be needed for repair of the urethra. Arrange for the plastic surgeon to see the baby, and explain to the parents the importance of not having circumcision done, whether they ask about this or not.

# Haemolytic Disease of the Newborn

The neonatal resident, or someone trained in resuscitation of the newborn should be present at the delivery of any woman suspected of having an infant affected by haemolytic disease (see p. 7). When a Rhesus-negative woman has had antibodies detected in pregnancy, or when her antibody titre has not been measured (or re-measured) in late pregnancy, the following investigations should be done on cord blood:

  (1) haemoglobin;
  (2) Kleihauer test for fetal cells when an intraperitoneal transfusion has been given;
  (3) direct Coombs test;
  (4) ABO and Rh grouping;
  (5) bilirubin.

  (1) and (2) are done on the same specimen in a sequestrene bottle, (3) and (4) on a clotted specimen, and (5) on another clotted specimen.

In Coombs-negative infants it will usually be unnecessary to have the bilirubin estimation done, unless the baby has had an intra-uterine transfusion.

Babies who are neither very pale nor hydropic require no immediate treatment other than routine resuscitation on the usual indications. The decisions about tranfer to the special care nursery, and exchange transfusion, can await the cord blood results (see p. 152 for subsequent management). Severely affected infants—those who are very anaemic and/or hydropic—require urgent treatment in the delivery room.

**The Severely Affected Baby**

Severe disease will usually have been anticipated before delivery. If possible, two neonatal residents should be present at the delivery. Two bottles of group O Rh-negative blood should be quickly available. Equipment for immediate exchange transfusions and an 'Angiocath' for paracentesis should be ready.

The signs of severe haemolytic disease are extreme pallor or greyish central cyanosis, generalised oedema with puffy face, ascites, and marked enlargement of the liver and spleen. Severe birth asphyxia is common.

Urgent treatment should be given in the following order.

(1) *Apnoea*. Unless effective spontaneous respiration is established at once, intubate and give intermittent positive pressure ventilation (IPPV). Intubation may be very difficult through an oedematous larynx, therefore do not remove the endotracheal tube too early. Wait until all immediate procedures are over, and the child's respiration is well-established. Once the umbilical venous catheter has been inserted (see below), inject 5-10ml of 7% THAM or 8.4% sodium bicarbonate, if you think the baby was in terminal apnoea (see p. 35).

(2) *Ascites*. Marked ascites will not only embarrass respiration but may even prevent it. Perform a paracentesis if there is obvious ascites and the baby does not breathe after IPPV, or if there has been a recent intraperitoneal transfusion. Paracentesis

65

should be performed in the left iliac fossa. (There is a serious danger of lacerating an enlarged liver in the right iliac fossa or midline.) Any ascitic fluid or blood should be allowed to drain freely.

(3) *Heart failure.* The severely affected baby will be in cardiac failure. Insert an umbilical venous catheter, and remove 20ml of blood. If the venous pressure is obviously high, remove another 20ml (less in cases of extreme immaturity). Give i.v. frusemide 2mg/kg (guess the bodyweight).

There are divided opinions as to whether digitalisation is necessary at birth. It is difficult to assess the dose—digoxin 0.02mg/kg has produced intoxication in a severely affected newborn baby—and as a rule we do not give it. However, if given, the first dose should be not more than digoxin 0.02mg/kg given slowly, by the intra-venous route, and we now know that digoxin may be given before the first exchange transfusion, because very little of the drug is removed by this procedure. There are no particular advantages in other digitalis preparations such as lantocide C.

(4) *Anaemia.* Give an immediate exchange transfusion, exchanging a total of 100ml, using group O Rh-negative blood (if possible packed cells). The purpose of this procedure is to raise the haemoglobin level—it is not intended to be a complete exchange.

After these emergency procedures have been done, see p. 154 for subsequent management.

(5) *Hypoglycaemia.* See p. 147.

# Hydrops Fetalis and Ascites

The term 'hydrops fetalis' has never been clearly defined, but is applied to infants showing generalised gross oedema and ascites at birth. As conditions associated with hydrops in one infant may be associated with ascites alone in others, it is convenient to consider these conditions together.

**Causes**

(1) Severe haemolytic disease of the newborn due to Rhesus iso-immunisation is the commonest cause in the U.K. The condition will, of course, normally have been anticipated before birth. Treatment is urgent (see pp. 65 and 66).

(2) Alpha thalassaemia. When homozygous for this condition, the baby is usually stillborn at 28-34 weeks gestation, and even if born alive the prognosis is hopeless. The heterozygous state in the parents can be identified by an estimation of Hb Barts. Parents are usually of Asian origin.

(3) Intra-uterine infections, *e.g.* toxoplasmosis, cytomegalovirus, syphilis.

(4) Lesions of the fetal cardiovascular system, *e.g.*:
  premature closure of foramen ovale or ductus arteriosus;
  other cardiac malformations;
  angioma within the fetus or placenta;
  thrombosis of renal or umbilical veins;
  feto-maternal or feto-fetal haemorrhage.

(5) Lesions of the fetal respiratory system:
  cystic adenomatoid malformations;
  pulmonary lymphangiectasia.

(6) Congenital nephrotic syndrome: an autosomal recessive condition described mainly in Finnish literature.

(7) Lower urinary tract obstruction causing urinary ascites: seeing an infant pass urine with a good stream excludes this.

(8) Achondroplasia.

(9) Congenital neuroblastoma.

(10) Unknown aetiology. When haemolytic disease due to Rh incompatibility has been excluded, the majority of the remaining cases do not have any of conditions 2-9 above, but have features in common which suggest a common but unknown aetiology.

The findings which are common to many of the above conditions are fetal heart failure, anaemia and hypoalbuminaemia.

**Investigations**

Do the following in any case of obscure oedema or ascites.

(1) Haemoglobin electrophoresis on blood of both parents.

(2) Kleihauer test on mother's blood for presence of fetal cells indicating feto-maternal haemorrhage.

(3) Test mother's blood for antibodies to fetal red-cells, for evidence of unrecognised isoimmune haemolytic anaemia.

(4) On baby's blood (before transfusion): Hb, P.C.V., white cell count, platelets, Hb electrophoresis, Coombs test, W.R. and tests for antibodies to cytomegalovirus and toxoplasmosis (see p. 23).

(5) Urine for protein, and culture for cytomegalovirus.

### Treatment

The following measures may be required.

(1) Immediate paracentesis, to aid the establishment of respiration. This should be done in the *left* iliac fossa, to avoid puncturing the liver if it is grossly enlarged.

(2) Intubation and IPPV.

(3) Exchange transfusion if the cord haemoglobin level is less than, say, 9g/100ml.

Hydropic babies usually die within three hours of birth due to hypoplasia of the lungs associated with massive pleural effusion.

Babies with congenital nephrosis may survive beyond the neonatal period and require renal biopsy to confirm the diagnosis suggested by heavy proteinuria, hypo-albuminaemia and hypercholesterolaemia.

### Chylous Ascites

This condition may present at birth as a result of congenital obstruction to lymphatic drainage from the lower half of the body (*e.g.* block at the level of the cisterna chyli), with consequent rupture of intestinal lymphatics and flow into the peritoneal cavity. The diagnosis is made from the milky appearance and high fat-content of the fluid. The condition usually remits over the course of several months, presumably due to the establishment of collateral lymphatic pathways.

# Examination of the Placenta

Examination of the placenta in the delivery room is usually considered a task for the obstetrician or midwife. Much of the information that may be gained from examining this organ is, however, more relevant to the health of the baby than to that of the mother. The paediatrician who sees the baby at delivery should therefore be prepared to examine the placenta himself and check for a few important features.

**Twin Pregnancy**

Examination of the placenta may allow determination of zygosity. The scheme to be followed is set out in the accompanying flow-sheet.

*Determination of Zygosity in Twins*

The only problem in this scheme is the determination of the number of chorions in a single or fused placenta.

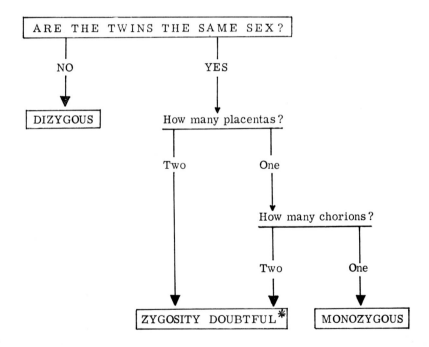

*Look at the twins! A marked discrepancy in facial features may enable one to diagnose dizygosity, provided there is not a marked discrepancy in birthweight. In this respect the colour of the hair, the shape and pattern of the pinnae and the shape of the hands are also relevant. Blood group and red cell and placental enzyme studies may enable one to establish dizygosity, but never to prove monozygosity with absolute certainty.

Examination of the fetal surface, in such a case, will usually show a double fold of membranes crossing the placenta, somewhere between the two umbilical cord insertions, and marking the line at which the two sacs were in apposition on the surface of the placenta (Fig. 5). If these membranes consist of amnion alone, they can easily be stripped off the placental surface, leaving no visible line of demarcation on it. If chorion is present in the membrane it cannot be stripped off, as it is continuous with the underlying tissue of the placenta, which is thus clearly demarcated into two parts. Rarely, a pair of monozygous twins are monoamniotic as well as monochorionic. In these cases there will, of course, be no membrane junction between the two cord insertions, and there is a very high incidence of congenital malformation and stillbirth.

If the facilities of a laboratory prepared to undertake enzyme studies are available, zygosity in dichorionic like-sexed twin pairs may be determined to a high degree of probability (although never with certainty) by examination of samples of tissue from each placental disk, and of blood from each cord and from both parents.

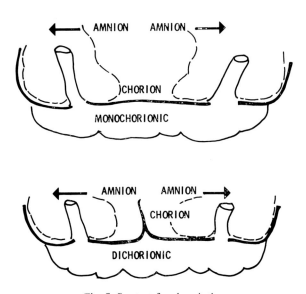

Fig. 5. See text for description.

## Placenta in Twin Transfusion Syndrome

In fused monochorial placentas, examination of the fetal surface often reveals large arterial or venous anastomoses between the two vessel systems. These appear to be of little functional importance. Paradoxically, however, these superficial anastomoses are inconspicuous in the twin transfusion syndrome, as the functionally important anastomoses are those where blood from an umbilical artery of one twin (the donor) perfuses the fetal placental villi before draining into the umbilical vein of the other (recipient) twin. These anastomoses are only seen on injection studies.

70

In severe cases of transfusion syndrome, the placental area associated with the anaemic donor twin may be large and pale, resembling that of a hydropic infant, whereas the placental area associated with the plethoric recipient twin is small and deeply congested.

## Fetal Haemorrhage

Antepartum haemorrhage may be confirmed as being of fetal origin if a vessel at the margin of the fetal placental surface is found to be torn. This is most likely to happen with marginal or velamentous insertion of the cord. The inability to find a torn vessel does not preclude the possibility of feto-maternal haemorrhage.

## Unexplained Birth Asphyxia

Placental examination may throw light on such cases.

(*a*) *Firm adherent retroplacental blood clot* indicates maternal ante-partum haemorrhage with partial placental separation. There may not always be a history of revealed ante-partum haemorrhage, or the clinical picture of *abruptio placentae*.

(*b*) *True placental infarcts*. These are firm lesions which are red when fresh, changing to brown, grey and white as they age. Sometimes infarcts are cavitated and contain masses of old clot (placental haematomas). However, it can be very difficult to distinguish old discoloured grey or white infarcts from a variety of common placental lesions of no significance. As a general rule, it can be assumed that lesions seen on the maternal surface over the central part of the placenta have played a significant rôle in any birth asphyxia, whereas lesions at the margin (usually perivillous fibrin deposits) or on the fetal surface (subchorial lake thrombi) are unrelated to any perinatal problems.

## Chorioamnionitis

The placenta affected by chorioamnionitis frequently smells offensive, with a cloudy appearance to the membranes. The condition is associated with prolonged rupture of membranes and, when diagnosed, should induce the suspicion that any symptoms developing subsequently in the baby may be due to infection (see p. 163). However, we do not consider that the diagnosis of chorioamnionitis of itself justifies antibiotic treatment of the baby and do not therefore perform routine histological screening of cord or membranes for this condition.

## Other Findings

Gritty white flecks seen over the maternal surface of a placenta are calcium deposits. These increase with lengthening gestation, but vary also with parity and vitamin D intake.

A statement by the midwife that a placenta is 'unhealthy' usually means either (*a*) that there is extensive calcification or (*b*) that there are a number of subchorial lake thrombi. Neither condition carries any significance for the health of the baby.

An unusually small placenta is commonly found in association with fetal growth retardation and is a feature of trisomy 17/18. Variations in placental shape, circumvallate placenta, etc., are seldom significant.

*NOTES*

72

# Section 3:
# Routine Care of the Normal Term Baby

*NOTES*

# Routine Procedures

Because this account of our standard practices in the care of normal newborn babies is brief, the reader should not conclude that we do not take this aspect of neonatal care seriously. As explained in the Introduction, this book is mainly about problems of illness in newborn babies.

Each newborn baby should be routinely examined as soon as possible after birth (see p. 40) and each baby is seen by the neonatal resident within 24 hours before his discharge (see p. 81). The paediatric consultant makes rounds once a week to see each newborn baby and to discuss his progress with the Ward Sister and the baby's mother.

**Labelling**

We have typed instructions on the labour ward and these instructions are reviewed regularly. Just because the risk of making a changeling (or rather two changelings) is so remote, one must never forget that it *is* a possibility where confinements are concentrated and is perhaps the greater risk when the baby's surname is something like Scopes, Tizard or Wigglesworth, rather than Davies or Robinson.

Our current instructions are that, when a mother is admitted to the obstetric department, a tape (on which her surname and given name has been written in block capitals) is tied to her left wrist and remains there until the baby is born. After the cord is clamped, the name-tape is removed by the midwife, the sex of the baby and the date of delivery is added to it, and the tape is then shown to and checked by the mother before being tied on the baby's right wrist. An 'Identiband' label (blue or pink according to sex) is then prepared with the same information and again shown to the mother before being clipped around the baby's left wrist. The 'Identiband' cannot be unclipped and is cut off just before his discharge from hospital. In the case of mothers having caesarean sections or other forms of delivery under general anaesthesia, the nurse accompanying the mother to the operating theatre removes the wrist-tape and shows it to the mother before anaesthesia is begun. The nurse is responsible for tying the tape and for preparing and clipping the 'Identiband' to the baby, checks being made by the senior midwife present.

**Bathing**

Babies weighing less that 2,200g, or otherwise needing transfer to the special care nursery, are not bathed. Babies born breech first, by assisted delivery or by caesarean section are kept for six hours in the labour ward before being bathed and transferred to the postnatal ward. Those staying with their mothers and who have had normal deliveries are usually bathed within one hour of birth, provided the rectal temperature is over 35°C (95°F) (see p. 105). The skin is then swabbed with cotton-wool soaked in about 2ml of 3% hexachlorophane detergent lotion, avoiding any raw areas and, of course, the eyes and mouth. The infant is rinsed immediately and thoroughly in a warm bath. He is then dried by dabbing, rather than rubbing, to avoid injury to the skin, and drying is done promptly to avoid a fall in body temperature. 1ml of phytomenadione (Vit.$K_1$) solution (containing 1mg) is given orally at this time. The baby is clothed in an open-backed nightdress, disposable napkin and flannelette wrapper, all of which have been pre-warmed.

The baby is bathed again on the fifth day with his mother watching, and is thereafter bathed by her daily until they go home.

## Feeding

We are very concerned about feeding practices, but have little influence over the most important decision, that of breast versus bottle-feeding. The decision has been made nine times out of ten before the baby is born—probably in most cases before he is conceived. It even seems likely that the mother's mother's own experience of infant feeding may have a bearing of her ability or willingness to feed her own baby from the breast. It needs a full-time doctor working in the antenatal clinic and postnatal wards (preferably someone like Dr. Mavis Gunther or the late Drs. Harold Waller or Charlotte Naish) to make a real impact on the declining incidence of breast-feeding. Nevertheless, the paediatrician—as well as the obstetrician—should show his satisfaction to the mother who is suckling her infant, without showing disapproval of the bottle-feeder in the next bed, and may sometimes help the wavering breast-feeder to struggle on through initial difficulties and discomforts (see p. 79).

We are not presenting the reader with a dissertation on the technical aspects of breast-feeding, or on its physical and emotional advantages and disadvantages, as others can and have done this better than we could hope to do. Neither are we including practical instructions on bottle feeding. We strongly recommend you to read the books and papers shown below*.

### The First Feed

We do not give water or glucose water. The first feed is either obtained from the breast or consists of a half-cream cow's milk preparation.

## Rooming-in

Obviously the baby's cot should be beside the mother's bed. However, not every mother will want her baby with her all the time. Thus there must be a nursery and the mother should be given the option of 'rooming-in' with her baby for as much or as little of the day or night as she wishes. Routine separation is old-fashioned and unkind.

## Avoidance of Cross-infection

Remember that a newborn baby may become seriously ill through infection with a micro-organism which is harmless or not very harmful to adults. Try to keep off the postnatal ward if you have a cold, any skin infection or diarrhoea.

*Gunther, M. (1970) *Infant Feeding*. London: Methuen.
Mac Keith, R., Wood, C. (1971) *Infant Feeding and Feeding Difficulties* (4th Edn.). London: Churchill.
Mitchell, R. G. (1970) 'Nutrition and feeding.' *In* Mitchell, R. G. (Ed.) *Child Life and Health* (5th Edn.). London: Churchill. p. 104.
Winnicott, D. W. (1969) 'Breast-feeding as a communication.' *Maternal and Child Care*, **5**, 147

We wear clean white gowns on the postnatal wards. We do not consider that the wearing of face masks is necessary or even desirable. We do consider it most important that doctors and nurses should wash their hands meticulously before and *immediately after* handling a newborn baby.

### Routine Measurements

The baby is weighed shortly after birth, on the third day after birth and daily thereafter. We do not carry out routine test-weighing of breast-fed babies.

Rectal temperature is taken before the first bath and once a day thereafter (see p. 105). The passage of urine, meconium and faeces is recorded on the temperature chart. Failure to pass urine or meconium within the first 24 hours is reported by the nurses (see p. 205 and p. 193).

### Communication with General Practitioner and Health Visitor

The printed discharge letter giving brief details about the baby's birth, general condition and feeding must be completed shortly before the baby leaves hospital. One copy is sent to the family's general practitioner. One copy is sent to the Medical Officer of Health responsible for the area in which the family lives. He in turn is responsible for seeing that the domiciliary midwife or the health visitor (Public Health nurse) makes contact with the family as soon as possible after discharge. One copy of the discharge letter is retained in the mother's case-folder.

# Mother's Worries

Enquire from Sister on the postnatal ward each day if there is any mother who wants to see you. Before seeing her, be sure you are adequately briefed about her home circumstances, whether she is married, and what has happened to her baby so far. Remember that a mother's specific worry may be but a cloak for a more general and deeply felt concern as to her baby's normality or her own capacity to care for him. When a mother is concerned about some aspect of her newborn baby's appearance or behaviour, first assume that there is good cause for her concern and do not be glibly reassuring without first having listened carefully to what she has to say. Remember that a mother is a far more constant and acute observer of her baby's behaviour than are the nursing or medical staff. The mother of a newborn baby is often very perceptive and accurate in her judgements: for instance if a mother says that her baby has had a fit and the nursing staff deny it, the mother is nearly always right.

Remember that if a mother overhears doctors or nurses whispering or sees them engaged in grave conversation she is apt to think that her own baby is the subject of it.

The attitude of the doctor should be both serious and at the same time light-hearted—an acknowledgement that the possession of a newborn baby should be a matter for joy rather than concern. If you cannot combine the two attitudes naturally, then stick to being serious.

## Minor Physical Peculiarities

(1) Cephalhaematoma. Tell the mother that this is quite harmless but warn her that it will take several weeks, or even months to disappear completely.

(2) The anterior fontanelle. This is not a part of the baby's body that need be handled any more gently than the rest; this especially applies to washing.

(3) Stork bites. These are sparse capillary haemangiomata on (a) the upper eyelids, (b) the nasium (where it is often v-shaped), and (c) the external occipital probuberance (where it usually escapes notice). Tell the mother what they are called; say that they nearly always disappear and that if they persist are not at all noticeable.

(4) White spots on the nose (milia). Show the mother another baby, they all have them.

(5) Nobbly head. Many babies have little elevated lumps in relation to the occipital suture.

(6) Subconjunctival haemorrhage, often taking the form of an incomplete ring around the iris. This is common and harmless and disappears in a week or two.

(7) Tongue tie. To some extent this is normal in every newborn baby and it should rarely interfere with either sucking or later speech development.

(8) Crumpled ears. They usually flatten out.

(9) Epithelial pearls. These are white spots, usually one on either side of the median raphe of the hard palate. Mothers do not usually notice them but they may be mistaken by the nursing staff for thrush.

(10) Breast engorgement. Physiological and usually harmless.

(11) Prominent xiphisternum. Normal.

(12) Cord won't come off. If treated by Polybactrin spray to prevent bacterial colonization, the cord may take two or three weeks to separate by dry gangrene rather than wet! The dry, horny object may be aesthetically displeasing to a mother until she understands the reason for it.

(13) Menstruation. A little bluish-red blood passed per vaginum usually from third to seventh day: explain why.

(14) Failure to straighten their legs—at first they cannot.

(15) Minor ankle deformities (see p. 57).

(16) Rashes. The common rash is urticaria of the newborn (*q.v.*).

(17) Peeling skin. This is common in post-term and in Negro babies; we do not know why. The skin will soon look normal.

(18) Jaundice. Explain that minor degrees of jaundice lasting a few days are seen in about one in three healthy newborn babies.

## Problems of Feeding and Behaviour

In reality a mother is more likely to worry about her newborn baby's behaviour than his appearance, so that feeding difficulties, regurgitation, crying and apparently excessive sleepiness are common causes of concern. Often there will be considerable anxiety and tension surrounding the problem, and the paediatrician's attitude can help to relieve this.

*Feeding Difficulties* (for gastro-intestinal disorders, see p. 192 *et seq.*).

Infant feeding, especially breast-feeding, is a huge subject and serious treatment of it would be out of place in this handbook. We refer the reader to Dr Mavis Gunther*, who is far better informed on the subject than we are. However, a few notes may be helpful.

In establishing the new relationship between a mother and her newborn baby there are always more than two individuals involved. The most important of the out-siders is the midwife, who has the delicate task of being a mother to the mother but, like all good mothers, not interfering overmuch. Some mothers will only be hindered in getting to know their babies by outside interference; other mothers will be absolutely dependent on the presence and support of the midwife, who has to try to give the *minimum* help which will be effective. However, the success or failure of breast-feeding is rather seldom determined by what happens after the birth of the baby.

In talking to the mother, we have found the following points helpful.

(1) If the mother is attempting to breast-feed, the paediatrician may say approvingly that it is nicer for the baby, but not imply that its future health or survival depend on it. Bottle-feeding is sometimes simpler, but always duller.

(2) He should ask when or if the baby has got the idea of breast feeding—a question which implies that the baby cannot be taught, but will learn in his own time.

*Gunther, M. (1970) *Infant Feeding*. London: Methuen.

(3) If things are going badly at first, he should explain that Nature has so arranged matters that no newborn human infant gets more than a trickle of milk for the first 36 or 48 hours and not much for a few days after that—perhaps adding that this may explain why we are all so miserable as adults.

The object of this small-talk is to indicate to the mother that she and the baby will manage all right and that there is no desperate urgency about the establishment of regular feeding habits.

### Regurgitation

The mother of a first baby is often worried about regurgitation of feeds, but almost all babies do this even when perfectly healthy and gaining weight satisfactorily (see p. 192).

### Excessive Crying

A crying baby may cause his mother to become anxious or depressed; conversely and more commonly, maternal anxiety or depression may lead to the baby crying (and there are good mechanistic explanations for this sequence of events). All babies cry sometimes, but it should naturally be regarded as a cry for help and the mother should not be dissuaded from an act of simple kindness—that is to pick up the baby and comfort him. She would need to be taught with her first baby how to sit him upright with his head supported and a firm hand on his belly to aid the passage of wind up and down.

### Excessive Sleepiness

This may be related to maternal sedation during labour, but we have the impression that, like fighting on the breast, it is sometimes a sequence of an initial conflict between feeding and breathing (see Dr. Mavis Gunther, 1970). It is best not to bully the baby to feed, but to let him sleep until he wakes hungry and then for the mother to nurse him in such a way that he can feed and breathe at the same time. The baby should be held horizontally with his chest pressed against the mother's chest, his chin touching the lower part of her breast so that the nipple is pointing to the roof of his mouth.

Sometimes a mother is concerned simply that the baby has his eyes closed most of the time: this is a normal state of affairs in the newborn.

# Routine Discharge Examination

**Doctor-patient Relationships**

You are the doctor and the newborn baby is the patient—an individual who is entitled to one's respect and forbearance. He is clearly not capable of rational thought, but he does have feelings to which one must be sensitive (not sentimental).

Unless pressed for time, do not wake the baby when he is in non-eye-movement sleep, as this seems liable to upset him. If respiration is regular, if no eye movements can be detected behind the closed lids, and if the baby is lying quite still, wait a quarter of an hour (when he is likely to have changed to eye-movement sleep) before rousing him. Examine him in a warm room on a soft surface and make sure your hands are warm. When examining the baby, talk to him in a soothing voice or sing quietly; if any one thinks you are an ass, let them. In picking up the baby, do not let his head move suddenly on his trunk; this is an action which elicits the Moro reflex—an experience which is clearly unpleasant for the baby. If you do hurt the baby, for instance in examining for congenital dislocation of the hips, or in doing a heel prick, pick him up immediately afterwards and comfort him. Before putting him back in his cot make sure that he is swaddled securely and then lie him on his side.

**Purpose of the Examination**

All babies should have been examined at birth (see p. 40) to exclude abnormalities which are an immediate threat to life or health. If the baby has developed untoward symptoms in the first week of life he should, of course, be examined at that time. Our discharge examination is normally carried out on the day before the baby goes home. In most cases at present this is on the seventh day of life; in cases where the mother was delivered by caesarean section it will be later (about the tenth day); in early (48-hour) discharge cases it will be on the morning of discharge.

The discharge examination has at least four important functions:
(1) to assess the baby's progress from birth (behaviour, feeding, weight, jaundice, etc);
(2) to exclude congenital malformations or trauma which have escaped notice at birth;
(3) to exclude signs of superficial infection;
(4) to reassure the mother about conditions which, though unimportant, may alarm her.

**Preliminary Arrangements**

Since this is not an emergency examination, the timing can be arranged to suit the doctor's working hours, but should also be arranged to suit the mother: for instance, meal times should be avoided.

The mother's presence is a decided advantage, for she can see for herself and voice questions as they arise. If anything abnormal is found the situation can be explained at once and uninformed fears and anxieties can be alleviated. At the same time, further details of the personal or family history may be elicited if it becomes apparent that they are important. Since the baby is to be examined naked, it is important that the room should be *very* warm, *i.e.* 25°C (75°F) or more, and that the examination is not unusually protracted.

Have the mother's notes, the baby's notes, and essential equipment handy, including tape measure and material for heel-prick (Guthrie test).

## The Examination

The following is a check list of examinations routinely carried out which, with certain information from the case notes, are routinely recorded.

---

*Condition on Discharge*

Date of discharge............................ Weight on discharge ............

Method of feeding      entirely breast-fed ....................................
          breast and complement...............................
          artificially fed......................................

Infections:   Eyes........Nails ........Skin ......Mouth ........Umbilicus........

Other abnormalities:    Hips...........    Feet.........    Skin...........
                      Skull...........    O.F.C........    cms.
                      Abdomen.......    Spine...........   Heart.........
                      Hernial orifices........                   Genitalia.......

Further notes      Diagnosis for coding
                1.
                2.
                3.
                4.

Guthrie test      done...........
                not done.........

---

The following are some brief notes about the examination.

### The General Appearance

The general appearance gives one an over-all impression of the baby's health, which is compounded of his size, maturity, colour, respirations, posture and activity. At the same time, certain abnormalities, *e.g.* skin lesions, defects in postural control, or abnormal or diminished movement in one limb can usually be detected.

### Infections

Systemic infection will have been discovered before this examination if the child has been ill. At this examination one looks for infection at specific sites: the eyes (? discharge), the nails (? paronychia), the mouth (? thrush) and the umbilicus (? discharge, redness or induration).

82

*Other Abnormalities*

*Skin.* Colour, including jaundice, petechiae, other rashes, birth marks, etc. (see p. 249). Breast engorgement is common and usually harmless.

*Feet.* Club-foot should have been noted before this age. Minor varus and valgus deformities are common. For varus deformities see p. 57. In general we do not believe that valgus deformities need treatment, unless associated with neuro-muscular abnormalities, but look carefully for congenital dislocation of the hip.

*Skull.* Examine for cephalhaematoma, forceps trauma, etc. Examine the suture lines for undue patency or ridges (see p. 174). Measure and record the occipito-frontal circumference.

*Mouth.* Apart from examining for thrush, look for a small cleft of the central palate which might have been missed at birth. (The inexperienced may mistake two epithelial pearls lying on either side of the median raphe for thrush).

*Spine.* Look for midline lesions over the spine and base of the skull. (See 'Neurological problems,' p. 180.)

*Eyes.* Look for conjunctivitis, glaucoma and other congenital abnormalities (see p. 241).

*Heart.* Symptoms of tachypnoea, sweating, cyanosis, etc. should have been noted before this (see p. 211 *et seq.*). Assuming none are present, this examination is to auscultate for murmurs.

*Chest.* In the apparently healthy baby, auscultation of breath sounds is a waste of time.

*Abdomen.* Examine the umbilicus for sepsis and for hernia *into the cord*. (The common type of umbilical hernia is not usually apparent at this age.) Examine the groin and scrotum for herniae. Palpate the belly for enlarged viscera. The liver edge is usually 1 to 2cm below the costal margin; the spleen and kidneys may be just palpable. If they feel enlarged, consider the possibility of infection. Rectal examination should not be done.

*Genitalia.* Inspect the genitalia carefully and explain any abnormality, even if trivial, to the mother. Record if a good stream of urine is seen. Look for the following abnormalities:
In the male:
   hooded prepuce and hypospadias (p. 64 and p. 60);
   undescended testicle (p. 246);
   hydrocele (p. 246).
In the female:
   vaginal discharge (p. 246);
   fused labia and/or enlarged clitoris (see 'Ambiguous genitalia', p. 60).
In examining the male do not retract the foreskin, and take the opportunity of telling the mother that this is not necessary for hygienic purposes and may be harmful.

*Hips.* Examination for congenital dislocation should never be omitted. Dislocated or dislocatable hips are usually, but not invariably, detectable at this age.

The baby should be lying supine on a flat surface. The hips are flexed to 90° with the knees bent. Take the thighs in your hands so that the bent knees are in the palms, the thumbs lying over the inner trochanters, and the middle fingers over the greater trochantar (Fig. 6a). Now test one hip at a time. Adduct the hip with slight internal rotation. Press laterally with the thumb and gently downwards with the palm along the line of the thigh (Fig. 6b) so that, if the hip is dislocatable, the femoral head is displaced onto the posterior edge of the acetabulum. Now abduct the hip until it is nearly flat on the surface, and as you do so press inwards (medially) with the middle finger. As the head of the femur returns to the acetabulum (in the abnormal case) a definite jerk and click is detectable. On returning the hip to the adducted position and pressing laterally with the thumb, the movement to the dislocated position is again discernible. The whole manoeuvre is carried out as a continuous movement, and should be performed firmly but gently.

If a definite jerk has been elicited, inform the orthopaedic surgeon. Keep the baby's hips abducted by a double thickness of napkins. We do not think x-rays are helpful in diagnosis at this age. The number of dislocatable hips is greatest shortly after birth and there are many fewer by the age of seven days. The condition is much more common in girls than in boys and is more common following breech delivery.

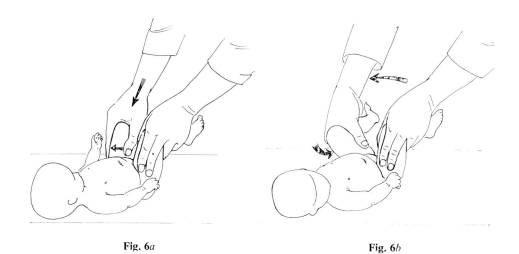

Fig. 6a          Fig. 6b

*Neurological Examination*

Formal neurological examination is not part of the routine discharge examination (see p. 173).

*The Guthrie Test*

This is a routine test, performed on every baby for the early detection of phenyl-ketonuria and other metabolic errors: explain it to the mother. It should be performed between the seventh and fourteenth day of life, *i.e.* the baby should have completed 6 x 24 hours from birth. If he is discharged younger than this, apply the sticker which says 'Guthrie test not done' to the notes, *and* to the discharge letter which goes to the appropriate Medical Officer of Health.

The blood is obtained by heel-prick. Before pricking, check if the baby needs some other investigation, *e.g.* bilirubin, Hb, that should be done at the same time. After cleaning and pricking the heel (see p. 269), apply the blood to the centre of the ring on the absorbent paper of the Guthrie Test Card. Enough blood must be applied to saturate through the paper over the *whole* area enclosed by the ring, and at least two rings (preferably three or four) should be saturated. Allow the card to dry, place in plastic envelope and post to the central laboratory. Apply the stickers 'Guthrie test done' to the baby's notes and to the discharge letter.

NOTE (1) Consider repeating the test in one week if the baby had been feeding badly or vomiting, especially if it is a girl. (The sex incidence of phenylketonuria is equal, but for unexplained reasons more affected girls than boys are undetected by the screening test).

NOTE (2) Postpone the test if the baby is on antibiotics.

**Reminder**
Tell the mother that the domiciliary midwife or the health visitor (Public Health nurse) will call upon her at home within a day or two of her discharge from hospital, and remind her that her general practitioner is available for consultation if she is worried about her baby. We will be happy to see her baby again at the general practitioner's request; if he is not immediately available she may, in an emergency, bring her baby to hospital. Many mothers need this reassurance.

*NOTES*

# Section 4: Major Problems of the First Week

*NOTES*

# Classification of Low-birthweight Babies

The term 'premature' was formerly used by international agreement to refer to all babies with a birthweight of 2,500g or less. It is now recognised that these low-birthweight babies are not a uniform group, since low birthweight may be the result of a short gestational period, or retarded intra-uterine growth, or a combination of the two. Low-birthweight babies must, therefore, be classified in terms of both birthweight and gestational age. The two basic terms used are 'pre-term' and 'small for dates'.

*Pre-term* defines those born before 37 completed weeks from the first day of the last menstrual period. These babies are truly 'premature' (*i.e.* born early) but because of the ambiguities surrounding this term it should not be used.

*Small for dates* defines those having a birthweight below the 10th centile for the gestational age (see birthweight-gestational age centile charts, p. 324 and p. 325).

Babies of birthweight 2,500g or less will always fall into one or other or both these categories. However, the classification can be extended to apply to babies of any birthweight and any gestational age (see Table III). The terms shown in the Table are used for coding purposes.

**TABLE III**

| Birthweight | Gestational Age | | |
|---|---|---|---|
| | Less than 37 weeks | 37-41$^6$/$_7$ weeks | 42 weeks and over |
| Below 10th centile | Pre-term, small for dates | Term, small for dates | Post-term, small for dates |
| 10-90th centile | Pre-term, normal weight for dates | Term, normal weight for dates | Post-term, normal weight for dates |
| Above 90th centile | Pre-term, large for dates | Term, large for dates | Post-term, large for dates |

Note that the adjective 'pre-term' refers simply to the baby's gestational age, and 'small for dates' refers simply to the relationship between his birthweight and gestational age. The term 'small for dates' carries no assumptions about the cause of low birthweight for gestation. There are undoubtedly many different causes of retarded intra-uterine growth, which can be broadly divided into those which primarily affect the embryo and its growth potential, and those which primarily affect intra-uterine nutrition of the fetus, including of course placental insufficiency. Note also that the decision on how early a baby has to be born to be called 'pre-term', and on how small he has to be at a particular gestational age to be called 'small for dates' are necessarily arbitrary. There is now a good measure of international agreement on the gestational age definitions we have given (Neligan 1970)* but no such agreement on definitions relating birthweight and gestation. Our use of the 10th centile as the dividing line between normal weight for dates and small for dates implies that 10 per cent of the infant population are classed as small for dates, and undoubtedly most of these babies are in no sense abnormal. The justification for using the 10th centile is that the great majority of babies who are at risk for hypoglycaemia will thus be recognised and treated accordingly.

TABLE IV

**Some problems of the low-birthweight baby**

| Normal weight for dates, pre-term | Small for dates, term |
|---|---|
| Respiratory problems ⟋ respiratory distress syndrome ⟍ apnoeic attacks | Respiratory problems — ⟋ severe birth asphyxia pulmonary haemorrhage ⟍ 'pneumonia' |
| Inability to suck and swallow | Symptomatic hypoglycaemia |
| Hypothermia | Hypothermia |
| Jaundice | Polycythaemia |
| Infection | Intra-uterine viral infection, *e.g.* rubella, cytomegalovirus |
| Intraventricular haemorrhage | |
| Functional intestinal obstruction | Congenital anomalies |
| Necrotising enterocolitis | |

It is obvious that babies who are born both pre-term and small for dates may show any combination of these problems

*Neligan, G. A. (Chairman) (1970) 'Working party to discuss nomenclature based on gestational age and birth weight.' *Archives of Disease in Childhood*, **45,** 730.

# Assessment of Gestational Age

The classification of low-birthweight babies on p. 89 obviously requires an accurate knowledge of gestational age as well as birthweight. Except in the very rare cases where the date of conception is known, there is no means of assessing gestational age that is inherently as accurate as an accurate menstrual history. All other methods of assessment provide an approximation which may differ from the true gestational age by at least two weeks in either direction.

### Assessment from the Mother's Menstrual History

The gestational age calculated from the first day of the last menstrual period may be relied on if the following conditions hold:

(1)   the mother's memory of the date is certain;

(2)   her menstrual cycle is regular and the situation was not confused by lactation or other factors affecting menstruation; and

(3)   her last period was normal in duration and amount of loss.

In the case of a low-birthweight baby, see the mother personally and ask about these three things. Do not simply rely on the obstetric notes and do not accept any obstetric revision of the mother's dates. (Such revisions may well have enabled the obstetricians to make a better-informed guess as to when the baby would be born, but at this point we are simply concerned with whether or not the mother was certain of her dates. If the dates were revised they were probably uncertain, but it is still worth checking this.)

The only piece of obstetric information which may be used to check the mother's history when there is uncertainty about the three conditions listed is the size of the uterus at booking, provided booking was done before the 16th week and bimanual examination was done (even this has sometimes misled us). Obstetric information obtained later in pregnancy, such as date of onset of fetal movements, uterine size, osseous development of the fetus on x-ray and staining of cells in the liquor amnii, is of value to the obstetrician in deciding when the baby will be or should be delivered, but gives a less accurate assessment of the gestational age than other methods available after birth.

When the mother's history is unreliable because of the three essential conditions being unfulfilled, a clinical method of assessing gestational age should be used. We suggest either the neurological method or the one based on physical characteristics, or a combination of the two.

### Neurological Assessment

The method we use is based on the presence or absence of five reflexes which have been found to have the most clear-cut times of appearance in terms of gestational age, these times not being affected by intra-uterine growth retardation. (Nor are they affected by whether the baby is maturing inside or outside the uterus.) The reflexes

91

**TABLE V**

**Reflexes of value in assessing gestational age**

| Reflex | Stimulus | Positive response | Gestation (wk) if reflex is Absent | Present |
|--------|----------|-------------------|--------|---------|
| Pupil reaction | Light | Pupil constriction | < 31 | 29 or more |
| Traction | Pull up by wrists from supine | Flexion of neck or arms | < 36 | 33 or more |
| Glabellar tap | Tap on glabella | Blink | < 34 | 32 or more |
| Neck righting | Rotation of head | Trunk follows | < 37 | 34 or more |
| Head turning | Diffuse light from one side | Head turning to light | Doubtful | 32 or more |

*Note:* 29 weeks means 203 days after the first day of the last menstrual period. If there is a conflict between two results, the reflex placed higher in the Table is more likely to give the true gestational age. (Reproduced from Robinson, R. J. (1966) 'Assessment of gestational age by neurological examination.' *Archives of Disease in Childhood,* **41,** 437.)

and the conclusions about gestational age which can be drawn from their presence or absence are shown in Table V. However, the neurological method may be inaccurate if the baby is ill.

*Notes on Elicitation and Interpretation of the Reflexes*

(1) Table V simply refers to whether the reflex is present or absent. *Any* positive response, however weak, indicates that it is present. For the first four reflexes the state is not really critical, but in doubtful cases it is best to have the baby awake with his eyes open.

(2) *Pupil reaction.* If the pupil is difficult to see, observe it through the +20 lens of the ophthalmoscope. The pupil contraction can be seen as the illumination is increased.

(3) *Traction reflex.* Some account may be taken of the strength of this reflex. If there is vigorous flexion of the arms or if the head is raised almost into line with the trunk, the baby is likely to exceed 35-36 weeks gestation.

(4) *Glabellar tap reflex.* Tap the baby just above the root of the nose. The positive response is just a blink. A generalised grimace, sometimes seen in very immature babies, does not count. The response can be elicited even with the eyes closed, but in babies in whom it has recently appeared, it is more easily seen with the eyes open.

(5) *Neck-righting reflex.* It is important that the baby should be on a fairly flat and hard surface and should not be encumbered by clothing or bedding. Any lifting of the shoulder on the side away from which the head is turned is a positive response.

(6) *Head turning to light.* State is critical for this response—it will only be elicited if the baby is awake with his eyes open. It is therefore less useful and reliable than the other reflexes.

### Assessment from Physical Characteristics

We have found the method of Dr. Valerie Farr and her colleagues (1966)* very useful. It is obviously better than neurological methods in babies who have neurological abnormalities, and it probably gives better discrimination at the higher gestational ages, but is less reliable below 35 weeks gestation.

In our population of babies, which includes a significant proportion of African and Asian parentage, Dr. Elizabeth Locard found that the best correlation between gestational age and physical characteristics score was obtained by using only eight of the physical characteristics, and their definitions are listed below. Give the baby a score for each character, add up the total score and then read off the gestational age against the score in Table VI (p. 95). Remember that, though the predicted gestational age is given to one place of decimals, the 95 per cent confidence limits are $\pm$ 2 weeks above 37 weeks gestation, and $\pm 3.2$ weeks below 37 weeks gestation.

*Definitions and Scores for Each Physical Characteristic*
(1) *Skin Texture.* Tested by picking up a fold of abdominal skin between finger and thumb, by inspection.
   0 = very thin with a gelatinous feel.
   1 = thin and smooth.
   2 = smooth and of medium thickness: irritation, rash and superficial peeling may be present.
   3 = slight thickening and stiff feeling, with superficial cracking and peeling, especially evident on hands and feet.
   4 = thick and parchment-like, with superficial or deep cracking.

(2) *Lanugo hair.* Examined over the back, holding the infant up to the light.
   0 = no lanugo, or very scanty short hairs present.
   1 = abundant; long and thick over the whole back.
   2 = lanugo thinning, especially over the lower back.
   3 = smaller amounts of lanugo, with areas of baldness.
   4 = at least half the back devoid of lanugo.

(3) *Ear form.* Assessed by inspection of the upper part of the pinna, above the external meatus.
   0 = almost flat and shapeless pinna, with little or no incurving of the edge.
   1 = incurving of any degree of part of the periphery of the pinna.
   2 = partial incurving of the whole of the upper pinna.
   3 = well-defined incurving of the whole of the upper pinna.

*Farr, V., Mitchell, R. G., Neligan, G. A., Parkin, J. M. (1966) 'The definition of some external characteristics used in the assessment of gestational age in the newborn infant.' *Developmental Medicine and Child Neurology*, **8,** 507.
Farr, V., Kerridge, D. F., Mitchell, R. G. (1966) 'The value of some external characteristics in the assessment of gestational age at birth.' *Developmental Medicine and Child Neurology*, **8,** 657.

(4) *Ear firmness.* Tested by palpation and folding of the upper pinna between finger and thumb.

0 = pinna feels soft and is easily folded into bizarre positions without springing back into position spontaneously.

1 = pinna feels soft along the edge and is easily folded, but returns slowly to the correct position spontaneously.

2 = cartilage can be felt to the edge of the pinna, though it is thin in places, and the pinna springs back readily after being folded.

3 = pinna firm, with definite cartilage extending to the periphery, and springs back into position immediately after being folded.

(5) *Genitalia*

MALES:

0 = neither testis in the scrotum.

$\frac{1}{2}$ = at least one testis low in the inguinal canal, so that it can be drawn into the upper scrotum.

1 = at least one testis high in the scrotum, though it may be drawn into the lowest position.

2 = at least one testis completely descended into the lower scrotum.

FEMALES: (examined with lower limbs half abducted).

0 = labia majora widely separated, with comparatively large labia minora protruding.

1 = labia majora almost cover labia minora.

2 = labia majora cover labia minora completely.

(The half score for grading the male genitalia is intended to keep the scoring for the two sexes the same—*i.e.* from 0 to 2).

(6) *Breast size.* Measured by picking up the breast tissue between finger and thumb.

0 = no breast tissue palpable.

1 = breast tissue palpable on one or both sides, neither being more than 0.5cm in diameter.

2 = breast tissue palpable on both sides, one or both being 0.5 to 1cm.

3 = breast tissue palpable on both sides, one or both being more than 1cm in diameter.

(7) *Nipple formation.* Estimated by inspection.

0 = nipple barely visible; no areola.

1 = nipple well-defined; areola present but not raised.

2 = nipple well-defined; areola edge raised above the skin.

(8) *Plantar skin creases.* Assessed by noting the creases which persist when the skin of the sole is stretched from toes to heel.

0 = no skin creases present.

1 = skin creases are faint red marks over the anterior half of the sole.

2 = creases are definite red marks over more than the anterior half of the sole, and indentation is present over no more than the anterior third.

3 = as (2) but the indentation is present over more than one-third of the sole.

4 = definite deep indentation present over more than the anterior third of the sole.

## TABLE VI

### Conversion of physical characteristics score to predicted gestational age

| Score | Gestational age (weeks) | Score | Gestational age (weeks) |
|-------|-------------------------|-------|-------------------------|
| 0 | 26.1 | 13 | 37.3 |
| 1 | 27.2 | 14 | 37.9 |
| 2 | 28.3 | 15 | 38.5 |
| 3 | 29.3 | 16 | 39.0 |
| 4 | 30.3 | 17 | 39.5 |
| 5 | 31.2 | 18 | 39.9 |
| 6 | 32.1 | 19 | 40.3 |
| 7 | 32.9 | 20 | 40.7 |
| 8 | 33.8 | 21 | 41.0 |
| 9 | 34.6 | 22 | 41.3 |
| 10 | 35.3 | 23 | 41.6 |
| 11 | 36.0 | 24 | 41.8 |
| 12 | 36.2 | 25 | 42.0 |

For use of this Table, see text.

# Feeding the Low-birthweight Infant

There is uncertainty about the precise nutritional requirements of low-birthweight infants in the first days of life, whether they are born early, small for dates or both; and the timing and amount of the first and subsequent feeds, the type of food and the route by which it is given are all controversial matters. We have taken the following into consideration when deciding our nursery routine.

(1) Brain growth normally proceeds at a very rapid rate in the last weeks of intra-uterine life, and there is increasing evidence that, if an infant is born early, this growth should be interrupted for as short a time as possible.

(2) The provision of adequate but at the same time readily utilised calories for such growth is probably most easily achieved by using maternal milk whenever possible; the newborn kidney functions most adequately and chemical homeostasis is achieved soonest when this is the food provided.

(3) Liberal amounts (see below) of breast-milk given in the first days of life will lessen the hyperbilirubinaemia of immaturity, obviating the need for exchange transfusion, and will largely prevent the symptomatic hypoglycaemia most commonly seen in the small-for-dates infant.

(4) We do not think there is sufficient evidence that a lower mortality results either from initial intravenous feeding of very low-birthweight infants, or from the use of smaller amounts than we have recommended by the oral route; and we do not believe that aspiration of feed into the lung is a significant factor in the neonatal mortality of our low-birthweight babies. Aspiration does seem to be a factor in an occasional neonatal death of a low-birthweight baby. However, since these deaths are by no means confined to babies of the lowest birthweight and, moreover, may occur when the baby is several days old, it is difficult to see how they can be avoided short of forbidding oral feeding for, say, one week in all babies of less than 2.5kg birthweight.

## Our Choice of Food

We always use undiluted human breast-milk for babies of very low birthweight in the first days of life and continue with it as long as it is available. We never have enough, so some larger babies have to have cow's milk early, sometimes from the start. This is given as a full-strength half-cream dried milk, reconstituted as 1 level, uncompressed scoop:30ml water. There is no point in giving glucose feeds initially.

## Method of Feeding

Feeds are given by indwelling polyvinyl nasogastric tube (Bardic No. 5 French) to babies of *very* low birthweight, or larger infants who are ill, especially with respiratory distress. The tubes are kept in position by strapping across the cheek. The indwelling tube can act as an irritant and may contribute to airway obstruction, so that orogastric feeding (see below) should be substituted when feasible, and used until the infant is able to suck and swallow adequately. Larger well babies are fed by orogastric tube passed at each feed. Bottle or breast-feeding is encouraged at the earliest opportunity, but when the nursery is full and the staff busy this is not often achieved before the baby has reached a gestational age of 35 weeks. It is very much easier for an immature infant to suck from a small bottle, for example a 20ml Universal container, than from the conventional 250ml feeding bottle. The same teats are used for all.

### Other Methods of Milk Feeding

*Nasogastric drip feeding* has some advantages in that hands do not go into the incubator so often and thus opportunities for infection should be less. All drips need very frequent supervision for adjustment, but the use of constant infusion pumps simplifies the procedure.

We have never felt *gastrostomy* to be warranted or necessary, except occasionally as an adjunct to surgical procedures (for instance repair of an oesophageal atresia).

### Timing and Amounts

Feeds are started within two to three hours of birth and milk is given in the following amounts:-

| | |
|---|---|
| 1st 24 hours | 60ml/kg birthweight |
| 2nd 24 hours | 90ml/kg birthweight |
| 3rd 24 hours | 120ml/kg birthweight |
| 4th 24 hours | 150ml/kg birthweight |

Infants of very low birthweight, or those who are ill, particularly with respiratory distress, are fed hourly by indwelling nasogastric tube so that relatively small amounts are put into the stomach at any one time with a minimum of disturbance. Our nursing staff like to aspirate babies' stomachs at four-hourly intervals before a feed. We are uncertain of the value of this, as the stomach is unlikely ever to be empty with frequent feeding in the early days of life when gastric emptying is slowest. It seems sensible, however, if there is obvious abdominal distension. Those in whom orogastric tubes are used are fed at three-hourly intervals.

### Positioning of Infants

Some regurgitation occurs in about one-third of normal newborns in the first days of life. It occurs more frequently in the immature, particularly when ill. Theoretically at least it should be lessened and the dangers of aspiration into the lungs minimised if such infants are nursed prone rather than supine whenever possible, or at least lying on the right side.

### Contra-indications to Oral Feeding

(1) Intravenous feeding may be essential for a period before and after surgery if a congenital anomaly interferes with normal gastro-intestinal function, or following surgery for abnormality in other systems. (See p. 99 for details of electrolyte requirements and long-term intravenous feeding.)

97

(2) Some low-birthweight infants, usually but not invariably those that are illest, develop a functional ileus which very occasionally progresses to an enterocolitis. Oral (or nasogastric) feeding should be stopped, and intravenous fluids given (see p. 99). Peripheral veins should be used whenever possible, and the umbilical vein avoided. Hypoglycaemia can occur very quickly if a drip stops, and residents should be prepared to put up another almost immediately. For this reason oral feeding must be satisfactorily re-established before intravenous therapy is stopped.

(3) If an infant is having repeated fits that cannot be quickly controlled, intravenous feeding may be safer.

(4) We use the intravenous route temporarily while an infant is being weaned from the ventilator, to cover the period of vigorous treatment necessary for removal of tracheal secretions (see p. 138).

**Prevention of Hypoglycaemia**

Symptomatic hypoglycaemia can and should be almost entirely prevented by adequate feeding in the first days of life. Small-for-dates babies should be fed the amounts given on p. 97, using breast milk whenever possible.

*Warning*

The relatively liberal amounts of food we use in the first days of life for the *low-birthweight* baby are intended for him alone. The healthy, well-grown newborn does not need a large amount of milk at this time and does not get it if put to the breast. He can safely be left to provide the extra energy necessary for life by breakdown of his own tissue glycogen, fat and protein, of which he has an adequate supply. Too much cow's milk in the first days predisposes to hypocalcaemia (see p. 190), to intestinal obstruction by milk curds, and possibly to later obesity by a conditioning of the appetite centre.

**Choice of Food After the First Days**

If infants born early are of normal weight for dates, it may perhaps be assumed that they have a normal growth potential. Many small-for-dates infants, particularly those who are also immature, grow more slowly—for reasons not yet entirely understood.

It is said that the protein content of breast milk is too low for optimal growth of the very small pre-term baby. However, early breast milk from lactating mothers still in the maternity unit has a higher protein content than has later milk. If given in adequate amounts, and providing the infant has reached a weight of 1500g by the age of one post-natal month, growth similar to that *in utero* may be achieved (Stevens 1969)*. Unfortunately, breast-milk is not always available in sufficient amounts and we resort to the use of cow's milk (see above).

*Stevens, L. H. (1969) 'The first kilogram: 2. The protein content of breast milk of mothers of babies of low birth weight.' *Medical Journal of Australia*, **2**, 555.

# Intravenous Therapy

Intravenous administration of fluid and food is a poor substitute for oral feeding. Nevertheless, long-term intravenous feeding is increasingly being practised in a number of special care nurseries and we can recommend articles by Harries (1971) and Heird and colleagues (1972) as useful reading*. On the other hand, intravenous (i.v.) fluid therapy is frequently necessary for short periods in the newborn. The most frequently encountered situations when i.v. therapy is indicated are:

(1) when disease of the intestinal tract precludes oral feeding, or when there is a special risk of aspiration (see p. 138);
(2) when it is essential that administered fluid (blood, saline, etc.) enters directly into the circulation; and
(3) when the i.v. fluid is an essential vehicle for a drug or antibiotic.

The practical procedure for setting up i.v. infusions is described on p. 271. We prefer always to use a peripheral vein rather than the umbilical vein for continuous infusions, although we do use the umbilical vein for a single injection of a drug or glucose in certain circumstances.

The choice of fluid and the rate of administration vary with the clinical situation and the following notes are guide lines.

## Maintenance Requirements

The basic needs that one tries to meet with i.v. therapy are for water, sodium, potassium and calories. After the first few days, a growing newborn baby needs: water 150ml; sodium and potassium 2-3mEq each; and calories 100 or more; all per kg per day. When a baby is ill and not growing he is not 'binding' water and electrolytes for growth of tissue and his needs are slightly less and the risk of overloading him rather greater. Also the risk of overloading seems to be greater in the first two days of life. It is difficult to fulfil nutritional needs intravenously; this is an important reason for returning to oral feeding as soon as circumstances permit.

*Fluid*

| | |
|---|---|
| *Age 0-48 hours:* | pre-term infants 60-70ml/kg/day. |
| | term infants 50-60ml/kg/day. |
| | small-for-dates infants up to 90ml/kg/day. |
| | Fluid 5% or 10% dextrose. |
| *Age 48 hours or more:* | increase to 100-150ml/kg/day. |
| | Fluid 0.18% sodium chloride in 4.3% dextrose. |

*Sodium*

The above regime gives 3mEq/kg/day to babies of more than 48 hours. In babies

*Harries, J. T. (1971) 'Intravenous feeding in infants.' *Archives of Disease in Childhood*, **46**, 855.
Heird, W. C., Driscoll, J. M., Schullinger, J. N., Grebin, B., Winters, R. W. (1972) 'Intravenous alimentation in pediatric patients.' *Journal of Pediatrics*, **80**, 351.

less than 48 hours we do not give sodium supplements unless there is evidence of abnormal loss.

*Potassium*

We do not give potassium supplements for an infusion lasting less than 48 hours unless there is diarrhoea, vomiting or intestinal fistula, or unless plasma K is low. A normal or even high plasma potassium does not always imply a normal total body potassium, especially if the baby is dehydrated. A low plasma potassium level usually means that the total body potassium is depleted. When potassium is indicated, it is only given if the baby is passing urine. We never give it in concentrations of more than 40mEq/litre, and unless the loss is exceptional, never more than 3mEq/kg/day.

*Calories*

We recognise that 5% or 10% dextrose provides inadequate calories. For hypoglycaemic babies we use 10%, or even 15%, dextrose. For babies in whom long-term I.V. feeding (more than five to seven days) is envisaged, proprietary solutions of amino-acid and fructose are used and the instructions in the manufacturer's literature observed. In babies who have had major portions of their gut resected, we have also used intravenous fat preparations, observing the manufacturer's instructions (see also p. 271 and references at foot of p. 99).

*Dehydration*

The correction of dehydration involves administering I.V. fluids above the maintenance requirement. The amount and composition of the fluids depends on degree of dehydration, plasma sodium and potassium levels, and acid-base status. In a seriously ill baby, take blood for Na, K, chloride, bicarbonate, urea and osmolality; set up an I.V. infusion and give 30ml/kg of 0.9% sodium chloride or plasma.

While this is going in, or in less urgent situations before deciding on a particular I.V. fluid, plan therapy based on these assessments.

(1) *Degree of dehydration.* Assess by the following.
    (*a*) Loss of body weight.
    (*b*) Clinical degree of dehydration: mild = 5% body weight = 50ml/kg; moderate
       = 10% body weight = 100ml/kg; severe = 15% body weight = 150ml/kg.
    (*c*) Plasma osmolality: mild dehydration = 295-300m osmol/kg water; moderate
       = 300-310m osmol/kg water; severe = >310m osmol/kg water.

(2) *Sodium status.* Assess by plasma sodium.
        Na < 130 = hypotonic dehydration;
        Na 130-150 = isotonic dehydration;
        Na > 150 = hypertonic dehydration.
In isotonic or hypotonic dehydration, plan to make up the deficiency volume with fluid containing about 150mEq/litre of sodium in the form of chloride or lactate, depending on acid base status; *e.g.* 0.9% sodium chloride or M/6 sodium lactate. In hypertonic dehydration, use 0.45% sodium chloride and correct the Na level slowly, *i.e.* over about 48 hours.

(3) *Potassium deficit.* Assess by the following.

(*a*) The history. (Dehydration caused by vomiting or diarrhoea will inevitably lead to loss of potassium.)

(*b*) Plasma K. (This is *unreliable* evidence until after rehydration.)

Do not give I.V. potassium until rehydration is largely complete and it is known that the baby is passing urine. If I.V. potassium is needed, never use solutions of more than 40mEq K/litre and only give 3mEq/kg/day.

(4) *Acid base status.* Assess by the following.

(*a*) The history: *e.g.* diarrhoea = loss $HCO_3$; pyloric stenosis = high $HCO_3$.

(*b*) Plasma bicarbonate.

(*c*) Blood pH.

If $HCO_3$ is less than 18mEq/litre, give some of the sodium (2 above) as bicarbonate.

The over-all plan should be to restore circulating volume within 2 hours, to complete the rehydration of the extracellular fluid volume in 24 hours and to complete correction of Na and K status by about 48 to 72 hours.

## I.V. Fluids as Vehicles for Drugs and Antibiotics

When an I.V. infusion is set up, injecting drugs and antibiotics via the infusion to save pricking the baby is worthwhile, provided certain precautions are strictly observed.

(1) Ensure that the drug or antibiotic can be given by the intravenous route. Check with the pharmacist or the manufacturer's literature.

(2) Ensure that the drug is compatible with the infusion fluid. Dextrose and fructose solutions are acidic and *not* suitable vehicles for most penicillins, or for heparin, sulphonamide and barbiturate. Benzyl penicillin and ampicillin lose their activity rapidly in dextrose, while methicillin is stable for only six hours. Sodium bicarbonate solutions are unsuitable vehicles for any calcium salt.

(3) If more than one drug is given intravenously, make sure they are mutually compatible. In neonatal practice, important incompatibilities are: (*a*) penicillins and sympatho-mimetic amines; (*b*) heparin and hydrocortisone; (*c*) aminoacid solutions or lipid suspensions and antibiotics; and (*d*) gentamicin and carbenicillin. If in any doubt, check with the pharmacist. (Tetracycline, which is rarely used in the newborn, is incompatible with a number of drugs.)

(4) Observe strict sterility. Organisms multiply in most sugar and electrolyte solutions.

(5) Whenever possible, add I.V. drugs yourself and observe these precautions. If a nurse is to add the drugs, *write down* clear and detailed instructions on the treatment sheet.

(6) Whenever possible, avoid 'home-made' mixtures and use drug/I.V. fluid mixtures made up in the pharmacy.

(7) *Injection into the drip-tubing near the needle.* Injecting thus obviates some of the problems above. However, strict asepsis is still important. Clamp the tubing above the injection site and give the injection very slowly (2-5 minutes). Intravenous steroid preparations and penicillins are best given in this way.

# Temperature Control

The baby, though physiologically warm-blooded (a homeotherm), has a relatively large surface area and a small mass to act as a heat sink, so that body temperature is frequently unstable, when he is very small. In temperate climates, environmental temperatures are usually less than body temperature so that the major clinical problem is to conserve the baby's body heat and provide adequate warmth.

The consequences of not providing enough warmth are these:-

(1) In the case of low-birthweight babies, mortality rates are higher. This has been established by controlled trials.
(2) The baby uses more oxygen in an attempt to keep himself warm.
(3) The baby uses more body fuel in an attempt to keep himself warm.
(4) If his own homeothermy is overwhelmed and his body temperature falls, he may suffer from the 'neonatal cold injury' syndrome, or from a bleeding diathesis (intravascular coagulation) and, not infrequently, dies while being rewarmed.

For these reasons, meticulous attention to temperature control is a vitally important aspect of newborn care.

### Situations When a Baby is At Risk

(1) At birth, when he arrives naked, wet and partially asphyxiated. Some fall in body temperature is inevitable at birth, especially if the baby has needed resuscitation, but it should be minimised. Practical instructions are given on p. 39.

(2) During the first bath, when even a lusty term-infant's body temperature often falls to 35°C (95°F). A healthy baby will survive this ritual, but the bathing room should be very warm (30°C, 86°F) and the bath should be quickly performed. Babies of low birthweight or babies who are ill for any reason should not be subjected to a bath.

(3) When the baby is being transported, either from one part of the hospital to another or from one hospital to another. Instructions are given on p. 114.

(4) During clinical examination when the baby is naked at room temperature (see p. 82).

(5) During minor or major surgery or procedures.

(6) During x-ray procedures.

(7) While he is being nursed naked in an incubator (see below).

### Prevention of Hypothermia

When there is a risk of hypothermia, one should monitor the baby's temperature to measure the end result of thermal balance (see below for details). Environmental temperatures which seem excessively hot to adults, such as 30°C (86°F), may be far too cold for a small naked baby. A single measurement of temperature such as room temperature or the air temperature in an incubator describes only one aspect of the thermal environment: heat is also lost by conduction, evaporation and radiation.

Keep room temperatures as warm as is consistent with the efficient performance of the staff, swaddle such parts of the baby as do not need to be seen (including the bonnet area of the head, which is an important site of heat loss), and make judicious use of warming pads and radiant heat sources (see below for dangers).

**Incubator-nursed Babies**

For the naked baby in an incubator there is a very narrow range of thermal environment within which there is no thermal stress.* It must be emphasized that there is no one temperature range appropriate for all babies, since they vary in size and maturity. The temperature range for a very small baby is dangerously hot for a fat term baby, and that appropriate for a fat term baby is dangerously cool for a small pre-term baby.

A reasonable estimate of the incubator temperature for a given baby can be obtained from Fig. 7 (p. 104). These temperatures apply when the baby is nursed in an incubator with a perspex heat-shield (p. 290) over his body. The heat-shield, in effect, provides a second skin of perspex which is warmed on both surfaces by incubator air, and thus makes the operative temperature to which the baby is exposed independent of room temperature outside the incubator. The environmental temperatures suggested are very warm compared with older estimates; the figures derive from studies in a metabolic chamber. They may not always be exactly correct for the baby in an incubator—even with the perspex heat-shield in position. In all cases it is essential to monitor the baby's temperature to ensure that the environmental temperature chosen has worked out well in terms of the individual baby. The rectal temperature should be maintained at 37°C (98·6°F) or, better still, the skin of his exposed abdomen should be 36.5°C (97·7°F).

From the point of view of temperature control, a baby who no longer needs to be seen naked should be lightly clothed, or swaddled in his incubator, or removed to a cot. The fact that a baby is in an incubator is not an argument for not clothing him.

*Cot-nursed Infants*

The infant who is clothed and wrapped in a cot-blanket is less a prey to changes in his thermal environment than is the infant in an incubator. The neutral range of environmental temperature for such a baby is wider, and the metabolic cost of mis-judging his individual requirements is smaller. Nonetheless, a cot-nursed infant needs a warm room. (See Fig. 7.)

**The Environment that is Too Warm**

The small pre-term infant does not sweat effectively, and even a term infant cannot lose more heat by evaporation alone than his basal metabolic heat production. Temperatures hotter than the baby are therefore dangerous. Reduce environmental temperature *at once* if the baby overheats.

---

*The neutral range of environmental temperature for a given baby with a normal rectal temperature is that within which his oxygen consumption is minimal, *i.e.* where he needs to do the least amount of metabolic work to control his body temperature.

103

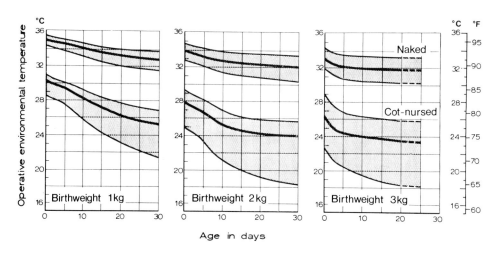

**Fig. 7** Neutral temperature ranges for newborn babies. The upper range is for babies nursed naked in an incubator and with a perspex 'heat shield' in position (see p. 290). The lower range is for babies who are clothed and in a cot, with light blankets. (This Figure was kindly provided by Dr. Edmund Hey and is redrawn from his illustration on p. 180 in *Recent Advances in Paediatrics*, 4th Edition (1971) edited by Gairdner and Hull, published by Churchill, London.)

Radiant heat sources and warming pads may be useful in certain circumstances but always carry a risk of overheating or burning a baby. They should always be carefully watched and the end result of their use in a baby must be monitored as a skin or rectal temperature. The skin of a collapsed baby with a poor circulation can easily be burnt by any contact with a surface, even a blanket, whose temperature is above 45°C (113°F).

**The Silver Swaddler**

This swaddler, developed at Hammersmith, occludes heat exchange by conduction convection, radiation and, most importantly, by evaporation. However, it carries three possible dangers: the baby in the swaddler could overheat; the plastic material could suffocate the baby if he turns his face into it; and cord haemorrhage might be undetected. It should, therefore, only be used in emergency situations and when the baby is under observation.

Some of our residents have argued that it is disadvantageous to wrap a cold baby in a silver swaddler, thus occluding any possible heat gain of a warm transport incubator. However, a baby who is alive is necessarily producing heat, and if the baby is insulated he will warm himself, albeit somewhat more slowly than if heat is poured into him artificially.

We do not know the optimum rate to warm up a very cold baby, though it has been said—and we would agree on general grounds—that this should not be done very rapidly.

**Taking A Baby's Temperature**

The instruction to 'monitor' the baby's temperature is frequently made above; the following are notes on the technique of measurement.

*Frequency*

Any baby who is put into an incubator, or is transferred from one incubator to another, or who for any reason is deemed to be ill enough to warrant special observation, should have his temperature recorded every hour until it has risen to within a degree of normal. Thereafter the temperature should be taken only every four hours to reduce handling of the baby. When no disturbance to the baby is involved, *i.e.* when an electrical thermometer is being used for continuous measurements, we record the temperature with any other half-hourly observations.

A baby who graduates from an incubator to a cot, or a normal term baby after birth, should have his temperature recorded every four hours until it is stable and normal. Thereafter temperature need only be recorded twice a day.

*Site and Techniques*

The sites from which we record temperature are (1) the rectum; (2) exposed abdominal skin; or (3) the axilla. Each has its advantages and disadvantages, and limitations. *Whenever a body temperature is recorded, the site must also be recorded.*

(1) RECTUM

*Depth:* The deeper the probe is inserted—up to a depth of 10cm—the higher the temperature recorded. The major changes occur in the first 4cm, and since it is undesirable and impracticable to insert very deeply, we recommend that the thermometer should be inserted 4cm. In particular, a stiff thermometer such as mercury in glass should not be inserted beyond 4cm. The baby should be lying on his side and the thermometer directed slightly posteriorly. However, when a flexible electrical probe is left in situ, it is less likely to come out with the next stool if it is inserted to 6 or 8cm, and strapped to the thigh with adhesive tape.

*Advantages.* Rectal temperature is a reasonable measure of core temperature. Other sites, *e.g.* oesophagus or tympanic membrane, are impractical in the baby.

*Disadvantages.* Perforation of the bowel is unusual, but it can occur, especially if there is bowel pathology such as Hirschprung's disease or enterocolitis. Clearly, rectal probes must be inserted very gently. There is always a risk of glass thermometers breaking. Removing the nappy and inserting a thermometer is an obvious occasion when hands can be contaminated, and the use of the rectal thermometer has cross-infection risks. For these reasons we recommend that temperatures should be taken less frequently when a stable situation is achieved (see above) and that axillary temperatures should be used when intensive care is no longer needed.

*Low-reading thermometers.* Any baby whose temperature is less than 35°C (95°F) should have his temperature checked using a thermometer which reads down to 30°C (86°F)—or even lower if necessary. Shake it down well, and do not expose it to an incubator temperature of, say, 33°C before inserting it.

*Normal rectal temperature.* We regard a rectal temperature of 36.8°C ± 0.2 (98.2°F ± 0.4) as normal in a baby.

105

(2) EXPOSED ABDOMINAL SKIN TEMPERATURE

Use electrical probes (thermistor or thermocouple) which are designed for the purpose, not a mercury thermometer strapped to the skin or an electrical probe designed for another purpose. Strap the probe to the skin of the abdomen above the umbilicus with a fairly long (10cm) strip of tape. A second short piece of strapping on the wire about 3cm from the tip of the probe helps stabilise it. The temperature recorded is not, in strict physical terms, a 'surface temperature'.

*Advantages.* This temperature will fall sooner than the core temperature if the environment is too cold and thus an adjustment to the environmental temperature can be made before the baby's deep body-temperature falls. The probe does not interfere with a baby's orifices. The electrical read-out box can stand outside the incubator, thus reducing handling and cross-infection, and the temperature can be read at any time.

*Disadvantages.* The probe is quite easily displaced and this can be dangerous if it is being used for servocontrol. We regard a skin temperature of the exposed abdominal skin of 36.5°C $\pm$ 0.3 (97.7°F $\pm$ 0.5) as normal.

(3) AXILLARY TEMPERATURE

This is taken using a mercury-in-glass or an electrical thermometer. It is a less reliable measure of core temperature than rectal, oesophageal, etc., since it is usually lower, but may (if brown fat is being stimulated) occasionally read higher. It has the advantages of minimal handling and of not involving a body orifice, and is satisfactory for routine monitoring where no obvious thermal problem exists. If an axillary temperature is unexpectedly high or low, it is best to check the rectal temperature.

We regard an axillary temperature of 36.5 to 37°C (97.7 to 98.6°F) as normal.

# Oxygen Therapy — General Principles

Giving oxygen-enriched air to a newborn baby in respiratory failure is sensible on theoretical grounds, and common experience suggests that it is worthwhile although it is difficult to prove its efficacy in terms of saving life or preventing brain-damage. On the other hand, excess oxygen is poisonous; any concentration above that present in air (20.93%) is unsafe if breathed for very long periods, and the higher the concentration the shorter the exposure needed to produce toxic effects. The pre-term baby is particularly at risk because of the danger of retrolental fibroplasia.

If the arterial oxygen content is too high for too long the retinal capillaries will be damaged; if the arterial oxygen content remains within normal limits the risk is far less, whatever the concentration of inspired oxygen. On the other hand, it seems likely that a high concentration of oxygen may damage the lungs even if the arterial oxygen content remains low.

The aim of oxygen therapy is to ensure an adequate supply of oxygen to the mitochondria. The adequacy of the supply will depend on the arterial oxygen saturation, the haemoglobin concentration in the blood, the cardiac output and the tissue diffusion gradient. As one cannot in practice measure all these variables, it is impossible to lay down precise indications for oxygen therapy. We observe the following empirical rules, which are designed (*a*) to limit oxygen therapy to those situations where it is really necessary, and (*b*) to control it by careful monitoring when it has to be given.

## Rules to Limit the Use of Oxygen Therapy

(1) Only give oxygen when there is a definite indication. The circumstances when oxygen therapy may need to be given are as follows.

    (*a*) Birth asphyxia—when we limit the concentration to 40% (see p. 32).

    (*b*) Pulmonary nitrogen washout tests, in which 100% oxygen is administered for 15 minutes for the measurement of pulmonary shunts (see p. 132).

    (*c*) The respiratory distress syndrome (see p. 123).

    (*d*) In some cases of recurrent apnoea (see p. 143).

    (*e*) In some cases of pneumomediastinum or pneumothorax, in which a high concentration of oxygen is used (see p. 140).

    (*f*) Pneumonia (see p. 119).

    (*g*) Severe anaemia and shock.

    (*h*) Heart failure.

(2) Give oxygen in the lowest effective concentration.

(3) Stop oxygen therapy as soon as possible.

(4) Avoid using 100% oxygen as far as possible. (This rule is made not solely on account of oxygen toxicity, but also because, when apnoea supervenes in a patient whose lungs have been inflated with 100% oxygen, pulmonary atelectasis quickly occurs.)

**Control of Oxygen Therapy**

Oxygen therapy should be controlled by measuring the concentration of oxygen in the inspired air and the oxygen content of the arterial blood. The first is always possible and must always be done, the second should be done whenever possible. Ideally, continuous measurements should be made. This is possible in the case of ambient oxygen concentration and we sometimes use an oxygen electrode in the incubator for this purpose. Continuous measurement of arterial oxygen tension is now, becoming a practical possibility.

*Oxygen Concentration of Inspired Air*

This ambient oxygen concentration is measured by an oxygen analyser: an indirect estimate based on the flow of oxygen to the incubator is far too inaccurate. Ambient oxygen concentration must be measured at hourly intervals, and ten minutes after any alteration in oxygen flow to the incubator.

The instrument we generally use for measuring ambient oxygen concentration is the Beckman paramagnetic oxygen analyser. It is important to observe the following precautions in using it.
(1) Squeeze the bulb ten times, take a reading, then squeeze another five times and check that the reading has not altered.
(2) Ensure that the bungs on the silica gel water absorber are tightly fitting; if they are not, room air may be entrained and a falsely low reading of oxygen content obtained. In any case....
(3) check the analyser daily by sucking in a sample of 100% oxygen, to make sure the instrument is not reading falsely low. Do not blow the sample through.

*Arterial Oxygen Content*

We use the arterial oxygen tension ($paO_2$) as an indirect measure of arterial oxygen content. Oxygen saturation would provide a more accurate indirect estimate at low levels of arterial oxygen content, whereas tension provides a more accurate estimate at high levels. We use tension, mainly because it is simpler to measure, but also because we are particularly concerned with avoiding unnecessarily high levels of arterial oxygenation which might lead to retrolental fibroplasia.

$PaO_2$ is measured by the oxygen electrode, using samples of arterial blood obtained from an indwelling catheter or by direct puncture (see p. 268).

The general rule is to keep the $paO_2$ between 60 and 90mmHg, by adjusting the ambient oxygen concentration to the level necessary to achieve this. This problem is discussed further under 'Respiratory distress' (see p. 123).

If there is an arterial catheter in place, measure $paO_2$ (*a*) at not greater than four hourly intervals; (*b*) after administration of alkali, which may raise $paO_2$; and (*c*) after raising ambient oxygen concentration. *It is particularly important to make regular $paO_2$ measurements during the recovery phase of respiratory distress when shunts will diminish spontaneously, and $paO_2$ may rise rapidly.*

If there is no arterial catheter in place, arterial puncture may be used*. The frequency of sampling must depend on its ease and practicability and also on how stable the clinical situation seems.

If arterial blood samples are not obtainable, it is reasonable to regard central cyanosis as an indication for oxygen therapy. Cyanosis occurs at an approximate $paO_2$ of 40mmHg (*i.e.* 65% saturation).

The situation in which it is most often necessary to give added oxygen without frequent arterial monitoring is in the very immature baby with recurrent apnoeic attacks. This problem is discussed fully on page 143, but it is important to emphasize that these are the babies most at risk for retrolental fibroplasia, and that not even small amounts of added oxygen should be given without arterial monitoring unless there are good grounds for thinking that the frequency of apnoeic attacks is being reduced.

*The use of the intra-arterial $pO_2$ electrode has shown us that $paO_2$ may fall temporarily during the procedure of radial artery puncture. Thus the danger of misleadingly low results must be borne in mind.

# Prevention of Infection

### Intranatal

Obstetricians generally prescribe antibiotics for the mother when the membranes rupture prematurely. Though eminently justifiable on maternal grounds, there is no good evidence that this prevents infection in the infant. But as he may become colonised with organisms from the birth canal resistant to the antibiotic used, always note what has been prescribed.

When the mother is known to have gonorrhoea, or has been treated for it earlier in the pregnancy, we instil silver nitrate drops into the baby's eyes after birth (see p. 22).

### Postnatal

*Main Sources of Infection*

(1) The hands of attendants (*i.e.* mothers, nursing and medical staff).

(2) Apparatus, especially that containing water (resuscitation apparatus, incubators, suction equipment and mechanical ventilators). Gram-negative organisms in particular flourish in the humidification units. Other equipment touched by hand, *e.g.* the blood gas apparatus, may also be contaminated, as are sinks, particularly overflow pipes.

(3) Feeds and medicaments can be infected during preparation (very rare with the standard techniques in use for sterilisation), or in distribution and administration.

(4) Airborne droplet infection from attendants.

The environment has to be scupulously clean to be safe for a baby, particularly in nurseries for sick and low-birthweight infants, where those working must not only have a clear understanding of aseptic techniques, but must practise them conscientiously and assiduously.

*'Barrier' Techniques in the Neonatal Ward*

(1) The use of cotton overshoes does cut down the dissemination of bacteria in dust brought from elsewhere by your shoes, but do wash your hands *after* putting them on.

(2) Masks need only be worn if you have any suspicion of an upper respiratory tract infection; remember to hold them only at the corners, preferably by the tapes or elastic, avoid touching them when on, and cover nose as well as mouth.

(3) Clean gowns are worn when working in the intensive care nursery. When wearing long-sleeved gowns, roll the sleeves up to the elbow to avoid their being put through successive incubator portholes, and wash forearms as well as hands!

(4) *Effective handwashing is probably the single most important measure in preventing the spread of infection.* We urge you to be obsessional about it. The use of a 3% hexachlorophane emulsion (active against Gram-positive bacteria, but only slightly so against Gram-negative) has a cumulative antibacterial effect. Povidone-iodine is an acceptable alternative.

*Other Measures to Keep Infection at a Minimum*

(1) *Infant skin care.* The use of 3 % hexachlorophane detergent lotion for bathing has probably contributed to the reduced incidence of staphylococcal colonization in the newborn. Hexachlorophane is absorbed through the intact skin and, if improperly used, may be toxic to the central nervous system. *The skin must therefore be carefully rinsed after its application, and the manufacturers' directions should be followed in detail.*

(2) *Treatment of the umbilicus.* We use Polybactrin spray at birth (see p. 30) and daily until the cord separates: this ensures a sterile stump in the great majority of babies. The proximity of the umbilicus to the perineum with its heavy bacterial contamination, and to the blood stream, makes this an essential procedure if umbilical vessels have to be catheterised. Moreover, the dying umbilicus provides a culture medium for bacteria. From the time we began to keep the umbilicus sterile, the incidence of infections in other parts of the body, especially conjunctivitis, was greatly reduced.

(3) *Surveillance of bacterial flora.* We swab the nose, throat, umbilicus and rectum of each infant in the special care nursery at weekly intervals, and record the current flora. Thus any build-up of organisms such as *Pseudomonas aeruginosa* or Klebsiella, which do not normally colonise the newborn, can be noted early and a search for the source made. Ideally, regular surveys of the environment (*e.g.* incubators, hand-cream dispensers, sinks) should also be made, but to reduce routine laboratory work we reserve these surveys for emergencies.

(4) *Screening of admissions.* As a rule, we do not admit to the special care nursery infants born elsewhere who are more than 48 hours old. However, on occasion we waive this rule, *but known cases of gastro-enteritis must never be admitted.* If more than one case of serious cross-infection occurs in the nursery at any one time, it must be closed to all further admissions until the source is traced and the situation is under control.

(5) *Cleaning of equipment.* We attach great importance to the thorough and frequent sterilisation or cleaning of equipment. For methods and references, see Davies (1971).*

(6) *Responsibility for control of infection.* The checking of weekly swab results, frequent critical review of techniques used for cleaning and sterilising apparatus, and close liaison with the hospital's Cross-infection Officer are the responsibility of one member of our staff, to whom infection in the nursery should be made known at once.

*Maternal Infectious Disease*

In the event of a mother developing an infectious illness after delivery (see also section on known infectious disease in pregnancy, p. 20 *et seq.*), the infant will of necessity have no immunity to it. This is one of the occasions on which separation of the baby from his mother may be necessary—particularly in the case of 'childhood' infectious illnesses and severe bacterial, *e.g.* streptococcal, infection.

*Davies, P. A. (1971) 'Bacterial infection in the fetus and newborn.' *Archives of Disease in Childhood*, **46**, 1.

*Antibiotic Prophylaxis and Immunoglobulin Administration*

There is insufficient evidence for, and some evidence against, the use of these in the prevention of infection: we do not use them, apart from the cord spray (see p. 30).

*Routine Bacteriology on Staff*

We have found that routine nose and throat swabs are unhelpful and involve the laboratory in unnecessary work. Appropriate swabs must be taken from members of staff if there is an outbreak of infection.

# Transport of Sick Newborn Babies

In our experience, the condition of a sick baby is seldom adversely affected by transport if the procedures described below are adopted (see Storrs and Taylor 1970*).

A neonatal resident and nurse are available to go in the ambulance to collect sick babies.

**Journey to Transferring Hospital**

An ambulance is called to the special care nursery to collect the doctor and nurse, emergency equipment and portable incubator, and then to go to the hospital requesting transfer. The incubator should always be kept warm and ready for use in the neo-natal unit so that it needs only to be plugged into the power point in the ambulance, where it remains until the baby is ready to be placed in it for the return journey. During the outward journey, keep the incubator covered with a metallized blanket to prevent heat loss.

**Arrival at Transferring Hospital**

On arrival at the transferring hospital, a history of mother and baby is taken on the standard 'baby-transfer' form (see Section 9 p. 316). A supply of these forms is given to all hospitals who regularly transfer cases, in the hope that many of the details can be filled in before the ambulance arrives. Full details must be obtained of the mother's obstetric history and drug therapy, the labour, and details of the baby's condition from birth, including the time of passage of urine and meconium, fluid intake, feeding, drugs, blood glucose estimations, apnoeic episodes, oxygen therapy and temperature. Try to obtain a sample of maternal blood. This is essential if the baby is affected by haemolytic disease. If possible obtain the placenta. Make it a rule to introduce yourself to the mother before leaving the referring hospital.

**Preparations for the Transfer**

The aim is to carry out all necessary resuscitation measures before transfer and to anticipate as far as possible the problems which may arise during the journey. Do a quick general examination of the baby and measure the rectal temperature.

*Intubation*

Apart from the usual indications (see p. 32), perform intubation also if it seems likely that artificial ventilation will be needed during the journey, *i.e.* in babies with a history of apnoeic attacks or with severe respiratory distress. Since intubation does not allow the baby to grunt, those with presumed hyaline membrane disease should have continuous positive airway pressure (CPAP) or be ventilated (by hand or with the portable ventilator) during the journey even if they are breathing.

*Storrs, C. N., Taylor, M. R. H. (1970) 'Transport of sick newborn babies.' *British Medical Journal*, **3**, 328.

Nasotracheal intubation is recommended, as the tube is easier to secure and is less likely to become dislodged than an oral one.

*Hypoglycaemia*

Estimate blood sugar by 'Dextrostix' in babies who are small for dates or who have been severely hypoxic, and give i.v. glucose if indicated (see p. 148), taking a blood sample in fluoride first for later biochemical estimation.

*Hypothermia*

To prevent the baby becoming hypothermic, or to help him warm up if he is already hypothermic, wrap him in a silver swaddler (folded to leave part of the chest visible) and transfer him to the pre-warmed portable incubator as soon as the need for other treatment will allow.

*Acidosis*

Rapid pH determination may not be possible at the time of initial assessment and it may be necessary to guess whether the infant is likely to be acidotic on the basis of any previous results available, together with the history. If the infant has been severely anoxic, give intravenous alkali on an empirical basis. Sodium bicarbonate in a dose of 2-6mEq/kg should be given unless the baby has had a high sodium intake or is oedematous. In the latter situations, THAM may be used instead (see p. 130).

*Umbilical Catheterization*

If an umbilical venous catheter has been inserted this may be used for giving alkali or glucose as indicated. Otherwise give these drugs into a peripheral vein. If this is found to be impossible and the drugs are needed urgently, catheterize the umbilical vein with full sterile precautions (see p. 263). Unless umbilical drips are essential, take them down before the journey starts, but leave the catheter in place, filled with a heparinized saline solution (10 units/ml). If no umbilical catheter has been inserted, make sure that the cord is securely tied or clamped.

*Bacteriology*

We take swabs from the baby's nose, throat, umbilicus and rectum into transport medium *before* the journey. In addition, if an endotracheal tube has to be changed before starting, the end is cut off with sterile scissors into transport medium.

**Management During Journey**

In most cases smoothness is preferable to speed for the return journey, as any necessary procedures (*e.g.* manual ventilation) are difficult to perform in a jolting ambulance. If a procedure needs to be carried out urgently, ask the driver to stop. In urgent surgical cases speed may assume greater importance: if really in a hurry, arrange for a police escort.

Before the journey is started, the baby, wrapped in his silver swaddler, should be placed in the portable incubator and well padded, *e.g.* with disposable napkins, to reduce movement.

Observation during the journey is difficult, heart and breath sounds are usually inaudible, and respiratory movements are not readily distinguished from vibration. Use an electrocardiographically activated heart-rate meter when possible.

Oxygen should be given at a sufficient flow-rate to keep the infant pink. During long journeys (more than one hour) oxygen concentration must be monitored.

If ventilation is required, perform manual IPPV with 100% oxygen or use a battery-operated ventilator. (40% oxygen would be preferable, but unfortunately we have not yet been able to organize a supply for routine use in the ambulance.) A blow-off valve must always be in the circuit.

# Respiratory Distress

We label as having 'respiratory distress' all babies who have at least two of the following signs after the age of four hours:
(1) respiratory rate greater than 60;
(2) costal recession; and
(3) grunting.

We also label as having had respiratory distress any baby who dies or needs artificial ventilation before four hours and who has already had these symptoms. The purpose of the stipulation about four hours is to exclude babies with evanescent tachypnoea lasting only an hour or so after birth.

In babies who survive respiratory distress, a precise diagnosis cannot always be made with scrupulous honesty. Thus, hyaline membrane disease can only be diagnosed with certainty at post-mortem examination. For coding purposes, we label all babies with the above signs as cases of respiratory distress, adding in brackets the presumptive pathology in survivors and the actual pathology in fatal and autopsied cases, *e.g.* 'respiratory distress (probable hyaline membrane disease)' or 'respiratory distress (pneumothorax secondary to probable meconium aspiration)' in survivors, and 'respiratory distress (hyaline membrane disease)' in a fatal case.

The great majority of cases of respiratory distress are due to hyaline membrane disease (definite or presumed) and most of the remainder are due to meconium aspiration (with or without pneumothorax), intrapartum asphyxia or cardiac failure. However, the check list in Table VII may be of use in cases in which the circumstances or clinical findings are odd or unusual.

The investigation, handling and supportive treatment of a case of respiratory distress is much the same whatever the aetiology. Specific treatment largely boils down to antibiotics in cases of pneumonia, aspiration in tension pneumothorax, and surgery in cases of congenital malformations. The following section deals with the general management of respiratory distress, which, as stated above, usually means hyaline membrane disease.

## TABLE VII
### Types of respiratory distress

| Condition | Gestational age | | Onset | | | Predisposing or other suggestive circumstances and associated conditions |
|---|---|---|---|---|---|---|
| | Pre-term | Term | 1st day | 1st week | Later | |
| Hyaline membrane | +++ | (+) | +++ | | | Intrapartum asphyxia, maternal diabetes, caesarian section, antepartum haemorrhage. |
| Meconium aspiration | (+) | +++ | +++ | | | SFD, intrapartum asphyxia. |
| Pneumonia | +++ | ++ | | +++ | ++ | Long-ruptured membranes, intra-uterine infection, intrapartum asphyxia. Complication of other respiratory distress. |
| Pneumothorax | +++ | +++ | +++ | +++ | | Complication of HMD, meconium aspiration, hypoplastic lungs and staphylococcal pneumonia. |
| Late resp. distress, inc. Wilson Mikity | +++ | | | ++ | +++ | |
| Massive pulmonary haemorrhage | +++ | ++ | + | +++ | (+) | SFD, hypothermia, severe Rh incompatibility. |
| Pneumocystis carinii | +++ | + | | | +++ | Agammaglobulinaemia and other immune deficiency. |
| Pleural effusion, inc. chylous | + | +++ | +++ | (+) | + | Haemolytic disease, idiopathic hydrops. |
| Cystic fibrosis | + | +++ | | | +++ | Family history, meconium ileus, SFD |
| Upper airways obstruction (1) | ++ | +++ | +++ | | | SFD |
| Oesophageal atresia | ++ | +++ | +++ | | | Polyhydramnios |
| Diaphragmatic hernia | ++ | +++ | +++ | + | + | |
| Cong. lobar emphysema | + | +++ | ++ | +++ | ++ | |
| Mediastinal tumour (2) | + | +++ | +++ | ++ | + | |
| Pulmonary agenesis or hypoplasia | +++ | ++ | +++ | | | SFD, Potter face, oligohydramnios, anuria, thoracic malformations, hydrops. |

*(continued)*

See p. 118 for explanatory notes.

| Condition | Gestational age | | Onset | | | Predisposing or other suggestive circumstances and associated conditions |
|---|---|---|---|---|---|---|
| | Pre-term | Term | 1st day | 1st week | Later | |
| Cong. cysts of lung | + | +++ | + | + | +++ | |
| Cong. pulmonary lymphangiectasia | + | +++ | +++ | + | | Total anomalous pulmonary venous drainage. |
| C.N.S. depression | + | +++ | +++ | | | SFD, birth injury, intrapartum asphyxia. |
| Intercostal or diaphragmatic paralysis (3) | + | +++ | +++ | ++ | + | Erb's palsy. |
| Cardiac failure | + | +++ | + | ++ | +++ | See p. 213. |
| Metabolic disease (4) | + | +++ | ++ | +++ | | |

SFD = small for dates; HMD = hyaline membrane disease; cong. = congenital.

(1) includes choanal atresia, Pierre Robin syndrome, pharyngeal tumours, tracheal webs, vascular rings (see pp. 51, 53 and 145).
(2) includes accessory lobe of lung.
(3) includes myasthenia gravis, poliomyelitis, Werdnig-Hoffmann disease, congenital myopathies. Also consider eventration of the diaphragm.
(4) includes uraemia, diabetes mellitus, maple syrup urine disease, other organicacidaemias, diarrhoea with alkalosis.

We feel we owe to the reader some explanation of the meaning attached to these plus signs. In respect of gestational age, the plus signs indicate whether the condition is commoner in pre-term or term babies. Where there is one plus in the 'Pre-term column' and three in the 'Term' we mean to indicate that the condition is not really influenced by gestational age, and is only commoner in term babies because they outnumber pre-term babies. A (+) means that the condition is seldom seen at the gestational age indicated. Having given this explanation we will leave it to the reader to work out what the plus signs mean under the age of onset. *Please read across, and not down the columns,* as the plus signs are not meant to indicate the relative frequency of the pathological conditions in terms of gestational age and onset.

# Causes of Respiratory Distress

The following are brief notes on some of the causes of respiratory distress. We recommend Professor Avery's book*.

**Hyaline Membrane Disease** (HMD)

The condition is essentially one of lung collapse due to lack of pulmonary surfactant. Collapse of air-spaces is associated with loss of terminal bronchiolar epithelium, exudation of plasma into the terminal airways and plastering of blood constituents around the dilated respiratory bronchioles and alveolar ducts to form the hyaline membranes. Pulmonary blood-flow is reduced, and right-to-left shunts may lead to severe hypoxaemia.

The low reserves of surfactant in the lung of the pre-term baby render him liable to this condition. There is some evidence that surfactant synthesis may be impaired or its destruction enhanced by birth asphyxia, although the sequence of events is not fully understood. The second of a pair of twins, babies born by caesarean section or after ante-partum haemorrhage, and the babies of poorly controlled diabetics, all seem to be at particular risk of developing hyaline membrane disease.

Most affected babies have signs of respiratory distress from birth, but in some these signs do not develop for several hours. In most babies, including those who recover, there is deterioration during the first 24 to 36 hours. Radiologically, a fine granular pattern with air bronchograms (extending beyond the cardiac shadow) is generally thought to be characteristic of this condition, but in practice the x-ray may vary from the normal to the completely opaque.

**Meconium Aspiration**

This condition is seen predominantly in term babies. The gasps of an asphyxiated baby *in utero* can cause inhalation of a mixture of meconium, mucus, and epithelial squames into the small bronchi and bronchioles where it cannot be cleared by suction at birth. When the baby makes violent respiratory efforts after birth, the impacted material sometimes has a ball-valve effect in the bronchi, resulting in interstitial emphysema, pneumomediastinum and pneumothorax. A similar result may follow positive pressure ventilation. If infected liquor has been inhaled, pneumonia may supervene within 48 hours of birth.

The clinical picture is of an asphyxiated baby who has respiratory distress from the time of birth.

**Pneumonia**

This may develop in an initially healthy baby or as a complication of HMD or meconium aspiration. Infections developing soon after birth may have been acquired

---

*Avery, M. E. (1968) *The Lung and its Disorders in the Newborn Infant* (2nd Edn.). Philadelphia and London: W. B. Saunders.

from infected liquor (prolonged rupture of membranes) or from organisms in the birth canal (see 'Infection', p. 162).

The possibility of pneumonia should be considered in any baby with signs of generalised infection, even without respiratory symptoms, and in any baby with respiratory distress or meconium aspiration who unexpectedly deteriorates. *Pseudomonas aeruginosa* pneumonia is a constant hazard to babies on ventilator therapy for respiratory failure of any cause. In infants who die in the first few hours of life, the pathologist may have difficulty in deciding at necropsy whether masses of polymorphs seen within the airways are due to reaction by the fetus to pre-natal infection or are merely maternal polymorphs inhaled from the liquor.

## Massive Pulmonary Haemorrhage

This is an ill-understood condition for which there is probably more than one underlying cause. It may form part of a generalised bleeding diathesis in *secondary* haemorrhagic disease of the newborn due to consumption of platelets and labile coagulation factors by disseminated intravascular coagulation. This condition usually develops within 24 hours of birth. In some cases the haemorrhage may be more in the nature of a haemorrhagic oedema, possibly due to left heart failure. Hb estimation on the blood welling up the trachea may help to distinguish the two conditions.

The clinical picture is of an infant with rapidly deteriorating respiratory distress, who may have localised or generalised crepitations. Occasionally the first sign of the illness is a generalised fit. Blood welling up the trachea a few hours after onset makes the diagnosis obvious. The condition may develop suddenly at up to 2 to 3 days of age, especially in small-for-dates, hypoglycaemic or hypothermic babies, or those with kernicterus. The chest x-ray shows granular opacities which are not readily distinguished from hyaline membrane disease.

The condition is almost invariably fatal.

## Transient Tachypnoea

The condition as described by Dr. Avery is one of tachypnoea in term babies without evidence of any known cause of respiratory distress. Chest x-ray shows prominent perihilar streaking. The tachypnoea and radiological picture return to normal over 2 to 3 days. The suggested mechanism is a delay in the resorption of fetal lung liquid. We believe that this represents the mild end of the spectrum of respiratory distress in term babies: babies at the severe end of the spectrum may present a picture resembling cyanotic heart disease (Roberton *et al.* 1967)*. The difference between these conditions and hyaline membrane disease in pre-term babies may be due simply to the greater maturity of the lungs.

Many pre-term infants, too, develop transient signs of respiratory distress lasting only a few hours.

## Heart Failure

Respiratory distress due to heart failure usually presents as tachypnoea and

*Roberton, N. R. C., Hallidie-Smith, K. A., Davis, J. A. (1967) 'Severe respiratory distress syndrome mimicking cyanotic heart disease in term babies.' *Lancet*, ii, 1108.

tachycardia with or without cyanosis. Other findings, such as rales over the lung fields, gallop rhythm, murmurs, a firm enlarged liver, and abnormal cardiac outline on chest x-ray should help to differentiate these babies from cases of hyaline membrane disease (see p. 213).

## Upper Airway Obstruction

This may result from abnormalities of the larynx, such as congenital stenosis or web-formation; tumours in the pharynx, including teratomas, dermoids, sub-glottic haemangiomas and cysts of the larynx; or external compression by vascular rings or by tumours of the neck, such as goitres, lymphangiomas and branchial cysts. If the obstruction is severe, respiration may never be established. Symptoms include stridor in addition to cyanosis and retractions.

In the case of pharyngeal tumours, the respiratory distress may be intermittent, and may be relieved by changing the baby's position. The tumour may not always be visible on inspecting the pharynx. Tracheostomy may be necessary.

See also Pierre Robin syndrome (p. 51) and choanal atresia (p. 53).

## Pulmonary Agenesis or Hypoplasia

Bilateral pulmonary agenesis is incompatible with extra-uterine life and affected infants die within a few minutes of birth. The condition is often associated with renal agenesis, which in turn is associated with absence of cartilage in the pinnae, and the 'Potter face'*. The length of postnatal survival of babies with pulmonary hypoplasia is dependent on the severity of the condition. Pulmonary hypoplasia is also the cause of death soon after delivery of many hydropic or malformed infants. The condition should be suspected in any such baby in whom the lungs cannot be readily inflated on intubation. If the lungs are less severely hypoplastic, the infant may survive with signs of respiratory distress which are not readily distinguished from hyaline membrane disease in life. For pulmonary hypoplasia in association with diaphragmatic hernia, see p. 50. See also 'Birth asphyxia', p. 32.

## Congenital Pulmonary Lymphangiectasis

This condition consists in gross cystic dilatation of the lymphatic channels in the lung septa and is usually associated with congenital heart malformations, particularly total anomalous pulmonary venous drainage. Affected infants develop respiratory distress with cyanosis from birth or soon after.

## Lung Cysts and Cystic Adenomatoid Malformations

Cystic malformations of the lung vary from simple cysts to complex cystic and solid adenomatoid malformations and may involve part of a lobe or replace the whole of one or both lungs. Symptoms and radiological appearance vary with size, site and degree of cyst formation. Cysts arising from bronchi can partially obstruct the bronchus and present as lobar emphysema. The infant may develop acute respiratory

---

*Dr. Edith Potter first drew attention to the peculiar squashed faces of these babies. The nose is flattened, the jaw recedes, the eyes have an 'anti-mongolian' slant, there are marked epicanthic folds, skin creases are exaggerated and the ears are low-set.

distress with tachypnoea and cyanosis, often associated with displacement of the trachea. Chest x-ray shows a cystic or solid mass. Treatment is surgical, and may be urgent.

**Cystic Fibrosis**

Infants with cystic fibrosis occasionally present with staphylococcal pneumonia in the neonatal period.

**Congenital Lobar Emphysema**

This condition results from a valvular bronchial obstruction to an upper or right middle lobe, which becomes distended and leads to mediastinal shift and collapse of other lobes. It may present in the early neonatal period with signs of respiratory distress, but the onset of symptoms can be somewhat later in infancy. (It is usually due to defective bronchial cartilage (bronchomalacia), but there are a number of other possible causes, including intraluminar obstruction.) Diagnosis of lobar emphysema is made on x-ray, which often shows herniation of the emphysematous lobe across the mediastinum. Inform the thoracic surgeon as soon as you make the diagnosis.

# Management of Early Respiratory Distress (usually Hyaline Membrane Disease)

**Immediate Action**

Although for coding purposes we do not normally diagnose 'respiratory distress' until after the age of four hours, we naturally do not postpone treatment of the symptoms of respiratory distress until that age if the baby is ill enough to need it earlier.

(1) Ensure that the airways are clear, that the baby is in a suitably warm environment (see p. 102 *et seq.*) and for the time being give oxygen in just sufficient concentration to keep him pink. (You will find that you rarely have to give very high concentrations in the early stages unless the situation is almost hopeless.)

(2) Consider the differential diagnosis (see above).

(3) Insert umbilical venous and arterial catheters (p. 264) and arrange a chest x-ray (PA and lateral). However, if the child is less than four hours old and the symptoms are comparatively mild, wait until the age of, say, four hours before deciding on the insertion of catheters—the respiratory distress may subside in the meantime. In any case, if the child is cold or has just been subjected to handling or transportation, we sometimes defer catheterisation for about an hour while the baby's body-temperature improves and he settles down.

**The Chest X-ray** (order a PA and lateral)

The chest x-ray is intended to exclude other causes of respiratory distress and to support the diagnosis. We are unimpressed with its use for prognosis. We feel uncomfortable if we have not taken an x-ray, but must admit that it is seldom valuable in the management of a straightforward case. We usually take the film after the catheters are inserted so that their position can be seen.

**Management**

*General*

There is no curative treatment for hyaline membrane disease but, provided the baby can be kept alive for two or three days, spontaneous recovery will take place. The most important factor in keeping the baby alive is skilled nursing with attention to warmth, feeding, asepsis and accurate observation. In addition, we are likely to give oxygen therapy, correct acidaemia, use continuous positive airway pressure (CPAP, see p. 125) and, in severe cases, we may use mechanical ventilation.

*Observations*

These should be written on the flow-sheet, which gives a good picture of progress.

(1) *On admission:* chest x-ray; Hb and PCV; nitrogen washout (see p. 131); and

123

bacteriological swabs from nose, throat, umbilicus and rectum.

(2) *Arterial samples* for $pO_2$, pH, $pCO_2$ at least every four hours until the arterial catheter is removed (see p. 265). During unstable periods, more frequent sampling will be needed (see also p. 108).

We stop measuring arterial blood gases 4-hourly when the baby is clearly recovering and the $paO_2$ is above 60mmHg in 30% oxygen. Further analyses should be carried out twice-daily while the baby is having oxygen therapy (see p. 109 and p. 130).

Although the amount of blood taken at each sampling is small, frequent estimations may lead to an excessive blood-loss. For every baby in our special care nursery, a record of each sample taken (the amount and time and the total taken to date) is kept. This is particularly important in small babies with respiratory distress. When the total taken approaches 10ml/kg, we usually replace this amount with a small blood transfusion.

(3) *Clinical observations* (see p. 131 for definitions and details).

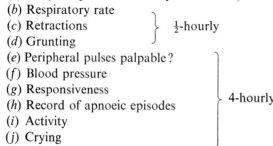

    (*a*) Body temperature—hourly until stable, then 4-hourly

    (*b*) Respiratory rate

    (*c*) Retractions           ½-hourly

    (*d*) Grunting

    (*e*) Peripheral pulses palpable?

    (*f*) Blood pressure

    (*g*) Responsiveness

    (*h*) Record of apnoeic episodes    4-hourly

    (*i*) Activity

    (*j*) Crying

*Warmth*

The baby should be in an incubator, with a perspex 'heat shield' in place, at an ambient temperature within the neutral range as assessed from the chart shown in Fig. 7 (p. 104). Subsequent adjustment may be necessary if body-temperature rises or falls. Preferably, temperature should be monitored from abdominal skin and this temperature should be maintained at 36.5°C (97.7°F). Alternatively, rectal temperature should be maintained at 37°C (98.6°F). As soon as the child is sufficiently recovered that the chest need not be seen, he should be clothed within the incubator.

*Feeding*

We aim to feed a baby with respiratory distress exactly as we would a baby of similar gestational age and birthweight without respiratory distress (see p. 96 *et seq.*). We nearly always feed by nasogastric tube, giving expressed breast-milk and starting as soon as the baby is admitted to the special care nursery. It is essential that the baby be positioned on his side or in the prone position. Indications for intravenous feeding, and the solutions and amounts, are given on p. 99.

*Oxygen* (See also 'Oxygen therapy' p. 107).

Our standard regimen is to adjust the oxygen percentage of the inspired air and, if necessary, to use CPAP so that umbilical arterial $pO_2$ is between 60 and 90mmHg.

The initial means of achieving this derives from the nitrogen washout (p. 131) which is performed routinely on all babies with respiratory distress syndrome (RDS), partly for prognostic purposes and partly as an initial measurement from which to plan oxygen therapy. The steps to be taken are shown in the flow-sheet on p. 126. The general principles are that if the baby needs more than 60% oxygen to maintain a normal $pO_2$, we also use CPAP; if the $pO_2$ is normal in less than 60% oxygen, we merely adjust inspired oxygen concentrations.

In all cases, frequent re-measurement may be necessary until a fairly stable normal $pO_2$ is achieved. Thereafter re-measure $pO_2$ every four hours and also after any alteration of oxygen flow to the incubator, change in CPAP or administration of alkali. In addition, re-measure $paO_2$ if there is any striking or obvious deterioration or improvement in the baby's condition. If an arterial catheter cannot be inserted, or blocks, arterial blood may be obtained from the radial, brachial or temporal artery (see p. 268).

Although our general rule is to keep umbilical arterial $pO_2$ between 60 and 90mm Hg, there are occasions when we do not observe the rule faithfully. When $paO_2$ is between 40 and 60 and can only be raised to the desired 60 by using very high concentrations of oxygen (80-100%) we elect to settle for the level of 40-60mmHg, provided (a) the child's clinical condition as shown by activity, blood pressure, etc., remains good, (b) there is no further fall in arterial pH. (Serial blood lactate levels are a useful guide to tissue oxygenation, but the measurement is too cumbersome for routine use.)

Unless there is clear evidence that the baby is suffering ill-effects from hypoxaemia, we believe that it is better to accept the hypoxaemia rather than to expose the lungs to a high concentration of inspired oxygen. Although we prefer to keep $paO_2$ between 60 and 90mmHg, we know that some pre-term babies may survive prolonged hypoxaemia (many hours with a $paO_2$ of about 40mmHg) without apparent brain damage.

As the baby recovers and $paO_2$ rises, ambient oxygen concentration must be cut down *pari passu*. Our aim is to stop oxygen therapy as soon as possible. There is no point in 'tailing off' oxygen slowly, *and low birthweight or gestational age are not in themselves indications for oxygen therapy.*

### Continuous Positive Airway Pressure (CPAP)

We think that CPAP is a rational treatment for babies with RDS and are impressed that it has been effective in the cases on whom we have used it, and by the results reported by Gregory et al. (1971).* We would emphasise that it is a treatment designed for babies with alveolar collapse and impaired compliance, and thus for babies with presumed HMD, rather than as a panacea for all forms of neonatal respiratory distress. The principle is that the continuous pressure will prevent collapse of some alveoli and terminal bronchioles, allowing gaseous exchange and thus improved oxygenation.

INDICATIONS

(1) For babies in whom inspired $O_2$ concentrations of more than 60% are necessary

*Gregory, G. A., Kitterman, J. A., Phibbs, R. H., Tooley, W. H., Hamilton, W. K. (1971) 'Treatment of IRDS with continuous positive airway pressure.' *New England Journal of Medicine*, **284**, 1333.

# OXYGEN THERAPY IN RESPIRATORY DISTRESS

NITROGEN WASHOUT (breathing 100% $O_2$ for 15 minutes)

$paO_2 < 100\,mmHg$

100 - 150 → Decrease $O_2$ ambient to 60% → Re-measure $paO_2$

150 - 300 → Decrease $O_2$ ambient to 40% → Re-measure

> 300 → Decrease $O_2$ ambient to air → Re-measure

Maintain $paO_2$ at between 60 and 90 by adjustment of inspired $O_2$ using 10 - 15% steps. After each step re-measure.

If it becomes necessary to increase ambient $O_2$ above 60%,

CPAP with 60% $O_2$. Increase pressure in steps to maximum of 15 cm (see text)

Re-measure $paO_2$

< 60 → Increase ambient in 20% steps to maximum of 95%. Re-measure

60 - 90 → Re-measure in 4 hours

> 90 → Decrease ambient to 40%. Re-measure

Maintain $paO_2$ at between 60 - 90 by adjustment of inspired $O_2$ using 10 - 15% steps. If and when inspired oxygen is <30%, reduce CPAP in 3 cm $H_2O$ steps. It is clear that some babies will need artificial ventilation *

*See 'Indications for ventilator treatment,' p.133.

126

to achieve paO$_2$ of greater than 60 (despite other supportive measures such as acid base correction).

(2) For babies with presumed HMD whose clinical condition is very poor and whose respirations are grossly irregular, with frequent apnoeic spells. In such babies, it should be tried before recourse to the ventilator.

TECHNIQUES OF APPLYING CPAP

We have two methods of applying CPAP, the first of which involves endotracheal intubation. This disadvantage is to some extent outweighed by the easier access to the upper airways and mouth, and by a rather simpler mechanical system. We prefer to use it for babies in the second category of 'Indications' above. The second system involves putting the whole of the baby's head into a box which can be pressurised, and is more suitable for a baby who is making good and sustained respiratory effort but not achieving good oxygenation (see Indication (1), p. 125).

CPAP WITH ENDOTRACHEAL INTUBATION (Fig. 8, p. 128)

Insert a nasotracheal tube and secure it using the 'harness' as described for ventilator (p. 134). Set the blow-off pressure (A) on the distal end of the system to 6cmH$_2$O and apply the suction pads which hold this valve and the emergency blow-off valve (B) to the wall of the incubator. Place the buffer reservoir (C) with its mano-meter (E) and whistling blow-off valve (D) on the top of the incubator where you can see the manometer needle easily. Connect the endotracheal tube to the U loop. Turn on oxygen slowly until a pressure of 6cm is generated and held; you will need a flow of 5 to 10 litres per minute. When you are satisfied that the pressure is stable, change over to 60% oxygen (unless the baby is still cyanosed) and set up the humidification infusion (see p. 134).

After waiting 15 minutes, during which you should again check that breath sounds are present and equal on both sides of the chest, measure blood-gas levels. If the desired pO$_2$ has not been achieved, increase the pressure (adjust valve A) by 3cm steps to a maximum of 15cmH$_2$O. You may have to increase the flow rate. If the desired pO$_2$ has still not been achieved, increase inspired oxygen by 20% steps (see oxygen therapy flow-sheet, p. 126).

If it becomes necessary to give artificial ventilation, apply your finger inter-mittently to the outlet of valve B until an assistant has fixed the two ends of the U loop to the ventilator (see Fig. 8 and p. 133).

CPAP USING THE HEAD BOX (Fig. 9, p. 128)

Open the neck-cuff to its maximum and pad the base of the box and the mattress with disposable napkins. Insert the baby's head through the opening and close the cuff carefully (keep a finger between neck and cuff to assess the pressure). The cuff should just be touching the circumference of the neck so that, as pressure is generated, it is pressed caudally and seals against the shoulders. A piece of sorbo rubber around the baby's neck improves the seal and prevents skin injury. Remember that some leak is inevitable. Adjust the blow-off pressure valve to 6cmH$_2$O as above. Apply the pressure-tight cover. Turn on the oxygen flow, watching the manometer needle. Since some

127

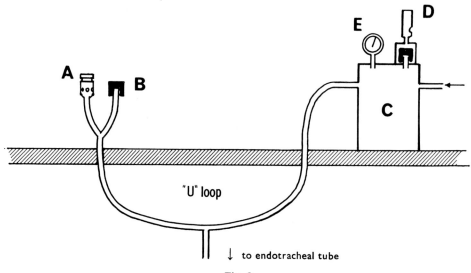

A
B
C
D
E

"U" loop

↓ to endotracheal tube

Fig. 8

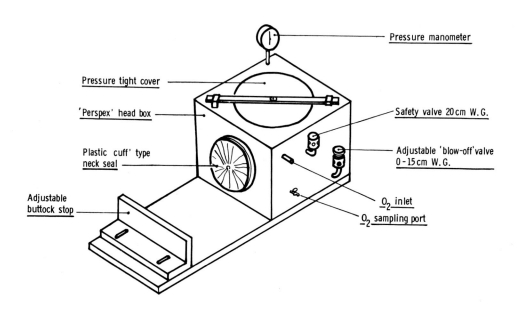

Pressure manometer

Pressure tight cover

'Perspex' head box

Safety valve 20 cm W.G.

Adjustable 'blow-off' valve
0 - 15 cm W.G.

Plastic cuff' type
neck seal

Adjustable
buttock stop

$O_2$ inlet

$O_2$ sampling port

C.P.A.P. HEADBOX

Fig. 9

leak is inevitable, flow rates have to be high (10 litres/min) to achieve a stable pressure of 6cm. If flow rates of 20 litres are needed, the leak at the neck-cuff is excessive and must be readjusted.

Inspect the child's chest movements and upper airways to make certain there is no airways obstruction.

When the pressure is stable, adjust the ambient $O_2$ to 60% and then re-adjust the pressure if necessary (see above, and oxygen therapy flow sheet, p. 126).

WEANING OFF CPAP

As the child improves it becomes possible to reduce ambient oxygen and CPAP. We prefer to reduce ambient oxygen to less than 30% as the first step and *then* to reduce CPAP by 3cm steps. However, it must be remembered that as surfactant activity returns (usually days 3 to 5), the CPAP is increasingly likely to affect venous return to the thorax. Thus, if the baby is more than three days old, and if the lungs seem not very stiff, we try to reduce the CPA pressure to $6cmH_2O$ or less, fairly rapidly.

When endotracheal intubation has been used, we follow the recommendation of Gregory *et al.* (1971)[*] that the CPAP should have been at zero, and the child's condition good for at least four hours before extubation. The reason for this is that when the cords have been intubated for any length of time, the baby may not be able to grunt, and it must be demonstrated that he can manage without grunting—which probably means the same as managing without CPAP.

*Acid Base Correction*

Try to correct pH to between 7.3 and 7.4 immediately after admission, using 8.4% sodium bicarbonate. The dose is injected into the umbilical venous catheter, taking 5 to 10 minutes over the injection, or into the arterial catheter or a peripheral vein if the umbilical venous catheter has been removed. The dead space of the catheter is then filled with heparinized saline. The dose of bicarbonate is adjusted to the arterial blood pH as follows:

| pH | give | mEq/kg |
|---|---|---|
| < - 7.0 | | 6.5 |
| 7.0 - 7.09 | | 5.0 |
| 7.1 - 7.19 | | 3.5 |
| 7.2 - 7.24 | | 2.0 |
| 7.25 - 7.3 | | 1.0 |

1ml 8.4% $HCO_3$ = approx. 1 mEq.

This dosage scheme is theoretically unsound (pH is a logarithmic scale) but it works fairly well in practice. It is designed to *undercorrect*. The pH should be measured 15 minutes later and a further injection given if necessary.

After the initial correction, further bicarbonate is given if pH falls below 7.25. We stop measuring pH when we stop measuring blood gases.

*See p. 125 for reference.*

129

Theoretically, THAM (trishydroxymethyl amino-methane) should be better than bicarbonate for correction of acidaemia, but we have abandoned its routine use because it may be associated with apnoeic episodes during or shortly after administration. We therefore only use THAM (a) when the total sodium administered exceeds 15mEq/kg in the first 48 hours, or (b) when the baby is already on a ventilator. As a practical guide, use 2ml 3.6% THAM as equivalent to 1ml 8.4% bicarbonate (this is *not* a precise equivalent, again erring on the side of under-correction).

*Antibiotics*

These are not given routinely but only when there is clinical and/or bacteriological evidence of infection or clinical grounds for suspicion—usually one or more of the following (see also 'Infection', p. 162):
(1) unexpected deterioration, including recurrent apnoea;
(2) localizing signs in the chest, either clinical or x-ray;
(3) purulent aspirate from the endotracheal tube;
(4) a history of prolonged rupture of membranes;
(5) spleen or kidneys not previously palpable which become enlarged.

*Ventilator*

Consider the use of the ventilator if:
(1) the baby is having serious apnoeic attacks;
(2) the $paO_2$ cannot be raised above 30mmHg;
(3) the $paCO_2$ is above 90mmHg.

For further details of indications for and management of ventilator therapy, see p. 133.

*Catheters* (see also p. 264)

We aim to remove the umbilical venous catheter after 24 hours. The umbilical arterial catheter is taken out after 48 hours if the disease process is assessed as being stable or improving *and* the $pO_2$ is more than 60mmHg in 30% oxygen. When the baby is very ill or on a ventilator, the need for the arterial line for monitoring outweighs the small dangers of infection and thrombosis, and the catheter has been left in for up to 18 days.

*Blood Sugars*

Do a 'Dextrostix' test on each four-hourly arterial sample taken. If low, see 'Hypoglycaemia', p. 147. We stop measuring blood sugar routinely when the baby no longer needs blood-gas analysis.

*Haematocrit*

Do micro PCV or Hb daily. Consider transfusion if below 40% or 13g/100ml respectively, especially in babies on IPPV or CPAP.

*Sudden Deterioration*

If a baby with respiratory distress suddenly or unexpectedly deteriorates, consider the following possible causes, listed in order of probability:

(1) intraventricular haemorrhage;

(2) pneumothorax (see p. 140);

(3) infection, especially pneumonia (see p. 119 and p. 162);

(4) pulmonary haemorrhage;

(5) hypoglycaemia.

See also 'Unexpected collapse', p. 218 and 'Problems and action to solve them', p. 135.

*Eyes*

All babies treated with oxygen have their eyes examined by our ophthalmologist (see p. 242).

APPENDIX I (Clinical Observations)

BODY TEMPERATURE (see pp. 102 to 106).

RESPIRATORY RATE. Record the rate counted over a half-minute *or* that displayed on the monitor.

COSTAL RETRACTIONS. Record as 0 = no retraction, + = intermediate, + + = gross retraction.

GRUNTING. Record 0 = no grunting, + + = audible without a stethoscope at the mouth and present on at least 50 per cent of breaths when not crying, and + = anything in between.

PERIPHERAL PULSES PALPABLE? Record as 'Yes' if you can feel the radial or dorsalis pedis pulse, or 'No'.

BLOOD PRESSURE. Take four-hourly by any of the means on p. 217 (record which method was used).

ACTIVITY. Record the activity reported in the last four hours: 0 = no spontaneous movement (other than respiration), + = intermediate movement, + + = normal movement.

RESPONSIVENESS. Does the child move or in any way respond to taking blood pressure or other handling (not pricking)? 0 = no response, + = diminished response, + + = normal response.

RECORD OF APNOEIC SPELLS. Every four hours, record the number of times the baby has been apnoeic in the last four hours. For this particular purpose, apnoea means an absence of breathing for 30 seconds.

CRYING. Has the child raised an audible cry in the last four hours? Record 'Yes' or 'No'.

APPENDIX II (Nitrogen Washout)

Place the child's head in the perspex head-box, allowing him to breath 100% oxygen, thus washing out nitrogen from his lungs. After 15 minutes, take an arterial sample for $pO_2$, pH and $pCO_2$. The result of the nitrogen washout is useful for (a) prognosis and (b) initial management of oxygen therapy.

*Prognosis.* In general, the baby who achieves a high $paO_2$ has a good prognosis. The generally quoted figures, which applied before CPAP was introduced, are that a baby aged 4 to 18 hours who achieves a $pO_2$ of more than 100mmHg during a nitrogen washout test has about an 80 per cent chance of surviving, and that those who achieve a $pO_2$ of less than 100mmHg have an 80 per cent chance of dying. There is no sudden cut-off point at 100mmHg and these generalisations are of limited value in an individual case. However, in a group of cases, the test is valuable in assessing the effect of a given line of treatment.

The initial pH and the highest lactate recorded (after the age of about four hours) also give a general indication of outcome: pH greater than 7.25 is good, as is lactate lower than 35mg/100ml.

*Initial Management of Oxygen Therapy.* From the $paO_2$ achieved in 100% oxygen, one can make an intelligent guess (see flow chart, p. 126) what ambient oxygen will be correct to achieve a $paO_2$ of 60-90mmHg. It will still be important to confirm by a measurement that one's 'intelligent guess' is working out in practice.

# Ventilator Treatment

Assisted ventilation is a rational means of treating certain babies with respiratory failure. Although we, like others undertaking ventilator treatment of babies, have cases where we are sure the baby would have died without assisted ventilation, there is little controlled evidence on its efficacy. Ventilation in babies has undoubted dangers, is expensive in equipment and personnel and is better not undertaken unless adequate facilities (skilled nurses and residents, blood-gas analysis, monitoring devices, x-rays, etc.) are always immediately available.

## Indications for Ventilator Treatment

Our indications are:

(1) *Apnoea:* (*a*) total absence of respiration failing to respond after 10 minutes of manual IPPV; (*b*) slow, gasping, obviously inadequate respiration which does not become regular after manual IPPV or CPAP.

(2) *Arterial* $pO_2$ *less than* 30mmHg, despite oxygen therapy (p. 107) and CPAP (p. 125). Either *two* readings half an hour apart, or a *single* reading of less than 30 if associated with a heart-rate falling below 100 per minute.

(3) *Arterial* $pCO_2$ *greater than* 90mmHg, associated with a pH that cannot be corrected to above 7.2 with alkali.

These are all circumstances in which we think the baby is very unlikely to survive without ventilator treatment. In general terms, the most rewarding results of ventilator treatment are found in relatively large babies ( > 2000g) who need assisted ventilation only after the age of 24 hours. We do not use the ventilator on babies in whom there is unequivocal evidence of severe brain damage. (See p. 185.) However, in very few babies at this age *is* such evidence unequivocal. Babies of less than 1000g and less than 28 weeks gestational age have a near-hopeless prognosis if they need assisted ventilation. One should not undertake ventilation of such a baby if the work load in the intensive care nursery is very heavy and if the care of other very ill babies with a more hopeful prognosis might be jeopardised.

## The Hammersmith Hospital Ventilator

This is a pressure-limited ventilator (see p. 293), in principle similar to such ventilators as the Bennett, the Sheffield and the Loosco. It has the very considerable advantages of cheapness, small size (it stands on the roof of the incubator and the tubing is a simple 'U' tube of 1cm polyvinyl tubing) and of simplicity (anyone trained in resuscitation of babies understands the principle of an 'automatic thumb'). We have no experience of negative pressure tank ventilators nor of volume-controlled ventilators.

The apparatus (p. 294) is essentially a 'U' loop of tubing into one end of which flows an oxygen-nitrogen mixture. At the other end a solenoid-activated valve provides intermittent occlusion (like a thumb during manual IPPV). This valve is activated by an electronic circuit bearing controls for rate and duration of occlusion.

With the valve in the closed position, the gas can only escape at the apex of the loop, thereby inflating the infant's lungs via an endotracheal tube. With the valve in the open position, expiration occurs passively. Inflation pressure is regulated by a spring-loaded blow-off safety valve adjustable within the range 10-70cmH$_2$O, the actual pressure being shown by a manometer mounted next to the blow-off valve. The blow-off valve and manometer are mounted on the box on the afferent limb of the 'U' loop. Humidification is maintained by a constant infusion pump which delivers water directly into the endotracheal tube.

### Variable Controls on the Ventilator
    (1) The gas mixture can be varied:
        (*a*) 100% oxygen;
        (*b*) compressed air (21% oxygen);
        (*c*) mixtures of above can be attained by a 'Y' connection having a flow
            meter on each supply.
    (2) Flow of gas mixture: usually 3 to 10 litres/min.
    (3) Period of occlusion of solenoid valve, within each respiratory cycle, *i.e.*
        inspiratory portion of cycle: 20-80%.
    (4) Pressure-limiting valves: 10-70cmH$_2$0.
    (5) Rate of constant infusion of humidifying water: usually kept at 1ml/hour.

### Intubation
    In an emergency, intubate and resuscitate as for birth asphyxia (p. 37).

When resuscitation has been achieved, insert a 3mm nasotracheal tube for connecting the baby to the respirator (see appendix—'Nasotracheal intubation', p. 139). If a 3mm tube is too large to pass the nostrils, do *not* use a 2.5mm tube; it is too narrow for efficient air movement. Use instead a size 12 or 14 orotracheal tube.

Secure a nasotracheal tube by adhesive tape at the nostril; cut off the excess tubing to 0.5cm and attach to the special nasotracheal adaptor (Fig. 17*a* and *b*, p. 291), which we call 'the harness'.

Check the breath sounds on both sides of the chest. If the endotracheal (ET) tube is too far down the trachea it usually passes to the right main bronchus and breath sounds are heard only on that side. The tube must be partially withdrawn.

### Initial Settings for the Ventilator Controls
    Set the controls to the following values, which are those which will adequately ventilate most babies; adjustments to other values may be necessary as indicated by chemical or blood-gas findings.

    *Rate.* 30-40 a minute (choose the higher rate if the baby is thought to have HMD
        and thus stiff lungs).
    *Inspiratory phase of respiratory cycle.* 30%.
    *Pressure limit.* 20-30cmH$_2$O (choose the higher pressure if the baby is thought to
        have HMD).

*Flow.* About 5 litres per minute. If the baby is thought to have HMD, increase the flow rate until the resistance of outflow achieves an end expiratory pressure of 5-10cmH$_2$O. It may be that with this flow the manometer reads higher than the selected blow-off pressure. Readjust the blow-off pressure limit so that the reading of the manometer does not exceed the desired limit.

*Gas mixture.* Set up with 100% oxygen because it is readily available, but reduce as soon as possible—being guided by pO$_2$ (see 'Oxygen therapy', p. 107).

*Humidity.* Infuse sterile water 1ml/hour.

*Artificial sighs.* Twice an hour, clamp the efferent loop of the U tube for 3 seconds.

*Subsequent Settings*

Adjustments from the initial settings are arranged to keep the baby's blood-gases and pH as near to normal as possible: *i.e.* pO$_2$ 75, pCO$_2$ 40, pH 7.3 -7. 4. Blood-gases are measured four-hourly and after adjustments have been made on the respirator controls.

We use the following guides for an initial assessment of the effects, to avoid too-frequent blood sampling:

*Clinical.* Is the chest moving? Is the colour good? Are breath sounds equal on the two sides?

*Monitoring.* Use the tracing of the impedance pneumograph (*e.g.* the Air Shields apnoea monitor) to get a crude assessment of tidal volume and minute volume and whether adjustments have increased or decreased these measurements.

But always have a final check by blood gases about 15 minutes after adjusting the respirator settings.

AT ALL TIMES, WHEN THE BABY IS ON A RESPIRATOR HIS CHEST SHOULD MOVE, THE MANOMETER NEEDLE SHOULD MOVE, AND THE RESPIRATOR SHOULD CLICK, WITH EACH BREATH.

## Problems and Action to Solve Them

*Blood Gas Problems*

pCO$_2$ too high. Increase flow-rate and/or increase blow-off pressure and/or adjust rate—a rate that is too slow or too fast leads to a poor minute volume. On rare occasions it will be necessary to reduce dead space by removing the T tube and harness and by attaching the limb of the U loop directly to the nasotracheal tube.

pCO$_2$ too low. Opposite of above. On rare occasions it will be necessary to increase dead space by adding more length to the T tube connecting the U loop to the harness.

pO$_2$ too high. Reduce the percentage of oxygen in inspired gas.

pO$_2$ too low. (1) Check that adequate ventilation is occurring, *i.e.* that the chest is moving and pCO$_2$ is normal.
(2) Increase the end expiratory pressure to 10-15cmH$_2$O by continuously increasing the flow.
(3) Increase the O$_2$ percentage in the inspired gas (to a maximum of 90%).

135

*Clinical and Mechanical Problems*

| | |
|---|---|
| Chest does not move. | (1) Auscultate both sides of chest for breath sounds. Is there any ventilation at all? |
| | (2) Is the ET tube blocked? It is sometimes difficult to tell; if in doubt, change it. |
| | (3) Is there any pressure being generated? (Manometer needle does not move.) |
| | (4) If any delay, ventilate by hand or mouth until the problem is sorted out. |
| One side of chest does not move. | (1) Is the ET tube in a bronchus? |
| | (2) Is there a pneumothorax? |
| | (3) Have secretions blocked the bronchus? |
| Baby's colour deteriorates. | (1) Is the chest moving? |
| | (2) Is there any pressure being generated; *i.e.* is the manometer needle moving? Check as below. |
| | (3) Is the ET tube blocked? Chest not moving, see above. |
| | (4) Is there a new pulmonary problem? Auscultate the chest. ?Pneumothorax or lobar collapse. |
| Manometer needle does not move. | No pressure is being generated. |
| | (1) Is there a leak? Check all connections. |
| | (2) Is the gas flow satisfactory? Check source. |
| | (3) Is the ET tube displaced? |

*The Infant Breathing Out of Phase with the Ventilator*

(1) The ventilator should be switched off, the ET tube disconnected from the ventilator, and the infant allowed to breathe spontaneously in the same $O_2$ concentration as when on the ventilator.

(2) If the baby fails to maintain adequate ventilation reconnect to the ventilator without delay. If he continues to breathe out of phase, the flow may be increased by increments to a maximum of 10L/min. When the flow in increased, however, the blow-off valve may require adjustment to prevent the manometer pressure rising beyond a maximum of 40cmH$_2$O.

(3) Sometimes altering the rate to that of spontaneous respirations solves the problem.

(4) If the baby breathes out of phase or is otherwise unduly restless, sedation with diazepam (1mg not more often than 12-hourly) should be considered if the baby is not jaundiced. We do *not* use muscle relaxants or morphine.

**Assessment of Progress**

(1) Blood gases should be measured four-hourly, and more often when adjustments are made to respirator controls.

(2) Chest x-rays. We try to keep these to a minimum, therefore chest x-rays are only taken when clinically indicated. (*N.B.* The resident should if possible be present at the time of x-ray to prevent mishap.)

136

(3) *Clinical observations* should be charted by doctors and nurses on the ventilator flow-charts.

**Chest Care**

(1) *Physiotherapy.* We do not carry out regular physiotherapy, other than turning the baby from one side to the other at about two-hourly intervals. However, the presence of coarse moist sounds on auscultation, or of moist sounds audible at each breath without a stethoscope suggests that secretions are accumulating. Under these circumstances the nursing staff suck out the posterior pharynx before and after applying chest percussion, with the baby lying on one and then on the other side.

(2) *Tracheal toilet* should be performed at four-hourly intervals. The suction pump is turned on. With a disposable plastic glove on the right hand, a catheter is passed down the nasotracheal tube as far as possible and then suction is applied while it is slowly withdrawn. The suction tube must not fit too tightly into the ET tube, otherwise massive atelectasis may ensue. The catheter should not be pushed up and down repeatedly; only if an excessive aspirate is obtained should the suction be repeated.

(3) *Tracheal suction* swabs should be taken every second day.

(4) *Systemic antibiotics* are only used as indicated (see 'Infection', p. 167).

(5) We have abandoned giving topical antibiotics down the ET tube.

**Weaning off the Ventilator**

An attempt should be made to get the infant to breathe off the ventilator at least once a day, choosing if possible periods of relative quiet in the special care nursery, and in any case if the baby is showing obvious efforts to take over.

*Stage I. Seeing if he can breathe adequately off the ventilator*

(1) If the baby is not already showing signs of breathing against the ventilator, turn down the rate to 15-20 per minute for about five minutes. If he still shows no sign of spontaneous breathing, the chances of getting him off at this stage are not good. If he does breathe:

(2) Switch off the ventilator and, in cases of respiratory distress, attach the CPAP (p. 125) to the endotracheal tube with pressure of 5-10cmH$_2$O. Use the same O$_2$ concentration as when on ventilator.

(3) If he breathes spontaneously but becomes cyanosed within five minutes, re-attach the ventilator and defer any further attempts for at least six hours.

(4) If he breathes for about ten minutes, preserving a good colour, but goes off by fifteen minutes it is reasonable to try him off IPPV for ten minutes each hour.

*Stage II. Extubation*

(1) If the baby breathes spontaneously for an hour and reasonable blood-gas measurements are obtained, he should be extubated at a convenient time in the next 12 hours.

(2) If CPAP is used, gradually reduce the pressure to 2-5cmH$_2$O.

(3) Set up an I.V. infusion from two hours before extubation to 24 hours after extubation and stop oral feeding to avoid the dangers of aspiration.

(4) Suck out the pharynx and remove the ET tube. Continue the CPAP with the head-box (p. 127) if the baby is thought to have hyaline membrane disease.

These instructions may have to be varied according to circumstances. For instance, an alternative to *Stage I* is merely to turn off the ventilator, allowing the baby to breathe spontaneously from the stream of fresh gas in the U loop. However, this may involve too much dead space and resistance in the harness and is not advocated as a routine.

A difficulty associated with weaning an infant after prolonged ventilation treatment is that of secretions, though this has been less of a problem in our unit since we found a satisfactory method of humidification. Physiotherapy, and suction to the posterior pharynx, are given as described above.

### Tracheostomy

Modern nasotracheal tubes are fairly well tolerated over a period of days. A tracheostomy has two advantages: (1) easier access to the trachea for suction; and (2) a small dead space. We are, however, more experienced in handling nasotracheal than tracheostomy tubes. We make it a rule to discuss the possibility of tracheostomy whenever a baby has been on the ventilator for more than a week, but so far we have never decided to do it in these particular circumstances.

# APPENDIX

**Nasotracheal Intubation**

Select a nasotracheal tube of a size that is likely to fit not too tightly in the trachea. In most newborn babies a 3mm tube will be big enough; in very large babies (more than 4kg) a 4mm tube may be better.

Insert the tube into a nostril. Push it to and fro to a depth of 1cm to lubricate it with nasal secretion. Push it in about 6cm. If it will not pass, try the other nostril; if you are still unsuccessful, lubricate very lightly with KY jelly. If nasal intubation is impossible, resort to orotracheal intubation (see p. 37).

With the laryngoscope blade, lift forward the tongue, inspect the cords, and suck out any mucus as in orotracheal intubation (p. 37). Locate the leading edge of the nasotracheal tube (if necessary by withdrawing the tube slightly), pick it up with Magill forceps and direct it through the cords into the trachea. Get an assistant to press slightly on the larynx if you cannot see the cords (see p. 37). Thread the tube about 1 to 2cm beyond the cords.

Attach a Y adaptor to the nasotracheal tube, and connect this to the wall supply of oxygen with a blow-off valve in the circuit. With the valve set to blow-off at $30cmH_2O$, apply IPPV by occluding the side arm of the Y adaptor, listen to both sides of the chest with a stethoscope; breath sounds should be equal. If the tube is inserted too far, it usually passes to the right main bronchus and breath sounds are faint on the left. If this occurs, withdraw the tube 0.5cm at a time until breath sounds are equal.

Fix the tube to the nostril and face, and then cut off excess tubing protruding from the nostril with sterile scissors (about 0.5cm should be left protruding). Arrange a chest x-ray to check the position of the tube.

# Pneumothorax

Pneumothorax and pneumomediastinum are most frequently encountered in the newborn when there is a history of meconium aspiration at birth. They also occur when the baby has aspirated mucus and when the bronchial secretions are excessively sticky, for instance when a baby is having ventilator therapy. They are a well-known complication of staphylococcal pneumonia. Pneumothorax is also said to occur after aspiration of blood. Although often attributed to over-zealous artificial ventilation, it is rarely caused by this alone provided that proper attention is paid to limiting inflation pressures with an effective safety valve; the sticky aspirate is a much more important factor.

Pneumothorax must be considered when any baby with respiratory difficulties deteriorates, but in particular, when one of the above situations has occurred. The clinical signs may be hard to detect and their absence does not exclude the diagnosis. Mediastinal shift is perhaps the most reliable and may be detected from the cardiac impulse or the position of the heart sounds. In cases of tension pneumothorax, the diaphragm may be pushed down, thus causing sudden apparent enlargement of the liver and abdominal distension. In some cases of pneumomediastinum the heart sounds become distant and difficult to hear. When the baby's condition is poor, action must be taken on clinical signs alone but, where possible, immediate x-rays—lateral as well as PA—should be arranged.

### The X-ray

In minor degrees of pneumomediastinum and pneumothorax, a halo of air may be seen around the heart. On the lateral film, air may be seen behind the sternum *before* there is an abnormality on the PA film. The classical findings of pneumothorax in the antero-posterior view are of a collapsed lung with a translucency beyond the lung border. (It is easy to mistake the border of *latissimus dorsae* for a lung border.) The thymus may be clearly outlined by air in a pneumomediastinum. Radiological signs of tension in the x-ray are a shifted mediastinum, herniation of the trans-lucency across the midline, bulging intercostal spaces and depressed diaphragm.

### Management

Unless there are signs of tension in the pneumothorax or pneumomediastinum, it is best to do nothing except to watch for signs of deterioration. Handling should be reduced to a minimum to prevent the child from crying.

In the term baby, a very high concentration of oxygen may be used in the incubator to facilitate absorption of the pneumothorax. In a pre-term baby, oxygen should not be used above 30% concentration, unless indicated on other grounds.

Where a tension pneumothorax is diagnosed, or where there is sudden deterioration in a known case of pneumothorax, the pleural space must be aspirated. A poly-vinyl tube is introduced by a needle (Angiocath or equivalent) at the fourth intercostal space in the anterior axillary line. After removing the metal needle so that only the polyvinyl tube is in the pleural space, allow the intrapleural gas under pressure to 'blow back' the syringe on which the catheter was inserted. Gently aspirate any excess air which comes freely from the pleural space, and then occlude the tube by pinching it until you have connected it with sterile tubing to an underwater seal; as a temporary measure, the free end of the tubing may be held 2cm under the surface of sterile water, but as soon as possible attach it to an intercostal drainage bottle. In the intercostal drainage bottle, the open end of the pleural drain, which is a glass tube, should dip 2cm under the water surface. Either a bubble of air blowing off or small excursions in the glass tube should be visible with each of the baby's respirations; it is not usual to see the large excursions one sees with pleural drainage in adults. This will suffice as an emergency treatment for most cases of tension pneumothorax. In some cases where the amount of air draining is large, or where blood occludes the small poly-vinyl tube, a thicker tube with at least two side holes will have to be inserted (using a trochar and cannula) to provide adequate drainage, and continuous suction using very low pressures—about minus 2cm$H_2O$—may be applied via the intercostal drainage bottle.

When air stops bubbling off, especially if the small excursions in the glass tube are no longer apparent, it may mean that the tube is occluded by blood or pleural fluid and that the pneumothorax is again accumulating. However, it may merely mean there is no more air to drain. Check the baby's condition and physical signs and, if necessary, get another chest x-ray to help you make the decision. This decision is very important, since inserting a fresh tube may either be life-saving or needless further trauma to the baby.

If it is necessary to transfer the baby, for instance from a trolley to an incubator, always clamp off the intercostal drain so that the baby's respiratory efforts do not suck air into his pleural space. However, try to arrange that the period of time that the tube is clamped (and therefore excluded from the underwater seal which is a safety valve) is only a matter of seconds.

Occasionally, air tracks from the mediastinal tissues causing subcutaneous surgical emphysema: the treatment consists of giving the child oxygen to breathe and draining any tension pneumothorax. Incising the skin to let out the air is unrewarding and dangerous for it will make the baby cry, thus aggravating the condition.

# Apnoeic Attacks

We make an arbitrary distinction between apnoeic attacks and periodic respiration. The latter commonly occurs in babies who are born early and who do not appear to be ill. Periods of rather rapid breathing lasting about 20 seconds alternate with periods of cessation of breathing lasting about 10 seconds. Babies with periodic respiration have been shown to have a higher arterial blood pH than control babies with regular respiration. Moreover, babies with periodic respiration will often breathe regularly if the ambient oxygen concentration is slightly increased. These observations suggest that periodic respiration may be due to hyperventilation consequent on slight hypoxaemia.

We define an apnoeic attack as cessation of breathing for more than 30 seconds. Apnoeic attacks are a common and serious problem in ill newborn babies and it is humiliating that we can speak with so little assurance about their aetiology and treatment.

The term 'cyanotic attack' must not be used as synonymous with apnoeic attack. There may be no cyanosis in an apnoeic attack lasting less than one minute, especially if the infant has been breathing oxygen-enriched air and if the pulse rate has not dropped. On the other hand, we sometimes find that an infant has become cyanotic with shallow breathing rather than apnoea. In the case of the infant in whom respiration is not being monitored and who has an unexpected but temporary episode of cyanosis with apparently normal respiration, it is not possible to exclude the occurrence of a spontaneous and temporary right-to-left shunt, but we cannot claim ever to have been sure that respiration preceding cyanosis has been normal.

There are two main circumstances in which apnoeic attacks are common: (a) in babies born very early (usually before 32 weeks gestation); and (b) in babies with severe respiratory distress, whatever the pathogenesis. In both situations, intraventricular haemorrhage is a common but not invariable finding in fatal cases. Regurgitation and aspiration of stomach contents may sometimes be the cause (or the result) of an apnoeic attack, and in some babies apnoea seems to be related to a tube-feed even when the baby has not aspirated. Indeed, any form of handling may precipitate apnoea in a very immature or very ill newborn baby. Excessive heat in the incubator may also predispose the baby to apnoeic attacks. We used to see apnoeic attacks commonly as a consequence of cerebral birth injury (often with subdural haemorrhage) and as a symptom of hypoglycaemia, but both conditions are to-day largely prevented. Maternal sedation may play a part in some cases of recurrent apnoea in the first day or two of postnatal life. Apnoeic attacks may also occur in the case of systemic infection, especially meningitis, in cases of subarachnoid haemorrhage and, rarely, they may be the sole manifestation of fits.

Newborn babies who are especially liable to develop apnoeic attacks need continuous observation of their respiration. We use apnoea monitors in this situation.

## General Treatment of Infants Who Have Had One or More Apnoeic Attacks

*The Very Immature Infant Without Respiratory Distress*

(1) Reduce handling to the minimum necessary.

(2) Check the incubator temperature: is it too high?

If the baby has more than one apnoeic attack which has not responded quickly to stimulation:

(3) give oxygen to raise the ambient concentration to 25 or 30%.

If apnoeic attacks are abolished or greatly reduced in frequency, reduce added oxygen after a few hours, and observe the effect. Sister Castle and her nursing colleagues at Hammersmith have long been convinced that raising the oxygen content of the incubator to, say, 30% may reduce the frequency of apnoeic attacks in some preterm infants. In some cases they have been proved to be right, but concentrations higher than 30% must not be given without starting routine blood gas analysis, and oxygen should be reduced after an apnoea-free period of about six hours. *Stop giving oxygen as soon as possible.*

(4) Consider the possibility of hypoglycaemia or infection. Examine the baby for signs of infection (see page 163). Take blood for glucose estimation, culture and white count. Consider whether a lumbar puncture should be done to exclude meningitis (remembering that positioning the baby and doing a lumbar puncture may provoke an apnoeic attack). If there is any supporting evidence of infection, or if the baby is more than two days old, take swabs and blood culture and start antibiotics.

*The Baby With Respiratory Distress*

(1) and (2) above still apply.

(3) Do not increase ambient oxygen unless this is indicated by a low arterial oxygen tension after recovery from apnoea.

(4) If the baby has more than one apnoeic attack, proceed as in (4) above.

*Term or Slightly Immature Babies Without Respiratory Distress*

Take steps to exclude hypoglycaemia and infection. Consult the senior paediatrician concerning lumbar puncture to exclude meningitis or subarachnoid haemorrhage. Do not forget the possibility of a congenital deformity affecting the respiratory tract (*e.g.* oesophageal atresia, Pierre Robin syndrome, choanal atresia). Consider the possibility that the apnoeic attacks are sole manifestations of fits. If possible, obtain an EEG, and when otherwise unexplained attacks persist, try the effect of anticonvulsants (see p. 190).

## Treatment of an Apnoeic Attack

Do not turn up the incubator oxygen *during* an apnoeic attack—it will not do any good while the baby is apnoeic, and may result in the baby receiving too much oxygen when he recovers from the attack.

When the apnoea alarm goes off, try to make the baby gasp by a physical stimulus. In babies who are having recurrent apnoeic attacks, our nursing staff sometimes tie a tape round the baby's ankle, so that they can pull it without opening the incubator. This may not be the most effective stimulus, but the method does have the advantage that hands go in and out of the incubator less often. When this is not successful, flicking the soles of the baby's feet, or a more painful stimulus such as pinching the skin of the abdominal wall should be used, or else the pharynx aspirated, since this is a powerful stimulus to respiration.

If the physical stimuli are unsuccessful, and providing the apnoeic attack has not taken place just after a feed, ventilate with 40% oxygen by face-mask. Ensure that the jaw is pulled forward, the mask firmly applied and the blow-off valve set at 20cmH$_2$O before occluding the escape tube rhythmically about 20 times a minute. Following the use of a face-mask, it may be necessary to aspirate air from the stomach.

If mask ventilation is contra-indicated or does not prove successful in restoring colour and respiration within about 2 minutes—or much sooner if the heart rate is below 60—intubate the trachea at once, aspirating larynx and trachea under direct vision. If adequate respiration (*i.e.* regular respiration sufficient to keep the baby pink and maintain the heart-rate) does not begin after about fifteen minutes of manual inflation of the lungs via the endotracheal tube, attach the artificial ventilator.

Finally, we have seen babies with respiratory distress (presumed hyaline membrane disease), complicated by recurrent apnoea, breathe regularly with CPAP when other indications for its use were not present.

# Stridor

By convention, the term 'stridor' is applied to noisy breathing coming from the larynx or the trachea. Laryngeal stridor is largely inspiratory, because the vocal cords approximate during inspiration; tracheal stridor is usually equally expiratory and inspiratory. In practice, it is usually easy to distinguish from noisy breathing arising in the nose or the bronchi. There are numerous causes for stridor in newborn babies in the form of lesions inside or outside the larynx or in the nervous system. The action to be taken depends on whether stridor is present at birth or develops later, whether it is constant or intermittent, and whether or not the baby shows signs of respiratory distress or respiratory obstruction.

**Stridor at Birth** (see p. 36)

Stridor at birth, accompanied by violent inspiratory efforts, will suggest a congenital malformation of the larynx or trachea, although the same symptoms will be seen if there is laryngeal obstruction with mucus. (Obviously where there is complete obstruction there can be no stridor.)

**Stridor Developing in a Baby Who Has Needed Resuscitation At Birth**

Babies who have needed endotracheal intubation or repeated pharyngeal aspiration at birth may develop stridor—presumably due to laryngeal oedema. It usually lessens and disappears within 24 hours. Provided the baby is not showing signs of respiratory distress, we take no positive action other than warning the nursing staff to be particularly careful about feeds since the risk of aspiration appears to be higher in babies with stridor of any origin. We see exactly the same thing happening in babies who have had prolonged endotracheal intubation for artificial ventilation—in this case obviously due to laryngeal oedema. In these cases, we have sometimes prescribed steroids but are uncertain of their efficacy. Occasionally re-intubation becomes absolutely necessary.

**Persistent or Worsening Stridor**

This suggests either an anatomical obstruction (see p. 37) or vocal cord paralysis of peripheral or central origin. The latter may be due to cerebral birth trauma or associated with a deformity such as the Arnold-Chiari malformation with myelomeningocele. Examine the neck for swellings and the skin for hemangiomata; arrange an PA and lateral x-ray of the chest and neck to detect narrowing and soft tissue swelling and call in the ENT surgeon with the object of obtaining an expert laryngoscopy. A barium swallow, preferably with cineradiography, may be helpful for diagnosing vascular rings. Apart from the neurological causes already mentioned, reflex precipitation of stridor (*e.g.* by feeding) has been reported to be responsive to anticonvulsants. Although laryngospasm is a recognised feature of tetany, it appears to be rare in newborn babies and we have not encountered it in cases of hypocalcaemia.

### Congenital Laryngeal Stridor

This is the term conventionally applied to a condition in which stridor appears to be caused by easy collapsibility of the aryepiglottic folds or the epiglottis itself. Despite its name, this condition rarely presents at birth, more usually appearing at the end of the first or in the second week of life. The important point of distinction between this condition and those already described is that stridor is intermittent. It may be influenced by the position of the baby and induced by feeding, crying or sleeping. Although this stridor disappears in the course of time, there is a higher proportion of CNS abnormalities detected in later infancy and childhood than one would expect on a chance basis. If the stridor fits with this clinical description and is not worsening, and provided the child is thriving, we do not always seek an ENT opinion.

# Hypoglycaemia

Blood-glucose concentrations in the newborn baby, whatever its birthweight or gestational age, are generally lower than those found in older children or adults. In general, we are not concerned unless blood-glucose concentration falls below 20mg/100ml in the newborn, and this should only occur rarely if the feeding instructions for low-birthweight babies (p. 96) are followed.

The definition of neonatal hypoglycaemia which we use for coding purposes is: 'A true blood glucose of less than 20mg/100ml which is *either* associated with symptoms attributable to hypoglycaemia *or* which is still present or recurs an hour or more after the first estimation'. However, it is usually best in practice to work out a programme of management when the first low blood-glucose concentration is discovered, without waiting for symptoms or for a second estimation showing a low concentration. The practical questions are therefore: (*a*) under what circumstances blood-glucose concentration should be measured in the newborn and how it should be measured; and (*b*) what to do if the concentration is low, *i.e.* below 20mg/100ml.

**Grounds for Suspicion of Hypoglycaemia**

This means grounds for measuring blood-glucose concentration (see flow-chart, p. 151). They can be divided into symptoms which might be due to hypoglycaemia and circumstances which put the baby at risk of developing hypoglycaemia.

*Symptoms*

(1) *Convulsions* (see p. 188). Blood-glucose concentration should always be measured in a baby having convulsions. (If the baby is small for dates and the convulsions occur in the first three days of life, intravenous glucose should be given as soon as blood has been taken for glucose estimation, and without waiting for the result.)

(2) *Apnoeic attacks* (see p. 142). Although symptomatic hypoglycaemia may present as apnoeic attacks, most apnoeic attacks are not due to hypoglycaemia; nevertheless, the blood glucose should always be checked.

(3) *Lethargy, hypotonia and shallow respiration.* Check blood glucose.

*Circumstances Predisposing to Hypoglycaemia\**

(1) *Smallness for dates.* All small-for-dates babies (*i.e.* those below the 10th percentile of birthweight for their gestational age) should have the blood glucose concentration checked between 12 and 24 hours of age, and again between 36 and 48 hours. Those who are grossly small for dates (more than 250g below the 10th percentile) or babies who appear thin and wasted, should have blood glucose checked at 12, 18, 24, 36 and 48 hours. Long, thin, 'scraggy' babies, even if above the 10th percentile of weight for gestational age, may be suspected of having suffered from postmaturity or placental insufficiency and should have blood glucose checked

---

*Symptomatic hypoglycaemia is commoner in boys than girls.

147

in the same way as small-for-dates babies. Of course, all small-for-dates babies should be fed early (see p. 96).

(2) *Maternal diabetes* (see p. 9). Infants of diabetic mothers commonly become hypoglycaemic in the first 8 hours of life, but the blood glucose concentration usually returns to normal levels soon after this. Check blood glucose at 6, 12 and 24 hours.

(3) *Haemolytic disease of the newborn* (see p. 154). Infants with severe haemolytic disease of the newborn—especially those who have had intrauterine transfusions or who are hydropic—often become hypoglycaemic. Check blood glucose six-hourly in the first 24 hours, and at 36 and 48 hours.

(4) *Birth asphyxia* (see p. 32). In babies who have been severely asphyxiated at birth—those who have been slow to establish spontaneous respiration after endotracheal intubation and ventilation, or who have required alkali during resuscitation —check blood glucose after resuscitation and at 6 and 12 hours.

(5) *Respiratory distress.* Check blood glucose when blood-gas measurements are done.

(6) *Very low birthweight* (below 1200g). Check blood glucose at 24, 48 and 72 hours.

(7) *Hypothermia* (see p. 102).

(8) *Inborn errors of metabolism* (see p. 225).

### Method for Measurement of Blood Glucose Concentration

'Dextrostix' provides a satisfactory screening test for low blood-glucose concentration. Follow instructions on the label, but cover only half the sensitive area of the strip with blood. (New residents should practise the 'Dextrostix' test on blood containing known low levels of glucose.) False positives occur (*i.e.* 'Dextrostix' indicates blood-glucose concentration below 20mg% when true blood glucose is higher) but false negatives are very rare (see Chantler *et al.* 1967).* Use 'Dextrostix' in the first instance wherever blood-glucose estimation is recommended, either in the previous section or on the flow-chart. If it shows a blood-glucose concentration above 20mg%, a formal laboratory estimation is not necessary; if below 20mg%, a laboratory estimation must be done.

### Management of Hypoglycaemia

This section deals with what to do when a newborn baby is found to have a blood-glucose concentration below 20mg%, whether or not we would define it as 'hypoglycaemia' (see above).

The management of hypoglycaemia is a complex subject, because it is influenced by many different circumstances. In general, the scheme which we follow is shown in the flow-sheet (p. 151). It would, of course, be much simpler to give intravenous glucose to all babies whose blood-glucose was below 20mg/100ml on two successive readings. We do not do this routinely because we believe the advantages of oral feeding with breast milk still apply in this situation. (Breast milk contains 67cals/100ml

*Chantler, C., Baum, J. D., Norman, D. A. (1967) 'Dextrostix in the diagnosis of neonatal hypoglycaemia.' *Lancet*, **ii**, 1395.

compared with 40cals/100ml in 10% dextrose). Furthermore, *symptomatic* hypoglycaemia is rare in the first 24 hours of life. We therefore reserve the use of intravenous glucose for babies with symptoms, babies who are not 'absorbing' oral feeds (see p. 150), and babies over 24 hours old in whom the risk of developing symptoms from hypoglycaemia is greater.

### Persistent Hypoglycaemia

The situation in which we have most often seen hypoglycaemia—or the tendency to hypoglycaemia—persisting after the age of 48 hours is in the baby who has been given an intravenous glucose drip, and who can only be weaned off it very slowly because of reactive hypoglycaemia. All that is needed is patience, and a very slow change-over from intravenous to oral feeds.

However, there are other causes of persistent hypoglycaemia which must be remembered, including hyperinsulinism due to islet cell hyperplasia (which may be due to Rh incompatibility or treatment of a diabetic mother with chlorpropamide) or tumour, leucine sensitivity, galactosaemia, hereditary fructosaemia, glycogen storage disease, and 'idiopathic' hypoglycaemia of McQuarrie type. The investigation and treatment of these rare disorders are complex: (see section on 'Inborn errors of metabolism', p. 225; also Cornblath and Schwartz 1966).* However, certain simple diagnostic considerations are worth noting here.

Hypoglycaemia will only occur in leucine sensitivity when the baby is receiving protein, in galactosaemia when the baby is receiving lactose, and in hereditary fructose intolerance when the baby is receiving sucrose or fructose. In all these conditions, therefore, hypoglycaemia is provoked by milk feeding, and does not occur if the baby is given glucose only. Milk feeding may also provoke hypoglycaemia in islet cell hyperplasia or tumour, since there is often some degree of leucine sensitivity.

### 'Transient Neonatal Diabetes'

We have had only one case of this puzzling condition. The following short account is a summary of the review by Gentz and Cornblath (1969)†.

The condition may be seen at any time in the first six weeks of life. The affected babies are usually small for dates, and may be hypoglycaemic before becoming hyperglycaemic. A family history of diabetes is common.

The infant usually presents with sudden weight-loss due to dehydration, accompanied by fever and failure to thrive, but without diarrhoea or vomiting. Hyperglycaemia (blood-sugar levels may go as high as 2000mg per 100ml) and glycosuria are marked. Ketonuria is mild or absent.

The diabetes should be treated with insulin, in doses sufficient to keep the blood-glucose down to about 200mg per 100ml (usually about 1.3 units per kg per day). Dehydration should be treated with intravenous fluids (*e.g.* 0.45% sodium chloride),

---

*Cornblath, M., Schwartz, R. (1966) *Disorders of Carbohydrate Metabolism in Infancy*. Philadelphia and London: W. B. Saunders.
†Gentz, J. C. H., Cornblath, M. (1969) 'Transient diabetes in the newborn.' *Advances in Pediatrics*, **16**, 345.

but care must be taken not to rehydrate too quickly if the serum sodium is high—which it sometimes is. (See also p. 99).

The majority of cases will stop needing insulin after a period of weeks or months, but in some cases diabetes is permanent.

Prognosis must be guarded, for many of these infants have shown neurological abnormalities later—though it is not clear to what extent these can be accounted for by hypernatraemic or hypoglycaemic brain-damage, which may be preventable with early diagnosis and adequate treatment.

---

### Explanatory Notes to the Flow-sheet

NOTE (1). *Symptoms of hypoglycaemia.* The only symptoms which we are convinced are sometimes attributable to hypoglycaemia are convulsions, apnoea and unresponsiveness, limpness and shallow respiration. Symptoms should not be attributed to hypoglycaemia unless they disappear when hypoglycaemia is corrected. 'Jitteriness' is probably not a symptom of hypoglycaemia; though it often occurs in hypoglycaemic babies, it is also common in small-for-dates or asphyxiated babies who are not hypoglycaemic. It is rarely corrected by giving intravenous glucose. If a baby showed definite neurological abnormalities other than these already mentioned, in the presence of a blood-glucose concentration below 20mg%, we would answer a provisional 'yes' to the question 'are symptoms present?' and give intravenous glucose. We would not *finally* attribute the symptoms to hypoglycaemia unless they disappeared quickly after intravenous glucose.

NOTE (2). *Single intravenous injection of glucose.* Give 1g glucose per kg body weight, as 10% or 20% glucose solution. Use a peripheral vein if possible, but if this is difficult or will cause delay, use a catheter in the umbilical vein. In that case we prefer 10% glucose unless there are special reasons not to give extra fluid to the baby. Follow the glucose injection into the umbilical vein with 5ml of 4% glucose in 1/5 normal saline.

NOTE (3). *Intravenous glucose infusion.* This is also best given into a peripheral vein, though the umbilical vein may be used in difficult circumstances. Give 10% glucose at approximately 75ml/kg/day (for further advice on intravenous fluids see p. 99), continuing oral feeds in half the previous quantities provided they were being 'absorbed'. Continue the drip for 24 hours, but (unless oral feeds are contra-indicated) aim to reduce and stop the drip in the second 24 hours, gradually replacing it by oral feeds. Check blood glucose four-hourly in this period: reactive hypoglycaemia may occur rapidly. If the drip stops, be prepared to set it up again at once. If hypoglycaemia recurs, see 'Persistent hypoglycaemia' (p.149).

NOTE (4). The point is that the exchange transfusion will provide a slow injection over the course of about 1½-2 hours of blood with a relatively high glucose concentration (about 200mg%). It is reasonable to wait and see if this corrects the initial low blood-glucose concentration, but it is essential to check for reactive hypoglycaemia after the exchange.

NOTE (5). The expression 'feeds being absorbed' is a convenient but inaccurate one used by our nursing staff. It really means that feeds are not pooling in the stomach.

*SUGGESTED SCHEME FOR TREATMENT OF HYPOGLYCAEMIA*

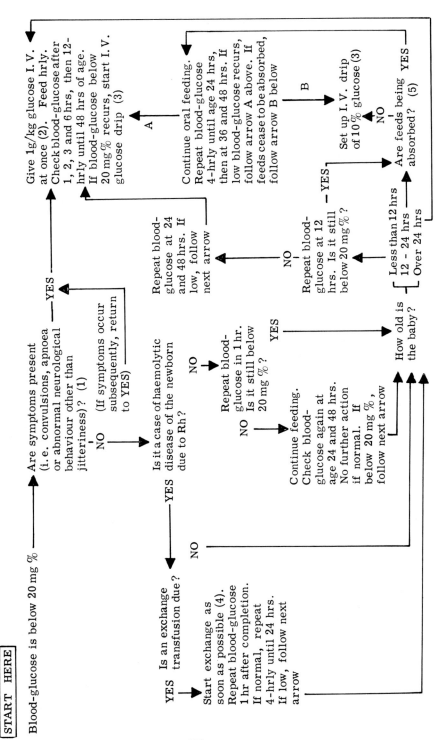

START HERE

Blood-glucose is below 20 mg %

Are symptoms present (i.e. convulsions, apnoea or abnormal neurological behaviour other than jitteriness)? (1) —— YES —— Give 1g/kg glucose I.V. at once (2). Feed hrly. Check blood-glucose after 1, 2, 3 and 6 hrs, then 12-hrly until 48 hrs of age. If blood-glucose below 20 mg% recurs, start I.V. glucose drip (3)

(If symptoms occur subsequently, return to YES)

NO

Is it a case of haemolytic disease of the newborn due to Rh? —— YES —— Is an exchange transfusion due?

YES — Start exchange as soon as possible (4). Repeat blood-glucose 1 hr after completion. If normal, repeat 4-hrly until 24 hrs. If low, follow next arrow

NO — Repeat blood-glucose in 1 hr. Is it still below 20 mg%?

NO — Continue feeding. Check blood-glucose again at age 24 and 48 hrs. No further action if normal. If below 20 mg%, follow next arrow

YES — How old is the baby?

Less than 12 hrs — Repeat blood-glucose at 12 hrs. Is it still below 20 mg%?
YES — Are feeds being absorbed? (5)
NO — Repeat blood-glucose at 24 and 48 hrs. If low, follow next arrow

12 - 24 hrs

Over 24 hrs

Are feeds being absorbed? (5)
YES — Continue oral feeding. Repeat blood-glucose 4-hrly until age 24 hrs, then at 36 and 48 hrs. If low blood-glucose recurs, follow arrow A above. If feeds cease to be absorbed, follow arrow B below
NO — Set up I.V. drip of 10% glucose (3)

A

B

# Haemolytic Disease of the Newborn

For instructions concerning the affected baby in the delivery room, see p. 65.

**Exchange Transfusions**

*Indications for the First Exchange Transfusion*

The purposes of the first exchange transfusion are to correct anaemia and to lessen the chances of subsequent hyperbilirubinaemia and anaemia. Usually the decision as to whether an exchange transfusion is necessary at birth is straight-forward, once the results of the cord-blood investigations are known. In some cases, the indications will be marginal, so the decision may be a matter of personal opinion and the consultant's advice should be sought.

As a rule, exchange transfusion will not be needed unless the direct Coombs test is strongly positive. However, it must be remembered that misleading negative results may occur:

(1) after an intraperitoneal intra-uterine transfusion, when the circulating cells are largely group O Rh-negative donor cells;

(2) when the cord blood is contaminated with Wharton's jelly; or

(3) due to faulty techniques in the laboratory.

If the decision is made not to transfuse, the resident should inspect the baby for jaundice within six hours and instruct the nursing staff to inform him if jaundice is visible at any time in the first 24 hours.

If the Coombs test is reported as strongly positive, exchange transfusion should be carried out if the cord Hb is below 12g/100ml, to correct anaemia. If the cord haemoglobin is above 12g/100ml, exchange transfusion should probably be done to reduce the amount of later hyperbilirubinaemia (by removing sensitised red cells) if any of the following conditions applies:

(1) duration of pregnancy less than 37 weeks;

(2) cord bilirubin more than 5mg/100ml;

(3) an intra-uterine intraperitoneal transfusion has been given (in fact, in these cases the cord Hb is very unlikely to be above 12g/100ml);

(4) marked enlargement of the liver and spleen.

We do not use a history of a previously affected baby as an indication for exchange transfusion, but one of the above conditions is likely to apply when a previous baby has been affected. Where the situation is borderline in respect of any of these conditions, the presence of more than one of them is an indication for exchange transfusion. If a baby has had a partial exchange done as an emergency in the delivery room, a further complete exchange should be done when the baby is settled in the special care nursery, provided the indications for exchange were confirmed by the cord-blood findings.

152

*Location for Exchange Transfusion*

Normally the transfusion will be carried out in the special care nursery. Exceptions are: (*a*) the emergency exchange transfusion of the hydropic baby (see p. 65); and (*b*) infection in the baby or in the special care nursery which might preclude transfer of the baby between that ward and the lying-in wards. (Provided he is big and mature enough, the baby is normally returned to the mother in the lying-in ward as soon as further transfusions are deemed unnecessary.)

*Consent for Exchange Transfusion*

A formal signed consent form is not necessary, but the mother, and where possible the father, should be informed of the necessity for exchange transfusion before it is carried out. If the parents refuse blood transfusion, follow instructions on p. 277.

*Timing of Transfusion*

In general, an exchange transfusion should take place as soon as possible after the indication has been established. However, if the child is in poor condition and there are reasons to expect an improvement in an hour or two, it may be delayed for this period of time. In particular, if the baby has a low body-temperature, he should be warmed to a normal body-temperature before the procedure.

*Donor Blood*

Wherever possible, one unit (500ml) of fresh heparinized, Rh-negative blood of the same ABO group as the baby and compatible with the baby's and mother's serum should be obtained. When the donor must be bled before the baby's ABO group is known, use group O Rh-negative blood from a donor whose blood has been tested for anti-A haemolysins. Once group O blood has been used in a group A, B, or AB, baby, it should be chosen again for any further exchange transfusion. For instructions on crossmatching, see p. 272. Requests for a donor are made through the Blood Transfusion department and if it is anticipated that blood will be needed between the hours of 10 p.m. and 9 a.m., an appropriate donor can be asked to remain available by telephone. Add 20ml of 5% dextrose to a pint of fresh heparinized blood before use. (Venous donor blood often has a low glucose concentration and Rhesus babies have a tendency to hypoglycaemia in the first hours of life.) Fresh blood should not be packed.

If it is not possible to obtain fresh blood, ensure that two pints of stored Rh-negative blood of the appropriate group, not more than three days old, are available. The potassium level should, if possible, be measured before the blood is used if it is more than two days old. A potassium level of more than 15mEq/litre precludes its use. Blood with raised levels up to 15mEq/litre may be used with caution (proceed *slowly* and keep watching the oscilloscope for high spiked T waves on the ECG). When it is known that exchange transfusion is imminent, ACD blood should be prepared as follows:
(1) add 1500 units of heparin;
(2) add 5ml 10% calcium gluconate;
(3) centrifuge and remove about 100ml plasma (to pack partially and remove some

of the citrate);

(4) add 6ml of 20% THAM (or titrate up to pH 7.4 using 20% THAM).

*Subsequent Exchange Transfusions*

The indications for subsequent exchange transfusions are related to dangerous bilirubin levels and apply also to jaundice for other reasons (see p. 156). The bilirubin level should be estimated again a few hours after the first or any other exchange transfusion. In general, bilirubin levels can be expected to rise for about three days (up to seven days in pre-term babies) and then stabilise and fall. A small 'rebound' rise occurs after the level estimated at the end of exchange transfusion. These factors enable some degree of prediction of the movement of bilirubin levels, and exchange transfusion is indicated if it appears that the unconjugated serum bilirubin level is likely to reach a dangerous level before the time an exchange transfusion could be arranged next morning. In general, the level considered dangerous is 20mg/100ml (but see also p. 156).

If the baby is ill, acidotic, dehydrated, infected, or has had severe asphyxia, levels a few mg lower may be dangerous. In a lusty term infant, levels up to 22mg/100ml may be acceptable. Also to be taken into account are age, plasma proteins and the neurological state of the baby. If we were to detect any signs suggestive of kernikterus we would do an exchange transfusion immediately.

## Other Methods of Reducing Serum Bilirubin

For a discussion of enzyme-inducing agents and phototherapy, see p. 159.

## Hypoglycaemia in Rh Babies

Infants with haemolytic disease tend to be hyperinsulinaemic and may become hypoglycaemic, hence the need for added glucose in venous donor blood (p. 153), and for checking blood sugars at about six-hourly intervals during the first 24 hours. This is most conveniently achieved by using 'Dextrostix' at each bilirubin estimation. See 'Hypoglycaemia', p. 147 and p. 151, for action to be taken. *An important aspect of preventing hypoglycaemia and of alleviating hyperbilirubinaemia is to institute early and adequate feeding.*

## Late Anaemia in Rh Babies

The Hb level of rhesus babies usually falls to reach its lowest point at about six weeks and then rises spontaneously. Inadequate attention to shaking the donor blood during an exchange transfusion may leave the baby relatively anaemic (10-11g/100ml) at the end of an exchange, at a time when a normal baby's Hb is 14-15g/100ml. This will aggravate the subsequent anaemia.

The folic acid content is higher in the red cells of a newborn baby than in adult red-cells, so an exchange transfusion removes the baby's reserves. Oral iron will not alleviate immediate anaemia, but will alleviate the late anaemia. We therefore usually:

(1) check Hb and reticulocytes weekly and plot out the curve on graph paper;

(2) give folic acid 0.1mg weekly;

(3) give oral iron from the fifth week (ferrous sulphate 30mg daily) if the baby is pre-term (see also p. 234).

**Simple Transfusion ('Top-up' Transfusion)**

No easy rules can be given for when to perform a top-up transfusion. For instance, a baby with Hb 6g/100ml (and no reticulocytes) at the age of two weeks will almost certainly need a transfusion. A baby with an Hb of 6g/100ml and 10% reticulocytes at the age of six weeks will almost certainly manage without transfusion. Some babies tolerate an Hb of 6-7g/100ml without symptoms; others become breathless, tire on feeding and may go into frank cardiac failure. Factors which help make the decision whether to transfuse are the Hb level after exchange transfusion, the rate of fall of Hb level, the reticulocyte count, the baby's symptoms and, occasionally, the *indirect* Coombs test on the baby's serum. A positive indirect Coombs test indicates that Rh antibodies are still circulating, and these may interfere with production of new Rh-positive cells or lead to their haemolysis. If the baby is in incipient or frank cardiac failure, intraperitoneal transfusion, rather than I.V. transfusion, may be preferable (see p. 274.)

**Persistent Jaundice in Rh Babies**

A proportion of seriously affected babies, especially those who have had intra-uterine peritoneal injection of blood, have a long-lasting jaundice (mostly direct reacting pigment) and persistently enlarged liver and spleen. Provided the baby survives the first week of life the prognosis is for gradual improvement, but one must consider infection, including virus infection (*e.g.* cytomegalovirus, Australia antigen) from the mother or from the blood donor as a cause for the jaundice.

# Jaundice

**General Considerations**

*In utero*, a baby's unconjugated bilirubin is removed by the placenta and at birth his total bilirubin is usually below 3mg/100ml. If abnormal haemolysis has been occurring *in utero*, the placenta may not have been able to clear the load and higher levels are seen (see 'Haemolytic disease', p. 152). After birth, conjugation must occur in the baby's own liver, and in every baby there is a rise of serum bilirubin in the first days of life, after which the level should fall. In pre-term babies the rise will continue for longer (and thus may reach higher levels). When haemolysis occurs, the rise is much more rapid and very high levels may occur unless treated. Conditions which interfere with, or compete with, the glucuronyl transferase system will aggravate jaundice (drugs, anoxia, infection and lack of fluid.)

Kernikterus (see p. 186) occurs in babies whose serum unconjugated bilirubin reaches high levels. However, bilirubin levels alone are not a precise determinant of the risk of kernikterus, for some babies with levels under 20mg/100ml are affected, while some babies with levels above 40mg/100ml escape. In our experience, kernikterus in a baby whose highest recorded serum bilirubin level has been less than 20mg/100ml has always been a postmortem finding—always in very immature babies in whom there has been another satisfactory explanation for death. The very few cases of kernikterus in survivors have usually been mild—consisting of partial deafness—and have been confined to babies whose serum bilirubin we could not prevent from rising well above 20mg%.

Our aim in general is to keep the unconjugated bilirubin level below 20mg/100ml, though individual circumstances may influence the decision. In a healthy term infant levels a few mg higher may be acceptable. If plasma proteins are known to be low or if the baby is ill, hypoxic, acidaemic or showing abnormal neurological signs (see p. 173 and p. 186), we plan exchange transfusions to keep maximum levels slightly less than 20mg/100ml—say 18mg/100ml. We never use exchange transfusion merely to prevent a bilirubin level exceeding 15mg/100ml, even in small pre-term infants. We have not routinely used a measure of albumen-binding capacity for bilirubin as a guide to treatment, although there are theoretical grounds for supposing it might be helpful.

For other details of planning exchange transfusions in order to keep bilirubin levels below the required maximum, see p. 153.

**Estimating Bilirubin Levels Clinically**

Not every baby who has a tinge of jaundice should be subjected to heel-prick for serum bilirubin estimation. With a little experience, one can usually judge if a bilirubin level is not more than 10mg/100ml, in which case laboratory confirmation is not necessary, since even if the clinical error is as much as 5mg/100ml, the baby is most unlikely to come to harm. A clinical impression of severer jaundice calls for aboratory estimation of the bilirubin level. There is no substitute for some experience

156

when assessing the lower ranges of bilirubin, and no substitute for serum *measurements* when assessing levels of 12mg or more. Measurement at any time of day or night has been much simpler since the residents have been using the 'Bilirubinometer' (American Optical Corporation, A.O. No. 10200).

Jaundice is not usually visible in a baby until the bilirubin level exceeds 5mg/ 100ml. The light used when assessing jaundice is vitally important: whenever possible use natural daylight, for artificial light may lead either to an underestimate or an over- estimate. The colour of walls and decorations may also influence one's assessment. (The special care nursery should not be painted yellow.) The yellow colour of the skin reflects the bilirubin imprecisely, especially when jaundice is rapidly deepening or fading. In our experience, the perspex 'Icterometer' adds no precision to the clinical estimate of jaundice. In African and Asiatic babies, look at the gums and at the conjunctivae, and beware that you may grossly underestimate the level of jaundice.

### Interpretation of Reported Bilirubin Levels

Bilirubin levels are reported as 'x'mg/100ml total, with 'y'mg of direct reacting pigment. If the value 'y' is the usual 1 to 1.5mg it should be assumed that *all* the total bilirubin value is in fact unconjugated. When the value 'y' approaches 6mg/100ml or more, one can assume that there really is some conjugated pigment present and that 'x' minus 'y' represents the unconjugated bilirubin level.

### Situations When Jaundice Requires Further Investigation or Action

(1) Jaundice visible in the first 24 hours of life: this suggests haemolysis.

(2) Jaundice that is severe (clinically or by bilirubin level) *at any stage*, or ap- parently mild jaundice in coloured babies, since this may in fact be deep.

(3) Jaundice that seems to be improving and then recurs, or jaundice which first appears after the fourth day: this suggests infection, dehydration, or one of a number of rare diseases.

(4) Jaundice which persists for more than seven days (unless rapidly fading).

### Action to be Taken When a Baby is Found to be Jaundiced

*If the baby is less than 24 hours old*, the likelihood is that this is haemolytic disease (either ABO, or Rhesus haemolytic disease missed in pregnancy). Take blood for bilirubin, direct Coombs test, haemoglobin, blood group (including Rh factor) and find out the mother's blood groups. When the results are known, consider the need for exchange transfusion (see 'Haemolytic disease', p. 152), but whatever your decision *repeat a bilirubin estimation* a few hours later. If the baby is small for dates or has petechiae and enlarged liver and spleen, early jaundice may indicate prenatal infection (see p. 162).

*If the baby is 2-5 days old*, the probability is that this is physiological jaundice, but other causes are possible. Always consider infection and if the history, circum- stances or clinical signs suggest infection, take appropriate cultures and start treat- ment (see 'Infection', p. 165). Find out the mother's blood group, although haemolytic disease is unlikely in jaundice presenting after the second day. In any case, if the jaundice looks more than a clinically estimated 10mg/100ml, take blood for bilirubin,

157

direct Coombs test, haemoglobin, blood film, and blood group, including Rhesus factor (and in infants of African, Asian or Mediterranean origin, for a G-6-P-D screening test).

Check the child's feeding history and weight loss. Look for bruising and cephalhaematoma, and consider the possibility of internal bleeding. Inadequate fluid and food seriously aggravate all forms of jaundice, and absorption from a haematoma increases the load of bilirubin.

If the bilirubin level is high (15mg/100ml), repeat an estimation in an few hours *no matter what the diagnosis you have made* and be on the alert for early signs of kernikterus (see p. 186). If the bilirubin level is 8-12mg/100ml and serious causes of jaundice have been excluded, come back and look at the child in a few hours. Clinical observation for deepening jaundice may be all that is necessary, but if in doubt get another bilirubin estimation.

### Prolonged Jaundice

Most physiological jaundice is no longer visible by about the seventh day, though it may last longer in pre-term infants or in babies whose peak bilirubin reached 15-19mg/100ml. Consider the following possibilities.

Is the jaundice rapidly fading? If the child is clinically well no further action is necessary.

Is the jaundice only fading slowly or not fading at all? Check on his history (especially feeding history) and weight chart for any suggestion that he is getting inadequate fluid or that he is not well. Examine him for signs of infection (see p. 163) and obtain a specimen of urine to exclude urinary infection and galactosaemia. Other possibilities to be considered are mentioned below under 'Notes on Causes of Jaundice' and include bruising, breast-milk jaundice, drugs, cretinism and obstructive jaundice. When prolonged jaundice is only one of the signs in a very ill baby, the most important considerations are sepsis and metabolic disease.

Although the causes of prolonged jaundice are many, and some of them serious, a not uncommon outcome is that the jaundice fades somewhat later than usual with no apparent ill-effect. Arrange an appointment at the hospital follow-up clinic or with the general practitioner.

Many seriously affected rhesus babies, especially those who have had intra-uterine intraperitoneal transfusions, have a prolonged jaundice, with a high proportion of direct reacting bilirubin, which persists for many weeks. Provided the baby survives the first few days of life, the prognosis is usually good and the jaundice will eventually disappear. No specific therapeutic action is needed.

### Methods of Reducing Serum Bilirubin

(1) *Exchange transfusion.* This is the most reliable and the only quick method of reducing bilirubin levels, but it carries a risk of death (about 1 in 200) and of disease (infection, circulatory problems from misplaced catheters, possibility of isoimmunisation, etc.). For technique, see p. 274.

(2) *Adequate fluid and food.* When serum bilirubin is rising slowly towards a dangerous level, ensuring that the baby receives adequate fluid and calories is a most

important aspect of supportive treatment. (See 'Infant feeding', p. 96).

(3) *Phenobarbitone*. Barbiturates induce the activity of glucuronyl transferase, and giving phenobarbitone to the mother before delivery or to the baby after delivery has been shown to reduce the ultimate peak bilirubin achieved. Phenobarbitone cannot be expected to prevent high bilirubin levels if the rate of rise is very rapid. It may be useful when rates of rise are low or in preventing the need for second or third exchange transfusions in cases of haemolytic disease. It is not known whether phenobarbitone has adverse effects, so our use of phenobarbitone in an attempt to alleviate jaundice has been confined to individual cases in which conventional measures, including exchange transfusions, were not adequately controlling hyperbilirubinaemia.

(4) *Blue light*. Light from the blue-green visible spectrum (not infra-red or ultra-violet) converts bilirubin to biliverdin, which is water-soluble and harmless. This occurs *in vitro* when a specimen of serum is exposed to light. *In vivo* exposure to light converts the bilirubin in the skin circulation, but the effect on serum bilirubin is slow. Blue light is therefore useful only in the situations in which phenobarbitone treatment might also be useful (see above). We do not use phototherapy prophylactically, but in selected cases we expose the baby to 2000 foot candles making sure the eyes are adequately shielded.

### Notes on Causes of Jaundice

(1) *Haemolytic disease* caused by rhesus incompatibility (see p. 152).

(2) *ABO incompatibility*. When a mother is group O and the baby is group A or B or AB it is possible, though unusual, for maternal haemolysins to cross the placenta and cause haemolysis in the baby. It is not usual to diagnose ABO incompatibility in the antenatal period, although it should be anticipated if there has been a previously affected baby or if a group O mother has IgG haemolysins. In the cord blood the Coombs test is usually negative (although occasionally weakly positive). The jaundice of ABO incompatibility not infrequently has a slower onset than that of Rhesus incompatibility, and late anaemia is less common. Thus ABO incompatibility presents only as the practical problem of jaundice in the newborn and, although the condition is uncommon, it provides one good reason for examining *all* newborn babies for an unusual degree of jaundice.

A diagnosis of jaundice due to ABO incompatibility can only be justified when the mother is group O, the baby is group A or B or AB, when the baby has neonatal jaundice and the mother's serum is shown to have IgG haemolysins to the baby's group. Spherocytes are commonly present in the baby's peripheral blood.

(3) *Infection*. Apart from the common bacterial infections, especially Gram-negative sepsis, one must also consider listeriosis, viral infection, syphilis, etc. (see 'Infection', p. 162).

(4) *Haematoma and bruising*. Large haematomata (for instance subaponeurotic haematoma, see p. 206) or extensive bruising (after a breech extraction in a very small baby for instance) or swallowed maternal blood all leave an added load of bilirubin to be cleared; and bilirubin levels may be expected to be higher and more prolonged in such cases.

(5) *Other haemolytic diseases.*

(*a*) GLUCOSE-6-PHOSPHATE DEHYDROGENASE DEFICIENCY. This occurs in Mediterranean, Asian and African peoples. It occurs as an x-linked condition, not always recessive, so that girls may be affected. The jaundice may be severe enough to necessitate exchange transfusion. The mother who is breast-feeding must avoid all drugs or food which are known to precipitate a crisis. Clothes stored in naphthalene moth-balls are a hazard to affected babies. A single 1mg dose of phytomenadione ('Konakion') may be given without harmful effects, if otherwise indicated.

(*b*) SPHEROCYTOSIS. There will be a family history of acholuric jaundice, unless the case is a new mutant. A blood film examined by an experienced haematologist for spherocytes is the most useful diagnostic test at this age, but spherocytes may be found in other conditions in the newborn. The jaundice may only rarely require treatment. Arrange follow-up.

(*c*) PYRUVATE KINASE DEFICIENCY AND OTHER RED-CELL ENZYME DEFICIENCIES may be associated with serious jaundice in the newborn period. The jaundice is treated to prevent kernikterus, and any subsequent anaemia is investigated at a later date. Most such diseases are inherited as autosomal recessive traits.

(6) *Breast-milk jaundice.* It has been suggested that some mothers excrete a steroid in their breast milk which aggravates jaundice by competing with bilirubin for conjugation. The clinical histories of a number of healthy breast-fed babies with protracted jaundice due to indirect-reacting bilirubin support the possibility. What is called 'breast-milk jaundice' may often simply be due to under-feeding. There is no evidence that breast-milk jaundice ever harmed a baby.

(7) *Drugs.* Certain drugs may aggravate jaundice by competing for conjugation, or increase the possibility of kernikterus by displacing bilirubin from albumen-binding sites (or both).

Examples of such drugs, which are therefore relatively or absolutely contra-indicated in the first week or two of life, are:

sulphonamides
vitamin K analogues (*e.g.* 'Synkavit')
oleandomycin
novobiocin
salicylates
diazepam injection.
(Steroids also compete for conjugation.)

(8) *Cretinism.* One of the manifestations of cretinism, usually recognised in retrospect, is neonatal jaundice prolonged for some weeks. In a baby with pro-longed jaundice who has a family or maternal history of hypothyroidism, or who is unduly lethargic and constipated, arrange a screening test for cretinism. The usual screening tests are an estimate of plasma protein-bound iodine or the $T_3$-uptake of red cells.

(9) *Galactosaemia.* Prolonged neonatal jaundice with mainly conjugated pigment is one of its early manifestations, which also include failure to thrive, poor feeding, vomiting, hepatomegaly and cataracts (see p. 226).

(10) *Other metabolic disease.* A number of other metabolic disorders (amino-

acidurias, organicacidaemias, etc.) may cause prolonged jaundice, usually in a seriously ill, acidotic infant. With such a presentation, collect urine for amino-acid and other organic acid measurements, and in the meantime treat the child with intravenous fluids for any dehydration, acidaemia, or electrolyte disturbance (see p. 99).

(11) *Hepatitis and bile duct atresia.* Both present signs of obstructive jaundice, sometimes as early as the end of the first week. They may be impossible to distinguish clinically and biochemically (see Thaler and Gellis 1968*). Intrahepatic bile-duct atresia may be an end result of severe hepatitis rather than a separate entity. The jaundice develops insidiously, and total bilirubin may not be high. The known causes of hepatitis to be excluded are: certain intra-uterine infections (see p. 162); inborn errors of metabolism such as galactosaemia (see p. 226); tyrosinosis (plasma and urinary amino-acid chromatography); cystic fibrosis (see p. 195); and $\alpha_1$ antitrypsin deficiency. The blood should be screened for Australia antigen; evidence of placental transmission has been reported and carrier mothers could infect their infants at delivery or later, in which case symptoms and signs of hepatitis might not appear for several weeks or months after birth. In the majority no cause will be found, and as two-thirds of the hepatitis cases recover completely, we favour conservative management. Only a very small minority of bile-duct atresias are operable and waiting for up to four months before exploratory laparotomy appears not to jeopardise the chances of success in the latter, and will avoid the risk of rapid deterioration and death which may occur if young infants with hepatitis are subjected to operation.

(12) *Crigler-Najjar and Dubin-Johnson syndromes.* These very rare diseases are due to defects of conjugation or of intrahepatic transport. We have yet to diagnose a case.

(13) *Dehydration*, on the other hand, is a relatively common cause of jaundice mentioned several times above and emphasized by being mentioned again.

*Thaler, M. M., Gellis, S. S. (1968) 'Studies in neonatal hepatitis and biliary atresia. I-IV.' *American Journal of Diseases of Children*, **116**, 257.

# Infection

Infectious illness in a newborn baby may have originated before, during or after birth.

**Prenatal and Intrapartum Infections**

When the mother is known to have had a disease in pregnancy, follow the instructions in Table II, p. 21 *et seq.* However, in most cases of intra-uterine infection, the maternal component has gone undetected. Many instances of maternal infection in pregnancy are retrospectively diagnosed because of what has happened to the baby. The obstetrician will consider the possibility of infectious disease in pregnancy in cases of abortion, premature birth, intra-uterine growth failure or stillbirth; in addition the paediatrician should consider this possibility when a baby shows certain abnormalities which are listed in Table VIII. Obviously many of these abnormalities may have a non-infective aetiology, but when in doubt, carry out the relevant investigations listed in Table II, p. 21 *et seq.*

Most of these infections are acquired prenatally, but some organisms may be acquired in passage through the birth canal, including *N. gonorrhoeae, Candida albicans*, bowel pathogens, cytomegalovirus and *Herpesvirus hominis*. Bacterial infection acquired in the birth canal may, on occasions, lead to overwhelming sepsis and death within 48 hours. In recent years this has most frequently been reported in cases of infection with group B, β haemolytic streptococci.

**Diagnosis of Prenatal Infection**

We routinely collect cord blood from all babies born at the Hammersmith Hospital and measure immunoglobulins in small-for-dates babies and others in whom intra-uterine infection is suspected. Most small-for-dates babies have normal levels, but remember that intra-uterine infection is a cause of growth retardation.

Because IgM is produced by the baby and not passively transferred, high levels (above 20mg/100ml) in cord blood may be indicative of intra-uterine infection. However, the level is sometimes normal where there is undoubted prenatal infection and must obviously be normal if the infection has been acquired during passage through the birth canal. In contrast, raised levels have sometimes been inexplicable in terms of intra-uterine infection. When high levels are found, repeat the test, and if the level is still high, collect specimens from the baby and his mother for culture and serology (see p. 21 *et seq.*).

A positive culture from the baby is diagnostic, but not all the infections listed in Table VIII can be thus diagnosed. When positive serological tests are obtained, indicate on the summary of the baby's case notes that he should be re-tested in three or four months time. A retrospective diagnosis of infection can only be sustained if specific antibodies persist in the baby's serum, which will not be the case if they have been passively acquired from his mother. On the other hand, *specific IgM* fluorescent antibody tests on the baby's blood do, when available, allow an *immediate* diagnosis of such infections as cytomegalovirus, rubella, toxoplasmosis and syphilis.

**Postnatal Infection**

The common ways in which infection may be acquired after birth are discussed on page 110.

In general, symptoms of postnatal infection are not likely to present before the third or fourth day, but very rarely bacterial invasion occurring immediately after birth (*e.g.* from contaminated resuscitation apparatus) may be so overwhelming that death will occur within 48 hours.

**Pathogens**

It is important to realise that virtually any bacteria are capable of causing disease in the infant. Some of those least disturbing to healthy adults (*e.g. Pseudomonas aeruginosa*) cause lethal illness in the pre-term baby. Many other antibiotic resistant Gram-negative organisms of this nature flourish in the humidification units of apparatus.

We diagnose non-bacterial infective illness less commonly, perhaps because we look for it less often, but epidemics of respiratory infection caused by respiratory syncytial virus and adenovirus type 7 may occur, and neonatal meningitis due to postnatally acquired Coxsackie and Echo viruses is known. We have not encountered *Pneumocystis carinii* infection.

**Suspecting and Diagnosing Infection**

Be on the alert for infection in babies of low birthweight, those with congenital anomalies, those born after prolonged rupture of the membranes or a protracted and difficult labour, those with any other serious non-infective illness, and particularly those who have had tubes inserted anywhere or who have been attached to moist apparatus. It is interesting, but diagnostically unhelpful, to know that male infants are more often the victims of infection than females.

Superficial infections may be obvious, and parenteral infection should strongly be suspected in any baby who is gravely ill. However, even serious infection in newborn babies may present with gradual, vague or non-specific symptoms, *e.g.* lethargic sucking or refusal of feeds, failure to gain weight or weight loss, vomiting and/or diarrhoea (which may be slight and intermittent), a late appearance of jaundice, 'cyanotic attacks', abdominal distension and fever.* In the absence of any of these symptoms, the first indication that a baby has an infection may be provided by the mother who is worried, or by the nursing staff who say that the baby has 'gone off' (see p. 240).

---

*Dehydration also may undoubtedly cause fever, but differentiation from an infective illness is usually not difficult. In cases of dehydration fever, the baby's weight will usually be less than 90 per cent of his birthweight; he will look well (red in the face); he will be vigorous and will drink water avidly, following which his temperature will fall to normal within a few hours. If you are in doubt, a measurement of plasma osmolality may be helpful, since it is usually above 300m osmol/kg water, which is seldom the case in infective fevers.

## TABLE VIII
### Neonatal signs of prenatal infection

| Possible clinical involvement | Infecting agents |
| --- | --- |
| **CENTRAL NERVOUS SYSTEM** | |
| Microcephaly | Cytomegalovirus (CMV), *Toxoplasma gondii*, rubella virus |
| Hydrocephalus | Bacteria, CMV, *Herpesvirus hominis* (HVH), *Toxoplasma gondii* |
| Abnormal CNS signs, fits | Bacteria, *Candida albicans*, Coxsackie virus, CMV, HVH, poliovirus, rubella virus, *Treponema pallidum*, variola virus. |
| Cerebral calcification | Bacteria, CMV, HVH, rubella virus, *Toxoplasma gondii* |
| **SPECIAL SENSORY ORGANS** | |
| Eye: cataracts | Rubella virus, *Toxoplasma gondii* |
| choroido-retinitis | CMV, HVH, rubella virus, *Toxoplasma gondii* |
| microphthalmia | Rubella virus, *Toxoplasma gondii* |
| keratitis and corneal opacity | HVH, rubella virus, *Treponema pallidum* |
| purulent ophthalmia | *Neisseria gonorrhoea*, or other bacteria *Mycoplasma hominis*, TRIC agent |
| Ear: eighth nerve damage (may not be detected even with special techniques) | Rubella virus, *Treponema pallidum* |
| **CARDIOVASCULAR SYSTEM** | |
| Congenital heart disease (patent ductus arteriosus, pulmonary artery stenosis, pulmonary valve stenosis, ventricular septal defect, aberrant subclavian vessels) | Rubella virus |
| Peripheral arterial stenoses | Rubella virus |
| Myocarditis | Coxsackie B virus, poliovirus |
| Pericarditis | Bacteria |
| **RESPIRATORY SYSTEM** | |
| Pneumonia | Bacteria, *Candida albicans*, Coxsackie virus, CMV, HVH, *Mycobacterium tuberculosis*, *Mycoplasma hominis*, poliovirus, rubella virus, *Treponema pallidum*, vaccinia virus, varicella-zoster virus, variola virus |
| **SKELETAL SYSTEM** | |
| Periostitis and/or defective mineralisation and growth disturbance | CMV, HVH, rubella virus, *Toxoplasma gondii*, *Treponema pallidum* |
| **GASTRO-INTESTINAL SYSTEM** | |
| Hepatosplenomegaly with or without jaundice | Coxsackie virus, CMV, hepatitis-associated antigen, HVH, *Mycobacterium tuberculosis*, plasomodia, rubella virus, *Toxoplasma gondii*, *Treponema pallidum*, vaccinia virus, varicella-zoster virus, variola virus |
| Enteritis | Enteropathogenic *Escherichia coli*, *Shigellae*, *Salmonellae* |

164

TABLE VIII (cont.)

| Possible clinical involvement | Infecting Agents |
|---|---|
| **GENITO-URINARY SYSTEM** | |
| Nephritis, nephrotic syndrome | *Treponema pallidum* |
| **HAEMATOPOIETIC SYSTEM** | |
| Anaemia, sometimes haemolytic with jaundice | Bacteria, CMV, HVH, rubella virus, *Toxoplasma gondii, Treponema pallidum* |
| Purpura, with or without disseminated intravascular coagulation (some haemorrhagic skin nodules are erythropoietic in nature) | Coxsackie virus, CMV, HVH, rubella virus, *Toxoplasma gondii, Treponema pallidum* |
| **SKIN AND MUCOUS MEMBRANE** | |
| Vesicular lesions, single, grouped or scattered, sometimes unilateral | HVH, varicella-zoster virus, *Treponema pallidum* |
| Large umbilicated lesions | Vaccinia and variola viruses |
| Macular or maculo-papular lesions | *Treponema pallidum* |
| Mouth - 'milk curd' lesions leaving raw area when removed | *Candida albicans* |
| Skin - papulo-vesicular and scaling | *Candida albicans* |
| Pustules, abscesses | Bacteria, *Mycoplasma hominis* |

In these circumstances, examine the baby for signs of infection, general and localised. An elevated or sub-normal temperature, jaundice of late onset (*i.e.* onset after the third day), pallor, raised pulse and respiration rate, unresponsiveness to examination, and enlarged kidneys, liver or spleen may be found as a consequence of infection at any site. Localizing signs of infection include skin pustules (including paronychia), discharging umbilicus, conjunctivitis, mastitis, infected superficial wounds and nasal discharge. Osteomyelitis may present with pseudoparalysis or an inflammatory subcutaneous swelling. The superficial infections and osteomyelitis are, for the most part, the work of Gram-positive organisms, especially *staphylococcus pyogenes*, and since we seldom see infection with this organism to-day, pay particular attention to the possibility of parenteral infection without localizing signs. Consider the possibilities of pneumonia (p. 119), meningitis, urinary infection, and septicaemia. The finding of definite but slight evidence of superficial infection should not of course blind you to the possibility of a more serious parenteral infection (it would be a pity to treat meningitis with local applications of gentian violet for oral thrush).

**Laboratory Diagnosis of Infection**
*Bacterial Infection*
The following are the routine laboratory procedures useful in the diagnosis of infection. Swab cultures must be made in every case of suspected infection. With the

occasional exception of CSF culture, the remainder must be carried out in every case of suspected *parenteral* infection. Consult the senior paediatrician if in doubt about the necessity for lumbar puncture.

(1) *Swab cultures.* Always take swabs from nose, throat, umbilicus and rectum, and any suspicious skin lesions. If there is likely to be delay in the plating out of the specimens, put the swab in a Stuart's transport medium bottle, breaking off the stick without touching the lower end.

Swabs from the first four sites mentioned will be sterile at birth in the great majority, but by the third day most infants will become colonised. Light growths are usually not important. Infection is more likely to occur in infants who are moderately or heavily colonised at nose, throat or umbilicus; and is commoner when this heavy colonisation is predominantly Gram-negative or predominantly Gram-positive, rather than mixed. Heavy colonisation, however, does not automatically mean infection; it is likely to be present in any sick infant, whatever the cause.

(2) *Blood cultures.* Whenever possible use peripheral veins, because falsely positive cultures may result when blood is drawn from an umbilical vein catheter. Although the amount of blood you withdraw will of necessity be small, try to get enough to inoculate three culture bottles, as this makes interpretation of results easier. A pure growth of one organism in all three bottles is significant; anything less should be considered doubtful. Blood-stream invasion by two different bacilli is known, but is rare. Remember that the growth of coagulase negative staphylococci may well indicate a genuine infection in the newborn.

(3) *Urine.* (See p. 283 for techniques of collection.) Normal clean-catch urines will have fewer than 10 leucocytes/mm$^3$ in both sexes, and bacterial counts of below $10^5$/ml. Use Trypan blue to differentiate renal tubular cells and leucocytes.

(4) *CSF.* Always ask the pathologist to make a Gram-stain because bacteria may be present without a raised cell-count at this age. Send even the smallest or most blood-stained amount of CSF collected for culture.

(5) *White cell count.* From 96 hours of age, the total neutrophil count varies little in healthy infants. The mean is 4100/mm$^3$ with a $\pm$ 2 S.D. range of 1400–6900/mm$^3$ (Xanthou 1970)*. Counts above or below this may therefore indicate infection, but are not absolutely diagnostic. An increase in immature and band forms, and the presence of toxic granulation, should also be regarded as suspicious. Repeat the WBC the following day.

(6) *Immunoglobulins.* A single estimation of IgM is of little immediate diagnostic help, but a sharp rise above mean for the age (see p. 330) over a seven-day period from the start of an illness would give confirmatory retrospective evidence.

### Viral Infection

We believe that acquired viral infection in the early neonatal period is much less common than is bacterial infection, but this may be because viral infection is more difficult to diagnose. However, viral infection should be thought of and looked for in cases of respiratory infection or diarrhoea, where no bacterial pathogen is isolated

*Xanthou, M. (1970) 'Leucocyte blood picture in healthy full-term and premature babies during neonatal period.' *Archives of Disease in Childhood*, **45**, 242.

(as well as in the case of symptoms or signs suggesting prenatal or intra-natal viral infection, see above). Consult the virologist about the collection and treatment of specimens. In the case of respiratory infection of possibly viral origin, ask him to use the direct fluorescent antibody technique on cells from nasal secretions—one of the very few viral investigations which gives a quick answer.

## Treatment of Bacterial Infection
### Indications for Antibiotics
It is rarely right to wait for the results of investigations for bacterial infection before starting treatment, for deterioration can be very rapid indeed in an infected baby. Thus we know that we over-prescribe antibiotics in the neonatal period: nevertheless we do not use antibiotics in a deliberately prophylactic sense.

We do not use systemic antibiotics routinely in babies having umbilical vessel catheterization or exchange transfusion, nor in cases of respiratory distress thought to be due to hyaline membrane disease, nor in an apparently well baby born after prolonged rupture of the membranes.

We do use antibiotics if there is definite evidence of a parenteral infection or if suspected as in any of the following situations.
(1) In infants who are known to have come from an infected intra-uterine environment (*i.e.* maternal fever and rigors during labour, purulent or foul-smelling liquor, etc.) *and who appear ill at birth.*
(2) In infants presenting with any of the vague symptoms listed on p. 163.
(3) In infants with respiratory distress who appear to be deteriorating or who develop moist sounds in the lungs.
(4) In infants with a discharging umbilicus, particularly if there is any local induration suggesting venous thrombosis.
(5) In infants with a profusely discharging eye, particularly if there is any periorbital oedema (see also p. 169 for local treatment).
(6) In infants suspected of having necrotizing enterocolitis (*e.g.* with abdominal distension, ladder patterning, bile-stained vomiting presenting after previously normal bowel function).
(7) In skin sepsis, including paronychia, if of more than a minor degree.

### Choice of Antibiotics
General policy will depend on prevailing bacterial flora and sensitivities, and changes every few years may be necessary. We use a combination of benzylpenicillin and kanamycin at present,* as staphylococcal colonisation is at a minimum and *Escherichia coli* strains are sensitive to kanamycin.

Other useful drugs in varying circumstances may be: gentamicin; chloramphenicol; ampicillin and kanamycin; ampicillin and cloxacillin; cephaloridine. (See p. 170 for dosage.)

---

*As we go to press the useful life of this combination, used by us now for over five years, may be coming to an end, as some kanamycin-resistant strains of *Escherichia coli* are appearing. Gentamicin will be substituted.

If infection with *Pseudomonas aeruginosa* or some of the other kanamycin-resistant Gram-negative organisms such as klebsiella is suspected, the antibiotics which may be effective are polymyxin, colistin, carbenicillin and gentamicin. If Pseudomonas infection is suspected, we usually start with gentamicin and penicillin, substituting carbenicillin for penicillin when proof is forthcoming*. *Listeria monocytogenes* and *Vibrio fetus* are both sensitive to streptomycin, and thus presumably to kanamycin and to chloramphenicol.

*Route of Administration and Duration of Treatment*

We have found blood levels of penicillin and kanamycin to be satisfactory, even in very ill infants, following intramuscular injection, and we nearly always use this route* at least in the first week of life, because of uncertainty of absorption from the gastro-intestinal tract, and always in serious infection. We usually give the drugs for at least five days, for as long as ten days to those with proven blood-stream infection, and for even longer if meningitis, osteomyelitis or urinary infection is present (see below). Before starting antibiotics, take the necessary specimens for bacteriology (see above). (For dosage, see p. 170.)

*Treatment of Specific Bacterial Infections*

(1) MENINGITIS

We see meningitis very rarely. Over 70 per cent of cases are due to Gram-negative organisms, mainly coliforms. Until definite identification has been made, we give penicillin with kanamycin†. Other drugs which may be used instead at present include chloramphenicol, gentamicin, carbenicillin and ampicillin. Give the first dose intravenously, and then continue with intramuscular treatment for at least three weeks. We are not convinced about the necessity for intrathecal treatment, particularly because it presents practical difficulties in the smallest babies, but have CSF antibiotic levels measured after 24 hours treatment and give intrathecal treatment if they are too low.** In meningitis associated with myelomeningocele and hydrocephalus, intraventricular treatment is necessary for good results, but we do not always treat. Kanamycin, gentamicin and polymyxin (for pseudomonas) are suitable intrathecal drugs, with penicillin probably useful only in streptococcal meningitis. A combination of trimethoprim and sulphamethoxazole ('Septrin') has been reported curative in a case of *Esch. coli* meningitis, after failure of other drugs, but we have no experience of its use and the manufacturers state that it must not be used in the first month of life. It *must* be avoided if jaundice is present. Carbenicillin given intrathecally is also effective in the treatment of pseudomonas meningitis, but if the case is one of myelomeningocele, we transfer the baby to the children's ward for fear of establishing a carbenicillin-resistant strain of pseudomonas in the special care nursery.

*Many I.V. fluids are unsuitable vehicles for drug infusion—especially acidic solutions such as dextrose, in which benzylpenicillin and ampicillin lose varying degrees of activity. Carbenicillin and gentamicin should not be mixed in solution. No drugs should be added to amino-acid solutions or fat emulsions. (See also p. 101.)

†See footnote on p. 167.

**To achieve adequate CSF levels considerably larger doses than those listed in Table IX are needed when hydrocephalus is present. See Lorber, J., Kalhan, S. C., Mahgrefte, B. (1970) 'Treatment of ventriculitis with gentamicin and cloxacillin in infants born with spina bifida.' *Archives of Disease in Childhood*, **45**, 178.

## (2) OSTEOMYELITIS

Gram-negative organisms may be assuming more importance in aetiology with the control of staphylococcal colonisation. To cover both possibilities, use methicillin or cloxacillin combined with kanamycin* or ampicillin. Give the drugs for three weeks, by the oral route after the first 10-14 days. Local aspiration of pus by wide-bore needle is now usually preferable to open operation.

## (3) URINARY INFECTION

In the first week, we give kanamycin* or ampicillin; once the period of physiological jaundice is over, the sulphonamides are still the drugs of choice. In most cases they can be given orally, but should be continued for six weeks. Nalidixic acid should be avoided in the neonatal period. Look for clinical evidence of urinary tract obstruction (poor urinary stream or dribbling, distension of bladder, abdominal mass which might indicate hydronephrosis or hydroureter, or ascites). Examine external genitalia for malformations which might predispose to urinary infection, *i.e.* intersex, abnormal position of anus or rectovaginal fistula. Look for spinal deformities and/or evidence of paraplegia. Measure blood urea. If all this is normal we do not usually do intra-venous pyelography unless follow-up of the baby is uncertain or the infection recurs after treatment.

## (4) GASTRO-ENTERITIS

(See p. 201.)

## (5) CONJUNCTIVITIS

A *profuse purulent discharge* from one, or more commonly both eyes is likely to be due to gonococcal infection, especially if it presents in the first 48 hours. A swab should be taken and sent at once to the duty pathologist who should be contacted by telephone and the likelihood that the infection is gonococcal explained to him. Even if gonococci are not identified on a smear, it is best to treat as if gonococcal and not to await the results of culture.

Give penicillin eye-drops (2,500 units per ml) very frequently for one hour, and gradually reduce the frequency as the discharge clears. Also give systemic benzyl penicillin (for dosage see Table IX). If this treatment is given assiduously, there is always marked improvement within six hours. If there is not, we suspect the presence of a coliform organism (see below).

A *sticky eye without purulence* should merely be washed with saline and observed, after taking a swab.

A *sticky eye with purulence* should be swabbed, and sulphacetamide 10% eye-drops instilled as frequently as possible for one hour, and then three-hourly until the result of culture is known. If only one eye is affected, lie the baby on the affected side.

A *sticky eye with purulence and evidence of periorbital extension or generalized illness* should be treated like any other systemic infection (see above). (Remember that osteomyelitis of the maxilla may present in this way.) Also give sulphacetamide 10% eye-drops until the results of culture are known.

Conjunctivitis caused by *Mycoplasma hominis* should be diagnosed on routine

*See footnote on p. 167.

## TABLE IX
### Suggested dosage

| Antibiotic or chemotherapeutic drug | Single intramuscular dose. (See p. 171 for frequency.)* | Single intrathecal dose. (See footnote **on p. 168) | Oral dose‡ per 24 hrs. (Give in 4 divided doses) |
|---|---|---|---|
| Cephaloridine[2] | 15mg/kg | | |
| Chloramphenicol | 12.5mg/kg (Max. daily dose should not exceed 25mg/kg for first week of life in term babies, first 4 weeks in pre-term). | | |
| Colistin | 25,000u/kg (Max. daily dose should not exceed 75,000u/kg.) | | 125,000u/kg |
| Erythromycin | 5mg/kg | | 25mg/kg |
| Gentamicin[1] | 2.5mg/kg | 1.0mg | |
| Kanamycin[1] | 5mg/kg (Increase to 7.5mg/kg after first 48 hours of life in term babies, and after first week in pre-term). | 1.0mg | |
| Neomycin | 2.5mg/kg | | 50mg/kg |
| Penicillins: | | | |
|   Benzylpenicillin | 15,000u/kg | 1000u | 40,000u/kg |
|   Ampicillin | 25mg/kg | | 60mg/kg |
|   Carbenicillin | 100mg/kg | 5mg | |
|   Cloxacillin | 12.5 mg/kg | 2.5 mg | 30mg/kg |
|   Methicillin | 20mg/kg | | |
| Polymyxin methane sulphonate | 20,000u/kg (Max. daily dose should not exceed 40,000u/kg.) | 5000u | |
| Streptomycin[1] | 7.5mg/kg (Increase to 10mg/kg after first 48 hours of life in term babies, and after first week in pre-term). | | 20mg/kg |
| Sulphadimidine | 7.5mg/kg | | 50mg/kg |
| Nystatin | | | 400,000 units |

EYE PREPARATIONS:     Sulphacetamide eye-drops, B.P.C. (10%)
Chloramphenicol eye-drops, B.P.C. (0.5%)
Chlortetracycline eye ointment, B.P.C. (1%)

SKIN PREPARATIONS:    Crystal violet paint, B.P.C. (0.5%)
Nystatin ointment
Hexachlorophane dusting powder, B.P.C.
Polymyxin B, Bacitracin and Neomycin (Polybactrin) Aerosol

ORAL PREPARATIONS:    Crystal violet paint, B.P.C. (0.5%)

*See p. 171 for notes.*

culture, provided the plates are kept for 48 hours. Treat with chlortetracycline eye ointment B.P.C. (1%).

The TRIC agent may also cause conjunctivitis, and this infection should be suspected when the onset of conjunctivitis occurs a few days after birth. For diagnosis, see p. 26. Treat with sulphacetamide eye-drops or chlortetracycline eye-ointment.

If there is a persistent discharge from one or both eyes, consider blocked naso-lacrimal duct (see p. 244).

(6) CONGENITAL OR POST-NATALLY ACQUIRED TUBERCULOSIS
Isoniazid 10mg/kg/day (given 6-hourly, orally)†.

## Treatment of Non-bacterial Infection
*Fungal*

| | |
|---|---|
| ORAL MONILIASIS | Crystal violet paint B.P.C. (the correct name for what we will continue to call gentian violet). Put 3-4 drops under tongue once or twice daily and the infant will probably get it around the mouth more effectively than if painted on individual lesions. We use this first unless we are talked out of it by the nursing staff. If it does not work after two days, try: Nystatin mixture B.P.C, 100,000 U (1ml) 6-hourly, orally. |
| PERINEAL MONILIASIS | Crystal violet paint B.P.C., *or* Nystatin ointment. |

*Protozoal*

| | |
|---|---|
| CONGENITAL MALARIA | We have never treated a case, but are always prepared for it to come our way. Nivaquine (chloroquine injection) 10mg of base (0.25ml) I.M. daily for five days. |

†Newer antituberculous drugs may be necessary, depending on infecting adult's drug sensitivity patterns, but we have no experience of their use in the neonatal period.

---

*\*INTRAMUSCULAR DOSAGE:*
*For term infants* (more than 37 weeks gestation), give above doses every 12 hours if in first 48 hours of life, 8-hourly if between third day and two weeks, and 6-hourly if over two weeks, unless otherwise indicated.
*For pre-term infants* (less than 37 weeks gestation), give every 12 hours if in first week of life, 8-hourly if between one and four weeks, and 6-hourly if over four weeks, unless otherwise indicated.

*INTRAVENOUS DOSAGE:*
No available guides to dosage based on serum levels—should probably not exceed two-thirds the intramuscular dosage.

*‡ORAL DOSE:*
Absorption from gastro-intestinal tract may be uncertain during first week of life in term infants, and during first two weeks of life in pre-term infants. Intramuscular dosage is therefore preferable during these periods.

1 Need not be given more than 12-hourly if I.M.
2 Need not be given more than 8-hourly if I.M.

TOXOPLASMOSIS*

We have rarely treated a case, and the correct course of treatment seems uncertain.

If treatment is begun after the first week of life, give sulpha-diazine 150mg/kg/day (given 6-hourly, orally) with pyrimethamine 1mg/kg/day (given 12-hourly, orally) for three days, and then 0.5mg/kg/day, together, for one month. The drugs have a synergistic action. In the unlikely event of treatment being started in the first week of life, do not give the sulphadiazine until the end of the first week because of the danger of bilirubin displacement from protein-binding sites. Watch for thrombocytopenic purpura and leucopenia as side effects of pyrimethamine.

*Spirochaetal*

CONGENITAL SYPHILIS

Procaine penicillin 150mg (150,000 units) daily (as single I.M. dose) for 15 days. (See also p. 23.)

*Viral*

HERPESVIRUS HOMINIS AND CMV INFECTION*

The treatment of these with idoxuridine is still experimental and convincing evidence of benefit has still to be accumulated. We have no personal experience to record. Idoxuridine 50mg/kg/day by continuous I.V. drip over four days or to a total dosage of 200-300mg/kg is said to be safe.

*There seems little be to gained by treating infants in whom extensive CNS involvement is already apparent at birth.

172

# Neurological Examination of the Newborn

Neurological examination provides less information in the newborn baby than in older people and, except in the case of certain peripheral lesions, it does not usually enable one to make an anatomical diagnosis. Neonatal neurological examinations are usually done for one of three purposes.

(1) To help in the diagnosis of a clinically evident illness.

(2) To help in predicting future neurological development, whether or not there is an evident illness. Our belief is that routine neurological examination of the apparently well baby is not at present worthwhile for this purpose in ordinary paediatric practice. There is no doubt that such examinations can have some predictive value, but we are concerned (a) about the reliability of short screening procedures, which are the only ones which at present might be practicable for routine use, (b) whether the return from the benefits of early diagnosis justifies the expenditure of medical manpower required, and (c) whether these benefits, which we believe are often exaggerated, outweigh the possible disadvantages of an incorrect diagnosis of neurological abnormality, which would undoubtedly be made in some cases. We therefore do not recommend a formal neurological examination as a routine in every newborn baby, though we are prepared to change our recommendation in the light of further evidence.

(3) To assess gestational age (see p. 91).

In the subsequent discussion, we assume that the purpose of the examination is (1) or a combination of (1) and (2).

*General Principles of Neurological Examination*

Observation of the baby may be more valuable than formal examination. The mother and nursing staff generally observe the baby for much longer than the examiner: enquire therefore about the pattern of sleep, activity and crying; feeding behaviour; whether the baby seems to look and follow with his eyes; whether there are any abnormal movements and whether the baby lies with his eyes open and staring for long periods. A baby who is reported by the nursing staff to be normal in all these respects is rather unlikely to have serious trouble in the CNS (though we have known a baby with hydranencephaly who reportedly behaved normally in the first few weeks).

It is essential to take into account the baby's 'state', and we use the classification of states of Prechtl and Beintema (1964).*

STATE 1: Eyes closed, regular respiration, no movements (other than an occasional whole-body jerk)

STATE 2: Eyes closed, irregular respiration, no gross movements

STATE 3: Eyes open, no gross movements

STATE 4: Eyes open, gross movements, no crying

STATE 5: Eyes open or closed, crying.

*Prechtl, H. F. R., Beintema, D. (1964) *The Neurological Examination of the Newborn Infant*. Clinics in Developmental Medicine, No. 12. London: S.I.M.P. with Heinemann.

The normal baby goes through a fairly regular cycle of states. During sleep, roughly 45-minute periods of State 2 (rapid-eye-movement sleep) alternate with 15 to 20 minute periods of State 1. Disturbance of the state cycle may be an early and important sign of CNS disturbance.

The results of many parts of the neurological examination are considerably influenced by the baby's state: most parts of the examination are best carried out in States 3 and 4. The state during the examination should always be recorded.

Ideally, the examination should be carried out on a surface with a slight curvature, on·which the baby is more secure than on a hard, flat surface. A mattress with some 'give', or a table with a slightly curved surface is suitable. The room must be warm (certainly not less that 22°C (75°F), and preferably warmer). Observe the baby first in whatever clothing he has on and do the visual tests if he is in State 3 or 4, but undress him for the remainder of the examination. The examination has to be somewhat limited when the baby is in an incubator. It should always be done with circumspection in ill babies. Remember in particular that babies with respiratory difficulty or apnoeic attacks withstand handling very poorly.

Simply for purposes of description, the examination may conveniently be divided into four main parts. It is not suggested that the individual items should necessarily be done in the order given here; on the whole, opportunism is the key to success in this examination.

(1) *General Observations Referable to the Central Nervous System*

(a) *Skull*—circumference (hydrocephalus or microcephaly—see OFC charts, pp. 326-327).

Anterior fontanelle (bulging or sunken?). Remember it is usually small in the first 48 hours.

Suture separation. In the first 48 hours, the vault bones may overlap. After this it is easy to appreciate that the vault bones are just separate, and the posterior and parietal fontanelles are easily palpable for the first few weeks. Even wide separation between the vault bones does not indicate hydrocephalus unless the skull circumference is increased. This delay in membrane bone formation *may* indicate osteogenesis imperfecta, hypothyroidism or congenital rubella, but usually does not. It is not uncommon for otherwise normal babies to have delayed ossification of the vault bones and thus persistent fontanelles and gaps in the suture lines.

Sutures ridging. A ridge at the suture line is easily distinguishable from overriding. A ridge at the metopic suture (anterior to the anterior fontanelle) is a normal, though unusual, variant. Ridges at the other suture lines imply premature closure (craniostenosis).

Auscultation is rarely informative, but a bruit may be heard in cases of angiomatous malformation, which may present with congestive heart failure and fits in the neonatal period.

Transillumination should be done in any baby whose head is abnormal in size and appearance, and in any baby who is neurologically abnormal. Transillumination must be done in a *totally* dark room, using a light which can be fitted closely to the baby's scalp. Allow yourself time for dark adaptation. There is normally a halo of light around the rim of the illuminator, about 1cm wide in the occipital region and 2.5cm wide frontally (more in pre-term infants). Abnormal transillumination is seen when there is an abnormal collection of fluid in the head which reaches to within 1cm of the skull. Such a collection may be ventricular, intracerebral, subarachnoid or subdural. Not too much importance should be attached to minor variations from normal—we have sometimes been misled into unnecessary investigations in these circumstances.

(b) *Spine*. Look for any midline abnormalities over it (see p. 180).

(c) *Fundi*. Retinal haemorrhages are probably of no special neurological significance, and papilloedema is a very unusual feature of increased intracranial pressure in the newborn. Don't waste too much time on the fundi. (See also p. 241.)

(d) *Pupils*. Pupil reactions to light are absent below 29-31 weeks gestation. They may be absent in cases of increased intracranial pressure, and especially posterior fossa compression.

(e) *Cranial nerves*. Certain tricks are useful for testing them.

2 and 8. See below, 'Vision' and 'Hearing.'

3, 4, and 6. To test eye movements, look for either the doll's eye phenomenon (rotating the baby gently through 90° side-to-side around its own long axis; the eyes tend to keep their position in space) or rotational deviation (holding the baby at arm's length, swing round and round until just before you get giddy): the baby's eyes deviate towards the direction of rotation, and in the opposite direction on stopping rotation, when nystagmus ensues. It is very common for normal newborn babies to show a few beats of nystagmus on lateral deviation of the eyes—whether this deviation occurs spontaneously or in carrying out tests of eye movement.

5 and 7. Glabellar tap, corneal reflexes, sucking and rooting reflexes. (For further details of these reflexes, see below).

9 and 10. Gag reflex.

12. Look at tongue. Rooting reflex.

Examination of the cranial nerves must obviously be done with great care in cases of suspected cranial nerve or nuclear abnormalities, *e.g.* Moebius's syndrome. In other cases it is likely to be uninformative.

(f) *Tendon jerks*. Not usually informative, except in cases of spinal cord lesions (especially myelomeningocele). They tend to be increased in deep (no-eye-movement) sleep, and are sometimes very brisk with clonus in normal babies.

(g) *Skin reflexes*. There are a very large number of these (see Vlach 1968).* They may be useful for localising spinal or peripheral nerve lesions.

(2) *Special Senses*

    (*a*) *Vision:* (i) Pupil reactions

           (ii) Blink response to light

           (iii) Head-turning towards diffuse light (*e.g.* a window)

           (iv) Following a moving object (*e.g.* 6cm red ball at 30cm); most likely
                  to be successful if the baby is sitting up)

*Vlach, V. (1968) 'Some exteroceptive skin reflexes in the limbs and trunk in newborns.' *In* Mac Keith R., Bax, M. (Eds.) *Studies in Infancy*. Clinics in Developmental Medicine, No. 27. London: S.I.M.P. with Heinemann. p. 41.

(v) Optokinetic nystagmus.

(i) and (ii) test perception of light only.

(iii), (iv) and (v) may test occipital cortical function.

These responses will only be present when the baby is in State 3 or 4. Try to catch the baby in these states or coax him into them: otherwise testing is a waste of time.

In general, we believe that a baby who shows responses (iii), (iv) or (v) in the immediate neonatal period is unlikely to have severe generalised neurological disturbance.

(*b*) *Hearing.* We are not sure how best to test hearing in the usual clinical setting without a soundproof room. We observe any change in the baby's activity in response to sound, but attach little importance to negative findings.

(3) *Motor Function*

(*a*) *Spontaneous movement.* Observe nature, amount and symmetry, and note in particular the presence and nature of any abnormal movements. The commonest are tremor (jitteriness) and fits, which are sometimes confused. It is normally possible to distinguish between them because in the case of tremor the rate of movement is the same in each direction, whereas fits (being caused by alternate rapid contraction and slow relaxation of particular groups of muscles) show a fast and slow phase of movement. Note how often the bursts of tremor occur and what parts of the body are affected. In the case of fits, note as carefully as possible what happens.

A rare form of abnormal movement is frequent or continuous clonus which may affect all four limbs, the jaw and sometimes the eye-lids. The distinction between these movements and those we have called 'tremor' is that they are much slower, *i.e.* of lower frequency, than tremor. The clonus appears to be due to grossly exaggerated stretch reflexes and occurs spontaneously (presumably elicited by gravity) or on slight handling of the baby. We have only seen this condition after gross perinatal hypoxia or trauma, and it has always been associated subsequently with death or very severe brain damage.

(*b*) *Muscle tone.* Observe the range of movement and resistance to passive movement individually in all four limbs, and in the trunk and neck. Record whether muscle tone is generally increased, generally decreased, or different between the two sides or between other parts of the body. Hold the baby in the prone and supine positions with one hand under the trunk. Observe how much the trunk and neck bend under the influence of gravity, and to what extent the limbs resist gravitational forces. Record the findings as a simple line drawing. With regard to generalized increase or decrease of muscle tone, the examiner needs to have some absolute standard of normality for comparison, and it is important to remember that muscle tone is strongly related to gestational age (increasing with increasing gestational age up to about 40 weeks) and is also influenced by state—for example it is increased when the baby is crying. Generalized increase or decrease of muscle tone must be very marked before it is regarded as unequivocally abnormal. In assessing apparent lateralized differences of muscle tone, it is important to have the baby's head held in the midline, if necessary by someone else, since if the baby's head is turned to one side, tonic neck postures may influence muscle tone unequally on the two sides.

(*c*) *Primitive reflexes.* The normal newborn baby has a very large number of primitive reflexes, *i.e.* reflexes which normally disappear during infancy. Too much importance is often attached to these reflexes in the neonatal neurological examination. As Dr. David Clark has remarked: 'It is not very difficult to compose long lists of reflexes which may be elicited from infants.... by scratching, tickling, thumping, spinning, or otherwise invading their privacy.' (Clark 1964).*

The primitive reflexes are of practical value in neurological examination for four reasons.

(i) In the assessment of gestational age (see p. 91).

(ii) Generalised increase or decrease of primitive reflexes may be seen in 'cerebral irritation' or 'cerebral depression' respectively (see below).

(iii) Particular reflexes may be used to test the activity of particular spinal segments, peripheral nerves or muscle groups when lesions of these parts of the neuromuscular system are suspected, *e.g.* in myelomeningocele.

(iv) (not neonatal). Delayed disappearance of certain primitive reflexes may be an early sign of cerebral palsy.

Test a limited number of primitive reflexes and record presence or absence, ease or difficulty of elicitation, and (where appropriate) symmetry.

(i) MORO REFLEX. Hold the baby supine with the right arm and hand supporting the trunk, and the left hand supporting the head. Allow the head to fall suddenly a few centimetres. A positive response is rapid abduction and extension of both upper limbs, followed by slower adduction and flexion. (The latter phase is frequently absent in normal babies up to 36 weeks gestation.)

The Moro reflex is one of the earliest to be depressed or disappear in cerebral depression. In cerebral irritation it is abnormally easily elicited, accompanied by tremor, and the total amplitude of movement may be decreased by hypertonia. In kernikterus the response may be stereotyped, with brisk extension of the arms but not flexion, and a downward movement of the eyes ('setting sun' sign), accompanied by lid retraction and a ghastly grin. The commonest cause of a lateralized Moro reflex is a local lesion—fracture of the humerus or clavicle, or brachial plexus palsy.

(*N.B.* We believe the Moro reflex is the single most useful reflex in the neurological examination, but we also think it is unpleasant to the baby. Do not test it without good reason and do not repeat it unnecessarily at a single examination.)

(ii) GLABELLAR TAP. Tap the root of the nose; the response is a blink of the eyelids (see also p. 92).

(iii) SUCKING AND ROOTING RESPONSES (much influenced by 'State'). Stroke the baby around the mouth and observe the movements of lips, tongue and head. Put a gloved finger in the baby's mouth and observe sucking movements.

(iv) ASYMMETRIC TONIC NECK REFLEXES (TNRs) An asymmetric tonic neck reflex is present if, when the baby's head is turned to the right, the right arm and leg extend and the left arm and leg flex (or *vice versa* with the head turned to the left). It is

*Clark, D. B. (1964) 'Abnormal neurologic signs in the neonate'. *In* Kay, J. L. (Ed.) *Physical Diagnosis in the Newly Born. 46th Ross Conference on Pediatric Research.* Columbus, Ohio: Ross Laboratories. p. 65.

177

important to distinguish between TNRs produced by the baby spontaneously turning its head and those elicited by the examiner passively turning the head: the latter (imposed TNRs) are more likely to signify neurological abnormality. It is also important to distinguish true TNRs from random movement. To do this, turn the head five times each way alternately, allowing about 15 seconds after each head turn. Observe each time whether the arms or legs move into TNR positions and record the score for TNRs from the 10 head turns. A score of 5 or more is unlikely to be due to random movement. Genuine imposed TNRs may be seen in normal babies, but if very consistently present they may indicate cerebral disturbance.

(v) TRACTION REFLEX. Pull the baby up by the wrists from the supine position: observe flexion of arms and neck (see p. 92).

(vi) PALMAR AND PLANTAR GRASP REFLEXES. Place a finger across the palmar surface of the fingers, or plantar surface of the toes. A positive response is flexion of the digits.

## (4) *Sensation*

Sensory testing is necessarily very limited in the newborn baby. Generally no formal sensory testing is performed in the neurological examination, though of course there is a sensory component to each of the primitive reflexes described. Where testing of skin sensation over particular areas is important, the skin reflexes described by Vlach (1968)* may be useful. Painful sensation can be tested by pinch or pin-prick: the baby shows a withdrawal response or other signs of displeasure. Clearly, however, this is an unkind examination which would not be done without good reason.

### General Interpretation of Findings

During the account of the examination, we have commented on certain findings which have specific significance. Much more commonly, the only conclusions which can be drawn from the examination are very general ones. The baby may be normal, or probably normal with one or two findings of uncertain significance. Alternatively, the baby may show one of the following syndromes suggesting cerebral disturbance.

(1) *General irritation or hyperexcitability.* Spontaneous movement and muscle tone are increased: tendon jerks and primitive reflexes are exaggerated. Tremor is frequent. The baby cries readily and the cry may be high-pitched.

(2) *Cerebral depression or apathy.* Spontaneous movement and muscle tone are diminished. Primitive reflexes, and sometimes tendon jerks, are depressed or absent. Tremor may occasionally occur but is not prominent. The baby tends to lie immobile with the eyes open.

(3) *Lateralized abnormality or hemisyndrome.* There is a definite and consistent asymmetry of spontaneous movement, muscle tone, tendon jerks or primitive reflexes.

None of these syndromes is characteristically associated with a particular anatomical or pathological lesion. They simply have to be recorded under the titles given. For a further account of their significance see 'Neurological Disorders' on the pages immediately following.

*See p. 175 for reference.

# Neurological Disorders

In the present state of knowledge of neonatal neurology, it is not possible to classify all neurological abnormalities into aetiological and pathological categories. It is therefore best simply to list the problems as they present.

## OVERT CNS MALFORMATIONS

### Hydrocephalus

The commonest cause of hydrocephalus is the Arnold-Chiari malformation associated with myelomeningocele (see p. 54). Congenital hydrocephalus may also result from aqueduct stenosis or atresia (sometimes secondary to toxoplasmosis), Dandy-Walker syndrome (obstruction to the outlet foramina of the fourth ventricle), or other congenital malformations of the ventricular system. Acquired hydrocephalus may result from obstruction to CSF flow caused by haemorrhage into the CSF (intraventricular haemorrhage with or without subarachnoid spread, or other forms of subarachnoid haemorrhage) or from meningitis.

The modern management of hydrocephalus is much the same whatever the cause and consists of a shunt operation (*e.g.* a ventriculoatrial shunt) if the head is expanding rapidly. In any case where hydrocephalus is suspected, measure the head circumference regularly and accurately—daily, if it appears to be increasing very rapidly, otherwise twice weekly. If the head-circumference plot has crossed two centile lines or gone above the 97th, consult the neurosurgeon. Generally he will not want to do a shunt operation until the head circumference exceeds the 97th centile, and spontaneous arrest of the hydrocephalus may occur before this. The rate of head expansion can sometimes be reduced by giving acetazolamide (50-100mg/kg/day) which reduces the rate of CSF production. Consider this, especially where the rate of head expansion is only moderately abnormal. (It is very unlikely to work in cases of myelomeningocele.)

The very small pre-term baby whose head circumference is crossing centile lines presents a particular problem. These babies generally have scaphocephalic heads, in which the ratio of head circumference to skull volume is higher than usual. Nevertheless, they may develop hydrocephalus due to a silent intraventricular or subarachnoid haemorrhage in the early days of life. We plot their head circumference weekly, but do not generally take any other action until this exceeds the 90th centile, or there are other signs of hydrocephalus, *e.g.* bulging fontanelle, separated sutures or 'setting sun' sign.

### Anencephaly

The infant is usually stillborn. If liveborn, it is unlikely to live more than a few days and we believe this is one situation where the parents should be discouraged from seeing their child. Nothing can be done for the infant, but study of these babies can still provide useful information about normal neurological and endocrine function.

**Microcephaly**

This simply means a small head, arbitrarily defined as below the 3rd centile. There are a number of known causes, including autosomal recessive inheritance, but most cases remain unexplained. Investigate the baby for congenital rubella, cytomegalovirus, toxoplasmosis and herpes (see p. 21 *et seq.*). Presumably you will already know if the mother has had therapeutic irradiation in pregnancy (p. 11). There is no evidence that diagnostic irradiation can cause this condition.

**Hydranencephaly**

In true hydranencephaly the cerebral hemispheres are absent—a fact which can readily be ascertained by transilluminating the head, when the whole cranial cavity glows brightly. Transillumination is not a routine part of the examination of the newborn, but should be done in any baby having a full neurological examination (p. 173) or who has an abnormally large or otherwise unusual head. What has usually led us to transilluminate the head in babies with hydranencephaly has been a slight enlargement of the head. No satisfactory treatment is available (though a shunt operation may reduce the rate of head expansion) and the prognosis for neurological and mental development is hopeless. No opportunity should be lost to study the behaviour of these babies, who provide an experimental model for understanding the role of cerebral hemispheres in the newborn.

**Myelomeningocele**

(See p. 54).

**Congenital Dermal Sinus**

This term is conventionally applied to one type of failure of closure of the neurenteric canal. It consists of a small (pin-head size) hole over the spine or skull. Whenever such a sinus is above the level of S2, it will inevitably communicate with theca and will thus provide a portal of entry for bacteria, which will eventually cause meningitis. It should be detected on routine examination (p. 83). Refer at once to the neurosurgeon.

A pit in the sacrococcygeal region, often several millimetres deep, is much commoner but harmless—at least in infancy. We believe these pits sometimes represent the origin of pilonidal sinuses in adult life.

**Other Midline Abnormalities Over the Spine**

Any abnormalities over the spine (*e.g.* a hairy patch or naevus) may indicate an underlying abnormality of the bony structure and/or spinal cord. X-ray the relevant part of the spine. The most important abnormality to look for is diastematomyelia. Whether or not an abnormality is found, record bladder and anal sphincter function and the neurological findings in the lower limbs very carefully, and arrange for the child to be seen monthly for the first few months and then less frequently. Even if an abnormality is present, neurosurgery is not usually indicated unless there is evidence of neurological deterioration.

180

## OVERT TRAUMA TO THE NERVOUS SYSTEM BELOW THE BRAIN

(1) Peripheral nerve palsies (see p. 48).

(2) Brachial plexus palsy (see p. 48).

(3) Spinal cord transection. This is hardly ever seen in modern obstetric practice. It results from very severe trauma to the cervical cord during delivery, often combined with bilateral brachial palsies. The baby's trunk and limbs are usually flaccid and there is bladder paralysis—an important point of distinction from other forms of flaccidity. Death in the neonatal period may result from respiratory failure. Prognosis for lower-limb function in survivors is very poor.

## ABNORMAL BEHAVIOUR, USUALLY FOLLOWING PERINATAL HAZARDS

This is both the commonest type of problem and the most difficult to classify and understand. There are, of course, certain readily recognizable forms of pathology found at post-mortem, but (except in the case of kernikterus) there are no clear-cut clinical syndromes which regularly correspond with these pathologies, nor is it possible to infer pathology from the clinical state in babies who survive.

The best recognized pathology in this group, apart from kernikterus, is intra-cranial haemorrhage. It is important to recognize that this is not a single or complete diagnosis—there are different varieties of haemorrhage which differ not only in their site but also in their causes, natural history and prognosis. The main features of the different varieties are summarized in Table X.

Whatever the underlying pathology, the baby whose brain function has been temporarily or permanently disturbed by perinatal hazard will usually show symtoms which fall into one or more of the following categories.

(1) Cerebral depression or apathy (see p. 178).

(2) Cerebral irritation or hyperexcitability (see p. 178).

(3) Lateralized abnormalities (see p. 178).

(4) Failure to suck and swallow (usually combined with (1) or (2) but occasionally the main or only abnormality).

(5) Respiratory failure (usually combined with (1)).

(6) Fits (see p. 188).

(7) Lack of attention: the most definite sign of this is lack of visual following (see p. 175), which is probably the most sensitive index of disturbance.

**Management of the Baby Showing Abnormal Behaviour Suggesting CNS Dysfunction**

There are three aspects to this: what investigations to do, what treatment to give, and what to say about prognosis.

*Investigations* (for technique, see 'Procedures', p. 279)

The place for special investigations is very limited, since they will rarely influence treatment and will not usually give additional information of prognostic significance.

181

## TABLE X
### Classification of intracranial haemorrhage
### (in approximate order of present-day frequency)

| Site | Source of bleeding | Associated or predisposing factors | Prognosis |
|------|--------------------|-----------------------------------|-----------|
| (1) Intraventricular | Ruptured subependymal haemorrhage (3 (a) below) | Immaturity, ?hypoxia, ?RDS. | Usually but not invariably fatal. Survivors may develop hydrocephalus |
| (2) Subarachnoid | Usually uncertain. (When secondary to intraventricular, subarachnoid spread is limited in extent.) | Various, ?hypoxia, ?RDS. | Good, but risk of hydrocephalus. |
| (3) Intracerebral | | | |
| (a) subependymal | Terminal veins in germinal layer | Immaturity, ?hypoxia, ?RDS. | We guess that survivors will show evidence of permanent brain damage, but a firm diagnosis can only be made in fatal cases. |
| (b) superficial | Various. Superficial vessels in cases of disseminated intravascular coagulation; ?mycotic aneurysms in cases of meningitis. | Secondary haemorrhagic disease, Rhesus incompatibility, hypothermia, etc. | Probably fatal in most cases. |
| (c) haemorrhagic infarction | | Gram-negative infection | Probably fatal in most cases. |
| (4) Subdural | Ruptured great cerebral vein or intraseptal venous sinus. | Trauma; e.g. breech, difficult forceps, especially in cases of intrapartum asphyxia, including small-for-dates babies. | Inevitably fatal when major vein is torn. |

Procedures such as subdural tap, which might be either diagnostic or therapeutic, or both, are also considered here.

(1) LUMBAR PUNCTURE. Its main value is in the diagnosis of meningitis where examination of the CSF is essential. The early signs of meningitis are usually non-specific signs of infection (see p. 163), rather than neurological signs. Lumbar puncture should nearly always be done when systemic infection is suspected, whether there are neurological abnormalities or not.

The other use of lumbar puncture is to reveal the presence of blood in the CSF, in cases of subarachnoid or other intracranial haemorrhage. Any abnormal neurological syndrome may be seen in any of the forms of intracranial haemorrhage (see above); lumbar puncture might therefore be expected to give information of some diagnostic value in any baby showing abnormal behaviour. However, absence of blood-staining of the CSF does not exclude subdural, intracerebral or intraventricular haemorrhage. Nor does the presence of blood in the CSF establish that intracranial or subarachnoid bleeding has occurred, unless it is certain that the lumbar tap was not traumatic: in cases of doubt, centrifuge the CSF and look for xanthochromia or macrophages, indicating that the blood staining has been present for more than a few hours. Xanthochromia is not diagnostic of subarachnoid haemorrhage, as it may result from hyperbilirubinaemia, especially when there is a high level of CSF protein. The only real practical importance of establishing the presence of blood in the CSF is that it warns the examiner to watch carefully for the development of hydrocephalus if the infant survives.

Lumbar puncture may also be of value in the measurement of intracranial pressure, but we have found it extremely difficult to make satisfactory and accurate pressure measurements in the newborn.

Normal CSF findings show a wide range of variation in the newborn. The fluid is very commonly yellow (see above). Protein levels are both higher and more variable than those found in older patients. Cell counts may be difficult to interpret, especially in pre-term infants if the fluid is bloodstained, when the normoblasts may be difficult to distinguish from white cells.

Naidoo (1968)* obtained the following figures from 135 normal newborns on the first day of life.

|  | Range | Mean* |
|---|---|---|
| Red cells per mm³ | 0 - 1070 | 9 |
| Polymorphs per mm³ | 0 - 70 | 3 |
| Lymphocytes per mm³ | 0 - 20 | 2 |
| Protein mg/100 ml | 32 - 240 | 63 |
| Sugar mg/100 ml | 32 - 78 | 51 |

*log. mean except in case of sugar.

In pre-term infants even higher protein levels may be found. Bauer *et al.* (1965)† found mean CSF protein levels in 'premature' infants of 180mg/100ml, with individual values very much higher, especially in very immature babies.

(2) CISTERNAL TAP. This is an alternative method of obtaining CSF if lumbar puncture is unsuccessful. It is only indicated where examination of the CSF is really important, *i.e.* in suspected meningitis.

(3) VENTRICULAR TAP. This is very rarely indicated. The main situations in which we have done it are (*a*) in suspected intraventricular haemorrhage, to establish the diagnosis and to remove blood, and (*b*) in rapidly progressive hydrocephalus, to relieve pressure. We no longer perform ventricular tap in situation (*a*) and in situation

*Naidoo, B. T. (1968) 'The cerebrospinal fluid in the healthy newborn infant.' *South African Medical Journal*, **42**, 933.
†Bauer, C. H., New, M. I., Miller, J. M. (1965) 'Cerebrospinal fluid protein values of premature infants.' *Journal of Pediatrics*, **66**, 1017.

(*b*) the proper course is usually an early shunt operation. Ventricular tap may be used to give antibiotics in cases of meningitis due to myelomeningocele.

(4) AIR STUDIES. We have never performed these in the neonatal period except, in consultation with neurosurgeons, to establish the site of blockage and ventricular size in hydrocephalus. Some authorities have recommended air encephalography in cases of suspected posterior fossa subdural haematoma, but we have never done this (nor subsequently wished we had).

(5) SUBDURAL TAP. We rarely do subdural taps in the immediate neonatal period. This is partly because subdural haemorrhage is rare in modern obstetric practice and partly because we have doubts about its efficacy in established cases. We have never seen at post-mortem a baby who appeared to have died of subdural haemorrhage which was not due to a tear of a major vein or sinus. Moreover, subdural tapping carries some risk of causing haemorrhage.

(We are in no doubt about the diagnostic value of subdural tapping in *chronic* subdural haemorrhage, after the early neonatal period. Incidentally, it is said that trauma at birth leads to chronic subdural haemorrhage: it obviously might do so but we have not seen it happen.)

(6) ELECTROENCEPHALOGRAPHY. The place of the EEG in the diagnostic assessment of a baby with neonatal fits is discussed on p. 189. Much the same is true in the case of other neurological abnormalities. The EEG may give information which, taken in isolation, would be of prognostic value, *e.g.* an EEG which is flat for more than 24 hours would suggest a bad prognosis, but the same conclusion would almost certainly be drawn from repeated neurological examinations. The EEG does not influence treatment.

*Treatment*

It is seldom that we can treat the underlying cause in newborn infants with neurological abnormalities (meningitis is an obvious exception); most treatment given is directed towards particular symptoms or complications.

*Fits.* Anticonvulsants should be given (see p. 190).

*Irritability.* In cases of excessive irritability, a sedative may be used. Try chloral 30mg/kg/day divided into four doses.

*Respiratory problems.* Serious neurological abnormalities may lead to apnoea or respiratory failure, which should be treated in their own right (see p. 133).

*Increased intracranial pressure.* This is very difficult to diagnose with certainty, since there is no really satisfactory method of measuring intracranial pressure in the newborn. Increased intracranial pressure may be suspected in a baby who has suffered severe perinatal hypoxia or circulatory arrest and who shows either profound cerebral depression or spontanous clonus (see above). We sometimes use dexamethasone, 1mg 12-hourly I.M. for two or three days, tailing off over the next three days. This is known to relieve cerebral oedema both in animals and adult human beings, and may stabilize lysosomal membranes, thus inhibiting further cell destruction. We do not use mannitol, urea, sucrose or magnesium sulphate.

*Prognosis*

*Future neurological progress can never be predicted with certainty.* At the best, one can only make an informed guess; and in talking to parents we acknowledge our uncertainty. In general, it is better to err on the side of optimism, since the expectation of abnormality may affect the way a baby is mothered and impair his progress, even if the expectation was originally incorrect. The opinion about prognosis will be based on three kinds of information: (1) circumstances, (2) happenings and (3) neurological findings.

(1) *Circumstances.* This means the factors believed to have led to the baby's neurological disturbance. The worst prognostic circumstance is circulatory arrest at birth. We have seen very few babies revived by external cardiac massage who survived neurologically intact; most of them died in the neonatal period or have survived with subsequent evidence of severe brain damage. Hypoglycaemia and hyperbilirubinaemia are both probably harmless in the long term if the baby shows no abnormal behaviour or neurological signs in the neonatal period, but in cases where such signs are present there is a very high risk of subsequent abnormality—deafness and choreoathetosis in the case of hyperbilirubinaemia; mental retardation, fits, or cerebral palsy in the case of hypoglycaemia.

Hypoxia and trauma in themselves have a relatively good prognosis, though the nature and duration of abnormal physical signs must be taken into account (see below).

(2) *Happenings.* These include fits and apnoeic attacks. Fits considerably worsen the prognosis (except those due to hypocalcaemia, which occur on the 5th to 10th day of life and are not associated with other neurological abnormality). Well over 50 per cent of babies with fits from other causes will die or subsequently be abnormal.

Apnoeic attacks may be either a cause or a result of neurological abnormality, but they are unlikely to cause brain damage if they are speedily dealt with and the baby does not suffer serious circulatory impairment. Regarded as a sign of pre-existing neurological abnormality, apnoeic attacks indicate that the abnormality is, at least, moderately severe.

(3) *Neurological findings.* From the prognostic point of view, the most helpful finding is a complete absence of abnormal neurological signs at any time. This, combined with a record of normal behaviour, justifies a very good prognosis even if the baby has had adverse perinatal circumstances. However the prognosis should still be guarded in a baby who has had fits other than those due to hypocalcaemia.

If one of the abnormal neurological syndromes is found, its prognostic significance depends on (*a*) the *duration* rather than the nature of the abnormal signs, and (*b*) the associated circumstances. Any abnormal findings in association with hypoglycaemia, or hypertonia and an abnormal Moro reflex in association with hyperbilirubinaemia, carry a bad prognosis. Abnormalities present for less than 48 hours following hypoxia or trauma carry a relatively good prognosis.

The nature of the abnormal syndrome present does not greatly affect the prognosis, though very prolonged cerebral depression is probably more serious than prolonged cerebral irritation and cerebral irritation has a more serious prognosis if preceded by depression. However, cerebral depression must be interpreted with care, since a similar picture can be produced by maternal drugs transferred to the fetus (the effect

185

may last for several days) or by sedatives or anti-convulsants given to the baby.

Even where it is feared that subsequent neurological abnormality is probable, it is difficult to forecast its probable nature.

*Subsequent Management*

Arrange follow-up examination for all babies who have had markedly adverse perinatal circumstances, happenings, or neurological abnormalities. If there has been blood in the CSF, watch particularly for the development of hydrocephalus. Follow-up includes, in particular, developmental assessment, testing of hearing and measurement of head circumference.

We advise the family doctor and welfare clinic to omit pertussis immunisation in all babies who have had neonatal neurological abnormalities.

## Kernikterus

We have tended to regard kernikterus as a disappearing condition, and we believe it should rarely, if ever, occur with ideal neonatal management. However, the experience of one of us in a neurological assessment centre shows that kernikterus still does occur.

*Clinical Features*

We do not have much experience of this condition in the neonatal period. We believe that what we have said in general about neurological abnormalities following perinatal hazards also applies to kernikterus, and there is no specific clinical picture regularly accompanying this specific pathology. The baby is likely to be lethargic and to suck poorly. There may be hypotonia, or hypertonia with opisthotonos, and convulsions may occur. Abnormal eye movements may be seen, especially downward rolling ('setting sun' sign). Two features which we have particularly noticed in newborn babies with kernikterus are:

(*a*) an abnormal Moro reflex, as described on p. 177; and

(*b*) very consistently imposed tonic neck reflexes.

If a baby with hyperbilirubinaemia shows signs suggesting kernikterus, exchange transfusion should be performed at once. Such signs are certainly not an indication to abandon treatment, which is likely to lessen or, in some cases perhaps, prevent neurological damage.

## The 'Floppy Baby'

The commonest causes of extreme hypotonia in a newborn baby are (*a*) extreme short-gestation, when hypotonia is a normal finding; (*b*) severe generalized illness. *e.g.* respiratory distress, septicaemia; and (*c*) intracranial disorders leading to 'cerebral depression' (see p. 178). Floppiness is not likely to present a difficult problem in differential diagnosis in any of these circumstances, because the history of the associated findings will suggest the cause of floppiness in most cases.

Occasionally, however, hypotonia is the main problem in an otherwise well baby. A number of rare disorders must then be considered in the differential diagnosis.

(1) Spinal cord injury (see p. 181).

(2) Spinal muscular atrophy (Werdnig-Hoffman disease).

(3) Poliomyelitis.

(4) Myasthenia gravis.

(5) Various congenital myopathies.

(6) Glycogenoses affecting CNS, heart and muscle.

(7) Organicacidaemias. The mode of presentation is distinctive: these babies appear normal at birth, but become profoundly hypotonic—usually within a few days—and develop signs of respiratory failure.

(8) Prader-Willi syndrome. These children present with hypotonia and feeding difficulties in the neonatal period. Later on they show mental retardation, become fat and may develop diabetes. Affected boys are likely to have undescended testicles.

(9) Down's syndrome. All babies with Down's sundrome are floppy, and we have known an unrecognized case of Down's syndrome to present in the neonatal period with the differential diagnosis of floppiness.

(10) 'Benign congenital hypotonia'. This label is really simply an admission that you do not have a diagnosis.

The following is a reasonable approach to making a diagnosis in the case of the 'floppy baby'.

(1) Enquire especially about family history. (Spinal muscular atrophy, glycogenosis and organic acidaemias are recessively inherited: there may be a history of affected siblings. Some congenital myopathies are probably dominantly inherited.) Enquire also about fetal movements (diminished fetal movement suggests that the disorder was present in intra-uterine life).

(2) Look for muscular wasting. Fibrillation of the tongue, which might suggest spinal muscular atrophy, is in practice difficult to be certain of, since the tongues of normal newborn babies may often be seen to quiver.

(3) Give edrophonium chloride to exclude congenital myasthenia gravis (see p. 13).

(4) Do plasma and urine amino-acids to exclude errors of amino-acid metabolism.

(5) Do an EMG and serum creatine phosphokinase (CPK). The EMG will probably help in the diagnosis of spinal muscular atrophy and myopathies; the CPK may help in the diagnosis of myopathies (but usually does not).

(6) Consider muscle biopsy. Though more of an assault than the other investiga- tions, it is the one most likely to lead to a diagnosis in a floppy baby in whom the diagnosis is not apparent from examination and simple investigations.

For further information, see Dubowitz (1969) and Tizard (1969).

Dubowitz, V. (1969) *The Floppy Infant*. Clinics in Developmental Medicine No. 31. London: S.I.M.P. with Heinemann.
Tizard, J. P. M. (1969) 'Neuromuscular disorders of infancy.' *In* Walton, J. M. (Ed.) *Disorders of Voluntary Muscle*. London: Churchill. p. 579.

# NEONATAL FITS

## Types of Fit and Their Recognition

Complete grand mal attacks are rare in the newborn; most neonatal fits are either (*a*) *tonic* with generalized stiffening, usually accompanied by apnoea and not followed by a clonic phase; or (*b*) *focal*—clonic twitching of some part of the body, usually unaccompanied by apnoea or other disturbance. Focal fits are often multifocal, *e.g.* twitching of the left leg may be followed by twitching of the right face.

Fits may occur in the course of another illness (*e.g.* in a low-birthweight baby with respiratory distress, where they may indicate that an intraventricular haemorrhage has occurred), or 'out of the blue' in a previously healthy baby. The following account of management applies mainly to the second situation, where fits are the major problem. It may be thought reasonable to omit some of the diagnostic and therapeutic measures proposed in a very ill baby, in whom fits may be merely an incident in the course of an already recognised illness.

## Causes and Associations of Neonatal Fits

*Factors present or operating before birth*

    Cerebral malformations.

    Intra-uterine infections, *e.g.* toxoplasmosis, cytomegalovirus, rubella.

*Factors operating during labour or at delivery*

    Birth trauma.

    Perinatal hypoxia.

    Local anaesthetics injected in error into the baby.

*Factors operating after birth*

    Transient biochemical disturbances:

        hypoglycaemia;

        hypocalcaemia;

        hypomagnesaemia;

        hyperbilirubinaemia.

    Infection—meningitis.

    Inborn errors of metabolism.

    Intracranial haemorrhage (which may be associated with birth trauma or perinatal hypoxia).

    Drug withdrawal.

## Diagnosis

Despite the large number of possible causes of neonatal fits, a diagnosis of the likely cause can very often be made on clinical grounds.

Fits associated with hypoglycaemia most commonly occur in small-for-dates babies and in the first three days of life. (However, hypoglycaemia may occur in other circumstances, and should always be excluded in *any* baby who has fits. See p. 147.)

Fits associated with hypocalcaemia usually occur between the fifth and tenth days of life in babies who have been fed on cow's milk, often in large quantities.

When fits are caused by perinatal hypoxia or trauma, this is usually apparent from the history. They generally begin in the first 48 hours of life, and the baby is unlikely to have been neurologically normal up to that time.

Fits occurring at any age and in any circumstances may be a sign of meningitis, although a fit is very rarely the presenting sign of this rare neonatal condition.

**Investigation**

*Investigations Which Should Always Be Done*

(1) Blood glucose.

(2) CSF examination. (We would only omit this in very ill pre-term babies with respiratory distress and apnoeic attacks, in whom there is no supporting clinical evidence of infection. Fits—usually tonic—in these circumstances are likely to be due to hypoxia and/or intraventricular haemorrhage.)

(3) Urine examination for smell, galactose (by 'Clinitest') and amino-acid chromatography.

(4) Transillumination of the head to reveal cerebral anomalies with abnormal or excessive fluid collections within or around the brain. Auscultation of the head for bruits.

(5) Where no other diagnosis is established, investigations for infections such as cytomegalovirus, congenital rubella and toxoplasmosis (see p. 21 *et seq.*).

*Investigations Which May Help*

(1) Serum calcium. The result may be difficult to interpret, since there is a considerable overlap in serum calcium levels between apparently normal babies and those who have the clinical picture of hypocalcaemic fits. On the negative side, we would regard fits as *not* being due to hypocalcaemia if the serum calcium level exceeded 8.5mg/100ml.

(2) Serum magnesium. Rarely, neonatal fits may be due solely to hypomagnesaemia. Less rarely, it may prove impossible to correct hypocalcaemia until the accompanying hypomagnesaemia is corrected.

(3) EEG. It is possible to manage neonatal fits entirely adequately without an EEG. The EEG may help assess prognosis: in general terms, the more abnormal the EEG and the more widespread the abnormality, the worse the prognosis.

(4) Diagnostic infusions. Many authorities recommend giving in succession intravenous pyridoxine, glucose, calcium gluconate and magnesium chloride, and observing the effect on fits, and/or on the EEG if this is abnormal. The results of this complicated procedure are rarely easy to interpret. We recommend giving I.V. glucose, calcium or magnesium as suggested below. In a baby with intractable and unexplained fits, we would give 25mg pyridoxine I.V. and observe the clinical effect (to exclude pyridoxine dependency).

**Treatment**

In summary, if an underlying cause is found, this is treated. If fits continue, whether or not an underlying cause has been found and treated, anticonvulsants should be given.

*Treatment of underlying cause*

HYPOGLYCAEMIA. If 'Dextrostix' indicates hypoglycaemia, or if for any reason this test cannot immediately be done and the circumstances suggest hypoglycaemia, give 0.5g/kg of glucose intravenously in 10% solution and observe the effect on fits if these are happening. For further treatment of hypoglycaemia, see p. 151.

MENINGITIS. See p. 168.

HYPOCALCAEMIA. Hypocalcaemic fits occurring on the fifth to tenth day of life are largely preventable. The hypocalcaemia is usually caused by overfeeding with cow's milk in the first week of life. Occasionally, however, hypocalcaemia in the baby is a sign of hyperparathyroidism in the mother. If the baby has not been overfed with cow's milk, ask the obstetricians to do a serum calcium, phosphate and alkaline phosphatase estimation on the mother, and to x-ray her hands to exclude hyper-parathyroidism.

A very rare cause of hypocalcaemia in the newborn is Di George's syndrome (thymic aplasia with absence of the parathyroids). The use of ACD blood for transfusion may also produce hypocalcaemia, but we avoid this by treating citrated blood before-hand with heparin and calcium gluconate.

The most important measure in correcting hypocalcaemia is to reduce the load of phospate given to the baby until hypocalcaemia is corrected. Either a low-phosphate-containing milk such as breast milk or S.M.A. may be given, or a dilute cow's milk feed, *e.g.* evaporated milk made up with 1 part milk and 4 parts water. If hypocalcaemia is suspected or confirmed and fits continue, 20mg calcium gluconate/kg (0.2ml/kg 10% calcium gluconate) followed by 0.3mEq/kg of magnesium (*e.g.* 0.1ml/kg 50% mag-nesium sulphate) may be given slowly intravenously. It is also reasonable to give oral supplements of calcium gluconate 400mg/kg/day in four or six divided doses, but the importance of this is secondary to the reduction of oral phosphate load. Rarely, a baby will have a persistently low level of serum calcium which will not rise until an accompaning hypomagnesaemia has been corrected.

**Anticonvulsants**

Neonatal fits will almost invariably stop during the neonatal period, whatever the ultimate prognosis may be. Further, except in the case of tonic fits occurring in acute hypoxia, they are not usually associated with disturbance of respiration. Never-theless, we feel that if fits continue (whether or not an underlying cause has been found and treated), anticonvulsants should be given.

For status epilepticus or very frequent fits, we recommend paraldehyde 0.1ml/kg intramuscularly. We have tried diazepam 0.4mg/kg, but have not found the same consistently good effect in the newborn as in older children with status epilepticus. We are also concerned about the risk of precipitating apnoea, and of bilirubin dis-placement from binding sites by the sodium benzoate component of injectable diazepam.

As an anticonvulsant for continuing use we recommend: chloral (30mg/kg/day in four divided doses); *or* phenytoin (4mg/kg/day in four divided doses); *or* phenobarbi-tone (5mg/kg/day in four divided doses).

**Prognosis** (see also p. 185)

The prognosis in cases of neonatal fits is that of the underlying disorder. Babies with hypocalcaemic fits occurring after the fifth day of life almost invariably do well. In all other forms of neonatal fits, the prognosis must be much more guarded. Continuation of fits for more than 48 hours, or marked bilateral EEG abnormalities, are discouraging signs, whatever the cause of the fits.

We recommend omitting the pertussis component of triple vaccine in all babies who have had neonatal fits.

# Gastro-intestinal Disorders

## VOMITING

Small vomits in newborn babies are usually called 'regurgitations' when the medical and nursing staff are not worried by them—although the mothers may be. They are relatively frequent in the first days of life, and are said to be associated with inco-ordinate oesophageal response to swallowing, with low tone in the inferior oesophageal sphincter, and with delayed gastric emptying. These factors may be accentuated in pre-term and ill babies. The vomits gradually become less frequent and stop, though in a small number of thriving babies they continue, often for many months.

Vomiting must be taken seriously if, in addition, the infant appears unwell, and/ or has diarrhoea; or if the vomits are large, very forceful and accompanied by abdominal distension; or if they are bile- or blood-stained; or if they are associated with static weight or weight loss. Vomiting associated with a steady weight gain is hardly ever a matter for concern.

Vomiting in the newborn may be the first sign of parenteral infections, the adrenogenital syndrome, or of metabolic disorders, as well as of intestinal infection or obstruction. The following is a guide to the clinical analysis of serious vomiting.

### History

Previous unexplained neonatal deaths should be noted, and enquiry made for any illness in the family which may be wholly or partly genetically determined. Hirschsprung's disease, cystic fibrosis and congenital hypertrophic pyloric stenosis are examples of gastro-intestinal disorders of this kind which may present in the neonatal period. Other inherited disorders which may have vomiting among the presenting symptoms are the salt-losing type of congenital adrenal hyperplasia—a condition likely to be overlooked in the male infant (see p. 61), and other inborn errors of metabolism such as galactosaemia (see p. 225).

The presence of maternal hydramnios may mean high intestinal obstruction in the baby, e.g. oesophageal or duodenal atresia, and an abnormally large amount of liquid (> 20ml) may be found in the latter condition if the stomach is aspirated at birth.

The timing of the onset of vomiting is of prime importance. It will occur as soon as feeds are given in high obstructions, and may be delayed beyond the first 24 hours in low obstructions.

Accurate recording of the passage of first meconium is also crucial. Onset of symptoms *after* the appearance of normal meconium, changing and milk stools may suggest peritonitis, necrotizing enterocolitis or malrotation with volvulus, though the latter more often presents early. The vomiting associated with cardiac failure or generalised infection may occur at any time.

**Examination**

Though particular attention should be paid to the abdomen, always make a complete examination to search for signs of generalised infection, congenital heart disease and congestive cardiac failure, and external anomalies. A shiny, oedematous and discoloured abdominal wall should suggest peritonitis. If distension is present, note whether it is primarily upper abdominal (suggesting a high obstruction) or generalised (suggesting lower small or large bowel obstruction). If an infant with a high obstruction is seen shortly after a large vomit, the abdomen may look normal.

Left-to-right peristalsis across the epigastrium may be seen in obstruction, but is occasionally present in normal babies. Ladder patterning (dilated loops of bowel running more or less transversely across the abdomen) is seen in small or large bowel delay, but is occasionally seen in normal pre-term infants with thin abdominal walls: listen for bowel sounds.

A mass may be palpable, for instance if perforation of the bowel has occurred with localisation of infection, or in the very rare cases of mesenteric cysts or bowel reduplication. Abnormal meconium is sometimes palpable. Rectal examination (with the smallest fifth finger available) may be informative; if it is followed quickly by a gush of meconium, flatus and relief of distension, Hirschsprung's disease should be strongly suspected. Note whether the anus is normally placed.

The hernial orifices should always be inspected—we have seen a strangulated hernia in an immature infant in the neonatal period.

**Feeding**

*A feed should be watched* and the forcefulness and timing of the vomit and its appearance noted. Quite forceful vomits can occur in normal babies as the wind is brought up, particularly if the feeds have been gulped down. It should be remembered that while congenital hypertrophic pyloric stenosis is usually not congenital, it may nevertheless present in the first week of life, and so the abdomen should be examined during a feed. Sitting at the infant's left side, and palpating with your left hand, you should be able to feel with your finger-tips the hypertrophied pylorus in the hypo-chondrium, deep in the angle between the lateral border of the right rectus muscle and the liver edge. It is usually an ovoid mass which feels about 2.5 x 1.0cm. Peristalsis will be seen best when the stomach is distended with a feed: even when pronounced, it is not invariably a sign of upper gastro-intestinal obstruction.

Vomiting occurring when the infant is put back in his cot is suggestive of hiatus hernia, and a small amount of fresh or altered blood due to oesophagitis is sometimes present in the vomit. Colostrum is occasionally a very deep yellow, but the green colour of bile should be unmistakable and should always be considered indicative of intestinal atresia until proved otherwise. Atresia of the duodenum can, however, occur above the entrance of the common bile duct. Swallowed meconium is a much darker, brownish-green colour.

**Stools**

The vast majority of newborn infants pass their first meconium within 24 hours of birth, but the first passage may be later in the immature, particularly those of low

193

birthweight who are very ill and in those whose mothers have been given large doses of certain antihypertensive drugs (see p. 17). Delay in the passage of meconium may also be associated with smallness for dates, intestinal obstruction, cystic fibrosis (meconium ileus) and Hirschsprung's disease. There may be a greyish sticky mucoid cast of meconium in cases of Hirschsprung's disease, cystic fibrosis and sometimes without obvious cause. Once this meconium plug is passed or removed it is followed by meconium of normal consistency, except meconium ileus due to cystic fibrosis.

Even in complete atresias some meconium may be passed, and though it is usually abnormal in appearance, consistency and amount, this is not invariably so. Prolonged delay in the passage of meconium may be accompanied by abdominal distension and vomiting. The passage of blood per rectum, even if not accompanied by vomiting and distension, should alert you to the possibility of malrotation with volvulus. Do not fall into the trap of attributing this to haemorrhagic disease of the newborn without first obtaining a plain x-ray of the abdomen; delay in diagnosis can result in ischaemic necrosis of a large segment of bowel. Blood in the stools with or without diarrhoea may occur in necrotizing enterocolitis (see p. 202).

**Further Investigation**

The history and examination should enable you to say whether vomiting is secondary to some other cause such as infection or congestive cardiac failure—in which case see the relevant sections—or primarily due to gastro-intestinal disorder. In the latter case, further investigation will be necessary.

(1) *Radiological examination* will be required, except in cases of congenital hypertrophic pyloric stenosis, in which a diagnosis can be made with confidence on clinical examination. The safest and most informative investigation is the plain abdominal film, taken in the supine and erect positions if obstruction is suspected. If a mass is palpable, a lateral view may be helpful. Air reaches the small intestines within 2 to 3 hours of birth, and has nearly always arrived at the anus by 12 to 24 hours, though sometimes later in the immature.

In duodenal atresia, one is likely to see an abnormally large fluid level in the stomach and a smaller one in the dilated proximal duodenum, with no further air apparent. When duodenal obstruction is incomplete, as in stenosis, annular pancreas or malrotation, dilated stomach and proximal duodenum will still be apparent, but air can be seen in the lower abdomen as well.

In small gut atresia (sometimes multiple), the site of fluid levels and the absence of air in the lower abdomen should help to localise the proximal site of obstruction. A mottled appearance (due to air in sticky meconium) with gross intestinal distension should suggest meconium ileus due to cystic fibrosis of the pancreas, but this granular effect is not pathognomonic and we have seen it with the abnormally viscid meconium passed by some small-for-dates infants.

Linear streaks of intramural air, most commonly present in the right iliac fossa, should suggest necrotizing enterocolitis, and air has also been reported in the portal tracts in this condition. Perforation may be diagnosed by the finding of free air under the diaphragm. Calcification may indicate an intra-uterine perforation (a rare condition possibly caused by occlusion of a mesenteric vessel in the fetus) and consequent meconium peritonitis.

Hypertonic contrast media (*e.g.* 'Gastrografin') are to be avoided; and barium is rarely necessary and can be dangerous, as it may become inspissated. Perhaps the only indications for it are as a swallow when hiatus hernia is suspected, or as a small and carefully given enema if malrotation or Hirschsprung's disease are thought to be the cause of symptoms. In malrotation the caecum may be seen in the right upper instead of the right lower quadrant. Remember how easily rectal perforation can occur in the newborn; catheters (and for that matter a thermometer or even a finger) should only be introduced into the rectum with extreme care and gentleness, always in a slightly posterior direction, preferably with the infant lying prone or on his side.

(2) *Abdominal transillumination.* If a mass is palpable (see below), cystic and solid lesions may be differentiated by the degree of translucence. Use a bright pencil torch and hold it at a right angle to the abdominal skin. Cystic masses will transilluminate readily; so of course will a full stomach, so the examination should be made before a feed. Normally the translucent halo round the torch should not exceed 1cm.

(3) *Protein content of meconium.*‡ Usually, but not invariably, high quantities of serum proteins are present in the meconium of infants with cystic fibrosis, whether or not they have meconium ileus. The test strip 'Albustix' can be used as a simple qualitative screening test for albumen (Schutt and Isles 1968)*, but a positive reaction is not diagnostic of cystic fibrosis, as we have found increased amounts of albumen in cases of intestinal obstruction not due to meconium ileus.

METHOD. Mix meconium and a few drops of distilled water well on a porcelain tile. Moisten one side of the strip with the diluted meconium. It may be difficult to detect a colour change, as 'Albustix' strips now have a plastic backing and it is therefore not possible to keep one side free of meconium in order to compare the colour. The presence of melaena would, of course, preclude testing. The laboratory will make a quantitative estimation.

(4) *Sweat electrolytes.* Their estimation may be necessary later to establish a diagnosis of cystic fibrosis if meconium ileus is present. The most reliable test is the determination of sweat chloride by direct reading electrode (Kopito and Schwachman 1969)† sweating being induced by pilocarpine iontophoresis. We have no experience of this method, and usually carry out a conventional sweat test. The diagnosis may have to be delayed in the pre-term infant in whom sweat will not be produced in adequate amounts at lower gestations. Values may be relatively high ($>40$mEq/litre) in normal newborns in the neonatal period.

(5) *Behaviour of the internal anal sphincter.* This may have to be investigated if Hirschsprung's disease is suspected. Normally, momentary distension of the rectum leads to reflex relaxation of the internal sphincter (smooth muscle) followed by contraction and increase in electrical activity of the external sphincter (striated muscle). In Hirschsprung's disease, there is contraction of the internal sphincter instead of relaxation. Recordings are made either by using an air-filled or strain-gauge system,

*Schutt, W. H., Isles, T. E. (1968) 'Protein in meconium from meconium ileus.' *Archives of Disease in Childhood*, **43**, 178.
†Kopito, L., Schwachman, H. (1969) 'Studies in cystic fibrosis: determination of sweat electrolytes in situ with direct reading electrodes.' *Pediatrics*, **43**, 794.
‡The protein content of normal meconium is less than 10 per cent.

and should be done by somebody adept at the technique (Howard and Nixon 1968)*. The normal or ill immature infant may give abnormal responses in the first weeks of life.

(6) *Rectal biopsy.* This will be necessary at some stage if Hirschsprung's disease is suspected. Discuss the timing of the biopsy with the paediatric surgeon.

### Further Management
*If Complete Intestinal Obstruction is Suspected*

(1) Ask the surgeon to see the infant.

(2) Stop all oral feeds, substitute intravenous therapy (a cut-down on the internal saphenous vein at the ankle—see p. 271—is preferable if the child is going to the operating theatre), and correct dehydration and electrolyte abnormalities before operation.

(3) Pass a nasogastric tube to allow relief of abdominal distension and aspirate frequently.

(4) Draw blood for electrolytes, blood grouping and cross matching.

(5) Give phytomenadione 1mg I.M. once pre-operatively.

(6) Always try to go to the operating theatre with the infant. He should be transported there and back in a heated incubator. See that adequate provision has been made for keeping him warm in the operating theatre (see p. 102) and keep an eye on his intravenous therapy.

*If Partial or Functional Intestinal Obstruction is Suspected*

(1) to (4) as above, without necessarily blood grouping and cross-matching.

(5) A period of intravenous feeding and gastric suction is commonly all that is needed in the functional ileus of the immature. If necrotizing enterocolitis is suspected *in the very immature* (functional ileus probably always occurs first), our view is that it is better not to operate unless signs of perforation and localisation have occurred (*i.e.* a mass, or area of increased resistance to palpation, usually in the right iliac fossa).

*Malrotation and volvulus.* Occasionally the obstruction resolves spontaneously, but waiting for this to happen once the diagnosis is entertained can be very dangerous and may condemn the infant to resection of a large amount of non-viable gut.

*Hirschsprung's disease.* Signs of obstruction tend to be intermittent and there is some controversy about treatment. The establishment of a colostomy is probably safest because of the dangers of necrotizing enterocolitis. Even colostomy does not completely safeguard against this.

*Meconium ileus.* We have no experience of 'Gastrografin' enema in the treatment of this condition, but preliminary reports suggest it may have a place (Noblett 1969, Waggett *et al.* 1970)†. About 60 to 90ml have been given, under fluoroscopic control, as it is essential to see the fluid reaches the distal ileum containing the inspissated meconium. Any dehydration must be corrected before the procedure, and intravenous

---

*Howard, E. R., Nixon, H. H. (1968) 'Internal anal sphincter. Observations on development and mechanism of inhibitory responses in premature infants and children with Hirschsprung's disease.' *Archives of Disease in Childhood,* **43**, 569.
†Noblett, H. R. (1969) 'The treatment of uncomplicated meconium ileus by Gastrografin enema. A preliminary report.' *Journal of Pediatric Surgery,* **4**, 190.
Waggett, J., Johnson, D. G., Borns, P., Bishop, H. C. (1970) 'The nonoperational treatment of meconium ileus by Gastrofin enema.' *Journal of Pediatrics,* **77**, 407.

therapy continued during it, for the large fluid shifts into the bowel resulting from the very high osmolality of 'Gastrografin' may dangerously deplete circulatory volume. Measure serum osmolality during and after the procedure.

### If Hiatus Hernia is Suspected

This is one of the few indications for barium examination for diagnosis. Medical management should suffice and consists in nursing and feeding the infant in the upright position in a special chair, and thickening the feeds, *e.g.* with Benger's Food. Occasionally intravenous fluid and electrolyte replacement is necessary initially.

## Post-operative Care

Intravenous feeding may be necessary for varying lengths of time, depending on the duration of ileus and on whether or not resection of bowel has been necessary. Scalp vein infusions can be used after the cut-down has stopped working. Remember the danger of hypoglycaemia occurring when drips stop (see p. 98). Oral or nasogastric feeds should not be restarted until distension has subsided, bowel sounds are present and the aspirate is no longer bile-stained. Remember that the treatment of post-operative pain is no less important in the newborn baby than in anyone else.

### Intravenous Fluids

Providing abnormal losses from the bowel are not occurring, the amounts and solutions for intravenous feeding are the same as for the normal infant (see p. 99). If such therapy has to be maintained beyond 3 to 4 days (as is often the case following massive small bowel resection), nutrition can be satisfactorily maintained parenterally for several weeks (for technique, see p. 271). Some advocate that fat solutions (*e.g.* Intralipid) should be alternated with protein solutions (*e.g.* Vamin), with electrolytes added: others believe fat to be unnecessary. For details of the solutions, amounts and methods used; see the papers by Rickham (1967), Filler *et al.* (1969) and Harries (1971)*.


## ABDOMINAL DISTENSION (see also 'Vomiting')

Abdominal distension may occur in the following situations, listed roughly in order of frequency.

(1) In the small pre-term infant, in whom it may be benign.

(2) In functional ileus which may occur in the ill newborn baby who has respiratory distress, enteral or parenteral infection, or who has had an exchange transfusion.

(3) In necrotizing enterocolitis, which may follow (2).

(4) In artificial ventilation due to inflation of the stomach.

(5) In cases of massive pneumothorax due to downward displacement of the diaphragm, liver and spleen.

*Rickham, P. P. (1967) 'Massive small intestinal resection in newborn infants.' *Annals of the Royal College of Surgeons of England*, **41**, 480.
Filler, R. M., Eraklis, A. J., Rubin, V. G., Das, J. B. (1969) 'Long-term total parenteral nutrition in infants.' *New England Journal of Medicine*, **281**, 589.
Harries, J. T. (1971) 'Intravenous feeding of infants.' *Archives of Disease in Childhood*, **46**, 885.

(6)  In gastro-intestinal obstruction.

(7)  In enlargement of one or more abdominal organs, ascites, cysts, malignant tumours (very rare in the neonatal period), and haemorrhage following damage to a viscus.

(8)  In cases of disaccharide intolerance (see p. 202).

(9)  In certain CNS disorders.

(10)  In absence of abdominal musculature.

(11)  In meconium peritonitis.

*If abdominal distension has occurred suddenly in a baby with respiratory distress (4) or (5) are likely and the appropriate action should be taken. Ensure that the endo-tracheal tube has not been displaced into the oesophagus. For the emergency treatment of pneumothorax, see p. 140.*

In cases in which the cause of the abdominal distension is not immediately obvious, the following is a guide to differential diagnosis. The most urgent of the various conditions to detect are ileus, either functional or associated with organic obstruction, and haemorrhage from or into an abdominal organ.

## History

Find out the following by consulting the mother, nursing staff and case notes.

(1)  Time of onset of distension.

(2)  Time of first passage of meconium and its appearance (any stools passed subsequently should be kept for inspection).

(3)  Time of first passage of urine. (If a boy, was the stream normal?)

(4)  Family history of possible relevance, *e.g.* Hirschsprung's disease or cystic fibrosis in a sibling.

(5)  Number of umbilical vessels.

## Examination

(1)  *Examine the abdomen.* Is the distension localised or generalised? Is there visible peristalsis? Does the skin of the abdomen wall appear normal? Is the distension tympanitic or dull? Is there a palpable viscus, tumour or crepitus? Is there localised or generalised guarding? Is there a fluid thrill or shifting dullness? Are bowel sounds audible on auscultation? Transilluminate the belly (see p. 195).

(2)  *Check hernial orifices.*

(3)  *Examine the scrotum for fluid—blood or ascites which has tracked down the processus vaginalis.*

(4)  *Do a rectal examination.*

(5)  *Do a thorough general examination.* Look especially for signs of shock or infection, for evidence of CNS disorder and for malformations.

(6)  *Examine the urine.*

(7)  *Ask for plain X-ray films of the abdomen—erect and supine.*

## Notes

(1)  *Generalised distension,* sometimes with ladder patterning, may be seen in very immature but otherwise healthy infants, but is also a feature of low small bowel or

large bowel obstruction.

(2) In necrotizing enterocolitis, *crepitus*—suggesting submucosal air—is occasionally felt and, with guarding, first noted in the right iliac fossa.

(3) Rupture of the liver or a subcapsular haematoma of the liver with haemorrhage into the peritoneal cavity is associated with difficult delivery. Rupture of the spleen is rare unless it is very large, as in severe haemolytic disease. Haemorrhage into one or even both adrenals may also be a consequence of difficult delivery or of septicaemia. Haemorrhage at these three sites is likely to occur within 48 hours of birth, but may be delayed for as long as one week. The baby will have signs of *shock, free fluid* (blood) in the abdomen in cases of ruptured liver, and a *large swelling* in one flank (or both) in cases of adrenal haemorrhage: a salt-losing syndrome may follow.

(4) The onset of *ascites* may be insidious over the first few days and weeks of life, unless of course it is associated with severe erythroblastosis fetalis (see p. 65) or with severe intra-uterine infection which may present a somewhat similar clinical picture (see p. 67), both of which are obvious at birth. Ascites may be chylous, urinary or biliary. Urinary ascites will be associated with lower urinary tract obstruction; biliary ascites with very slight jaundice but colourless stools and bilirubinuria. Also see p. 161.

(5) *Inflation of the stomach* is a fairly common feature of oesophageal atresia with tracheo-oesophageal fistula.

(6) *Masses in one or both flanks* are usually renal, commonly hydronephrotic or cystic kidneys, but mesenteric cysts, duplications of the gastro-intestinal tract, ovarian tumours, Wilm's tumour, neuroblastoma and adrenal haemorrhage have to be borne in mind. Lobulated swellings are often renal, and although usually palpated deeply, they may occasionally be unusually mobile and superficial. Renal vein and, very rarely, renal artery thrombosis may occur in the neonatal period. The former is more common in the infants of diabetic mothers, and occasionally thrombosis of the inferior vena cava accompanies it, in which case dilated venous channels may be obvious on the anterior abdominal wall. These infants are usually, but not invariably, ill, shocked and dehydrated, and haematuria will differentiate the condition from massive adrenal haemorrhage. Congenital anomalies of the renal tract may be associated with other defects such as congenital heart disease and anomalies of the ears, genitalia, or gastro-intestinal tracts.

(7) *Enlargement of the bladder* may be seen in myelomeningocele, spinal cord transection, urethral obstruction and as a terminal phenomenon in infants with massive intracranial haemorrhage. The bladder usually empties easily with gentle pressure in the last circumstance.

(8) In cases of *hypotonia*, the distension is only obvious when the infant is held erect. If hypotonia is generalised, look for other signs of CNS disorder. Localised distension may be seen with congenital absence of part of the abdominal musculature, or associated with paralysis of nerve supply to a particular muscle as in some cases of myelomeningocele. Generalised absence of abdominal musculature may be associated with wrinkling of the abdominal skin, often described as 'prune belly', and renal tract dilatation almost invariably accompanies this. The condition occurs most frequently in males, who usually have undescended testicles.

(9) *Meconium peritonitis* is due to intestinal perforation before birth and is usually, but not invariably, associated with meconium ileus and cystic fibrosis. Abdominal distension is present at birth but worsens because of intestinal obstruction.

**Radiography**

*Plain films of the abdomen*, erect and supine, should be done in suspected ileus or if a mass can be palpated—in which case a lateral may be useful. See section on Vomiting ('Radiological examination', p. 194) for details of the findings in intestinal obstruction. If you have palpated a mass, the films may help you to make a more accurate assessment of its size and position by showing displacement of bowel shadow. Calcification is very occasionally seen in certain tumours (*e.g.* teratoma, neuroblastoma) and in meconium peritonitis, and has been known to occur quite soon after large adrenal haemorrhages.

*Contrast radiography* should be done in consultation with the paediatric surgeon. If a single renal or suprarenal mass is palpated, an intravenous pyelogram may be the most helpful, and it will reveal whether the kidney is excreting adequately and/or whether it is displaced by a suprarenal swelling. If both kidneys and bladder are thought to be enlarged (*e.g.* as in partial urethral obstruction by valves, or in association with congenital absence of abdominal musculature—both largely confined to males), a cystogram is much more helpful. Pictures taken during voiding should show the typical cylindrical dilation of the prostatic urethra when obstructing valves are present. It should be possible to outline ureters and renal pelves with a cystogram, as well as demonstrating a patent urachus. Note that the earlier in life an intravenous pyelogram is done the poorer the definition is likely to be.

**Further Management**

See p. 196 if complete or partial or functional intestinal obstruction is suspected.

The treatment of abdominal distension secondary to ruptured liver (p. 218), adrenal haemorrhage (p. 219), or infection (p. 162) is that of the underlying disease.

The nature of ascitic fluid should be found by diagnostic paracentesis (p. 68). Chylous ascites is best treated by repeated aspiration, and appears to have a good prognosis. In biliary ascites, exploration of the common bile duct or bypass may be necessary, but we know of recovery without operation after repeated aspiration. The treatment of urinary ascites is that of the underlying urinary tract obstruction.

For the treatment of malignant disease see p. 220.

Renal vessel thrombosis has in the past been treated by nephrectomy or by embolectomy. However, many cases recover without operation. Careful attention is needed to fluid and electrolyte balance. Treatment of a renal mass such as cystic kidney is usually surgical. Relief of urinary obstruction should be undertaken urgently as soon as the diagnosis is made. An effective method is to insert an 'Intracath' into the bladder. Bilateral nephrostomies are the most effective form of drainage and the prognosis is by no means as hopeless as it may seem initially.

Always remember that any abnormality or instrumentation of the urinary tract may be accompanied by urinary infection. Long-term antibacterial therapy may be necessary.

# INFECTIVE DIARRHOEA

Stool frequency and consistency vary between individual infants, as well as with the mode of feeding. Any change in a baby's established bowel pattern towards greater frequency and looseness should be taken seriously. If the usual feeds are being accepted and retained, significant weight loss (*i.e.* more than five per cent of bodyweight) is due to fluid loss from the bowel in most cases. This fluid is sometimes mistaken for urine on the napkin—when a small amount of apparently formed stool is surrounded by a sizeable damp area—and infants may become seriously dehydrated if steps are not taken to replace it.

## Treatment

In mild diarrhoea, substitute 1/5 normal saline with dextrose for the usual milk feed for a 24-hour period, and follow with dilute milk feeds, gradually returning to full strength.

If clinical examination, weight-loss, electrolyte and osmolality determination suggest serious dehydration and/or hyper- or hyponatraemia, stop all oral feeding and feed intravenously (see p. 99) for 24 to 48 hours, then introduce small dilute oral feeds and stop the drip as soon as 150ml/kg is being tolerated by mouth, and electrolytes are normal.

In a very few cases, re-introduction of feeds leads to recurrence of diarrhoea. Sometimes a brief period of feeding with a low lactose milk will obviate the need for prolonged intravenous therapy in these infants.

If the diarrhoea is caused by enteropathogenic *Escherichia coli*, Salmonella or Shigella species, start parenteral treatment with gentamicin in view of the risk of septicaemia in sick and low-birthweight infants.

## Precautions to be Taken to Stop the Spread of Infection*

Diarrhoea should be regarded as due to a transmissable bowel pathogen (*e.g.* enteropathogenic *Escherichia coli*, Salmonella or Shigella) until proved otherwise by culture of several stools.

Ensure that as few people as possible handle the baby; in particular, arrange for nursing care to be restricted to nurses who do not deal with other infants, nor work in the milk kitchen.

'Isolation' in a cubicle within the nursery may serve to remind staff of the necessity to take extra precautions with handwashing, but is useless in preventing spread if aseptic techniques are not assiduously practised throughout the 24 hours.

Immediately one of the above pathogens is reported in a stool culture, steps should be taken to remove the infant from the nursery altogether to some other ward or hospital where there are no sick or low-birthweight newborn infants.

The ward should be closed to outside admissions.

The source must next be traced and, after consultation with the bacteriologists,

*The Department of Health and Social Security. 'Memorandum on the ascertainment and control of outbreaks of infantile gastro-erteritis.' May 1972.

rectal swabs from the mother and all nursing, medical and auxilliary staff on the ward should be examined, preferably on more than one occasion. If no carrier is found, do not forget that enteropathogenic organisms may be harboured in equipment.

Failure to take these steps may lead to a protracted epidemic causing mortality as well as considerable morbidity.

Family doctors of infants being discharged home should be told of the nursery infection: *no* infant in the nursery should be sent back to the lying-in wards.


## NON-INFECTIVE DIARRHOEA

Although neonatal diarrhoea should be regarded as infective (*e.g.* due to entero-pathogenic *Esch. coli*, Salmonella or Shigella species) until proved otherwise, remember that it may be among the presenting symptoms in certain other conditions, some of which need early diagnosis for successful treatment. These conditions are listed more with importance of recognition in mind than in frequency of occurrence.

### Hirschsprung's Disease
See below, and p. 192 *et seq.*; 196 *et seq.* for diagnosis and management.

### Necrotizing Enterocolitis
This occurs in three main circumstances: (*a*) in low-birthweight infants, particularly those who have a complicated early neonatal course with frequent apnoeic, cyanotic episodes; (*b*) among infants who have had exchange transfusions (usually multiple); and (*c*) among infants with Hirschsprung's disease. Its development is probably caused in all three categories by a period of intestinal stasis (in (*a*) and (*b*) bowel ischaemia may be preceding or contributory), during which bacteria multiply excessively in the gut lumen and later invade the bowel wall. Possible toxicity of polyvinyl used for umbilical vessel catheterisation has also been invoked as a contributory cause. True infarction due to primary thrombosis or embolism of mesenteric vessels seems rare, though there is often blood in the stools. The condition usually occurs after the second day, and the other clinical features are abdominal distension, bile-stained gastric contents or vomit, and signs of generalised illness including apnoeic attacks. Occasionally, instead of diarrhoea, there is ileus with cessation of bowel action. The radiological features are described on p. 194. We prescribe antibiotics when this condition is suspected, in addition to the measures outlined on p. 196.

### Congenital Adrenal Hyperplasia of the Salt-losing Variety
See p. 61 for diagnosis and management.

### Disorders of Carbohydrate Metabolism
Lactose is the carbohydrate present in both human and cow's milk. Sucrose is commonly added to evaporated and some dried milks. Thus, though all these disorders are rare, those associated with disaccharides will predominate in the neonatal period; some are genetically acquired. A detailed description is not possible here, but

see review article by Holzel (1967)*. Diarrhoea, with frothy, sour-smelling stools and associated abdominal distension may be seen in lactase deficiency ( ? primary, secondary), sucrase-isomaltase deficiency (only when sucrose and starch are being fed), and monosaccharide intolerance (due to malabsorption of glucose and galactose, and occasionally fructose).

*Screening Tests*

(1) Test the stool with a universal indicator strip: pH is commonly less than 5.5.

(2) an excess of reducing substances may be present in the stools, and can be detected using 'Clinitest' tablets (see below for method). False negatives may occur, particularly if the fluid part of the stool is not tested. False positive tests also occur since reducing substances are found in the stools of many normal newborns. Nevertheless, if these tests are positive with serious symptoms persisting, further investigations will be required for precise diagnosis, including paper chromatography of stools and urine, tolerance tests (proceed with great caution if the child is very ill), and possibly intestinal biopsy and enzyme assay.

Once the offending substances have been identified, management consists of feeding with a suitable diet (complete vitamin supplements are necessary with the synthetic diets), and treatment of underlying precipitating causes such as infection, which may be primarily intestinal, or elsewhere in the body. (See Clayton *et al.* (1966) and Harries and Francis (1968)† for details of dietary management.)

**Chloride-losing Diarrhoea**

This has been reported as occurring from birth or within a week or so of it, and after gut surgery in the neonatal period. It is characterised by the passage in the stool of unusually large amounts of chloride ion (greater than the sum of the stool potassium and sodium ion concentrations), absence of chloride in the urine, and a metabolic alkalosis. Stool samples for electrolyte estimation should be collected by nursing the infant on a metabolic frame, or using polythene-lined napkins. Potassium depletion may play a part, and chloride loss can be reduced as the alkalosis is corrected by replacing potassium. Associated disaccharidase deficiency may be present (see Aaronson 1971)**.

**Enterokinase Deficiency**

This is a very rare primary defect of protein digestion, presenting with diarrhoea, and treated with oral pancreatic extract. For necessary diagnostic steps, see Hadorn *et al.* (1969)‡.

*Holzel, A. (1967) 'Sugar malabsorption due to deficiencies of disaccharidase activities and of monosaccharide transport.' *Archives of Disease in Childhood*, **42**, 341.

†Clayton, B. E., Arthur, A. B., Francis, D. E. M. (1966) 'Early dietary management of sugar intolerance in infancy.' *British Medical Journal*, **2**, 679.

Harries, J. T., Francis, D. E. M. (1968) 'Temporary monosaccharide intolerance.' *Acta Paediatrica Scandinavica*, **57**, 505.

**Aaronson, I. (1971) 'Secondary chloride-losing diarrhoea. Observations on stool electrolytes in infants after bowel surgery.' *Archives of Disease in Childhood.* **46**, 479.

‡Hadorn, B., Tarlow, M. J., Lloyd, J. K., Wolff, O. H. (1969) 'Intestinal enterokinase deficiency.' *Lancet*, **i**, 812.

**Congenital Thyrotoxicosis**

See p. 10 for diagnosis and management.

**Maternal Drug-addiction**

See p. 222 for diagnosis and management.

**Cystic Fibrosis**

The stools may be bulky and very offensive in addition to being frequent, but cystic fibrosis does not usually present with diarrhoea in the neonatal period. Diagnosis will be easier if there has been a preceding meconium ileus (see p. 195), or if a sibling is known to have the disease, in which case an abnormal protein content of the meconium may already have been established. Analysis of duodenal juice may give a presumptive diagnosis, but demonstrations of a raised sweat sodium chloride content may have to wait until the second or third month of life (see p. 195).

**Maternal Laxatives**

If absorbable laxatives are being taken, the amount transmitted in breast milk may be enough to cause diarrhoea in the infant.

**Feeding Disorders**

Over-feeding occasionally leads to diarrhoea. Disaccharide intolerance may be responsible in some cases, but of course mild infective diarrhoea may be wrongly attributed to over-feeding. Feeds of 150/ml/kg/day should suffice for most infants in the first weeks of life, though very low-birthweight babies will need more earlier. If the infant is not thriving and diarrhoea is pronounced, hypernatraemia must be excluded, oral feeding should be stopped and intravenous therapy substituted (see p. 99) until the stools return to normal.

Small, green, watery stools may be passed when the infant is being seriously under-fed—a situation likely to be met, in hospital at least, only in the breast-fed. Supplementary or complementary artificial feeds will be necessary until supply improves, but if it does not, breast-feeding is best abandoned.

**Method for Detection of Reducing Substances in Stool with 'Clinitest'**

The stools should be collected by nursing the infant on a metabolic frame or using a polythene-lined napkin, and should not be contaminated with urine. Testing should be carried out as soon as practicable after the stool has been passed. Add two volumes of water to one volume of stool and mix thoroughly. Put 15 drops of this suspension into a clean test tube and add a 'Clinitest' (Ames) tablet. The reaction is the same as that in urine testing, and the colour standard provided is used to gauge the amount of reducing substance present.

NOTE: Glucose, galactose, lactose and other reducing substances may be found in the stools of normal infants in variable amounts. In the neonatal period, therefore, while a low result (below 0.5 per cent) is good evidence against sugar malabsorption, a high result is not diagnostic of it.

# Failure to Pass Urine Within the First 24 Hours

Nursing staff not infrequently report that an infant has failed to pass urine within the first 24 hours of life. It is easy to miss the passage of urine at or shortly after birth, but assuming the observation to be correct, serious abnormality in the infant is very rarely a cause. The urinary output in the first 28 to 48 hours is normally low. About 93 per cent of term infants have passed urine within 24 hours of birth, 98 per cent by 30 hours and 99.5 per cent by 48 hours.

Examine the infant's abdomen to exclude the marked renal enlargement and/or bladder distension which might suggest urethral obstruction, almost without exception in males only, and due most commonly to urethral valves (see p. 200). Inspect the external genitalia for anomalies. Remember that the prepuce of the male infant is so adherent that it may be difficult to see any orifice. This is *not* by itself an indication for probing or catheterisation, for in the vast majority the problem is resolved on the second day by the normal passage of urine. Serious malformations, such as urethral atresia, are exceptionally rare, but would of course need surgical intervention. Infants with renal agenesis or dysgenesis will not present in this way, for death normally occurs within an hour or so of birth.

# Haemorrhage

**WARNING.** SEVERE HAEMORRHAGE IS ONE OF THE MOST URGENT OF NEONATAL EMER-
GENCIES. IF THE BABY HAS BLED AND IS PALE OR BREATHLESS, HE PROBABLY NEEDS
IMMEDIATE TRANSFUSION TO PREVENT IRREVERSIBLE SHOCK. TURN AT ONCE TO p. 209,
BUT REMEMBER, TOO, THAT IF A SAMPLE OF BLOOD IS NOT OBTAINED FOR INVESTIGATION
BEFORE TRANSFUSION (see p. 207), RETROSPECTIVE DIAGNOSIS OF THE CAUSE WILL
PROBABLY BE IMPOSSIBLE.

## Causes and Varieties of Haemorrhage

The baby may bleed before or after birth.

### Fetal Haemorrhage

This may be associated with twinning, antepartum haemorrhage, and caesariean
section (where the placenta may be cut). When none of these conditions is present but
the baby is pale at birth, consider the possibility of feto-maternal haemorrhage and
examine the mother's blood for fetal cells. The physical signs and the treatment of a
baby who has bled before birth are described on p. 37. Transfusion may be needed
urgently, but is given on the same indications as for other forms of haemorrhage.

### Neonatal Haemorrhage

The causes of haemorrhage after birth fall into three main categories:

(1) local causes;

(2) bleeding tendencies;

(3) other types of less certain aetiology. These include intrapulmonary and
intraventricular haemorrhage.

In this section we are concerned with situations where blood loss *per se* is the
main problem. This is not usually so in category (3), which will not be considered
further here.

(1) *Local causes.* These include inadequately applied or displaced cord clamps
or ligatures, and birth trauma leading to internal or external bleeding. Some forms of
internal bleeding due to birth trauma, such as cephalhaematoma and subcapsular
haematoma of the liver, may not be apparent for many hours after birth, and a
bleeding tendency may be an added factor. (See also 'Unexpected collapse', p. 218).

In subaponeurotic haemorrhage, the bleeding is between the epicranial
aponeurosis (galea aponeurotica) and the periosteum. Blood can, therefore, spread
through the soft areolar tissue of the scalp and cover the whole calvarium. The condition is much commoner in negro than white babies. Blood loss may be substantial
and cause severe symptoms. Unlike the subperiosteal haemorrhage (see p. 254), this
may be a symptom of haemorrhagic disease of the newborn.

Bleeding into the gastro-intestinal tract may occur without any bleeding tendency.

206

Sometimes the cause is acute gastric erosion or duodenal ulceration, but we have seen a baby lose the equivalent of nine times its blood volume into the upper G.I. tract with no demonstrable bleeding point and normal blood coagulability. Surgical problems such as volvulus sometimes present with G.I. bleeding. *In cases of bleeding from the bowel, one must not assume the cause to be haemorrhagic disease of the newborn, even when the prothrombin time is prolonged: a plain X-ray of the abdomen must be taken and the baby observed carefully for signs of intestinal obstruction.*

(2) *Bleeding tendencies.* Classical haemorrhagic disease of the newborn due to deficiency of vitamin-K-dependent factors (II, VII, IX, X) largely occurs in breast-fed babies who have not been given prophylactic vitamin $K_1$ (phytomenadione). Babies born to mothers on anticoagulant therapy are especially at risk. We now give phytomenadione routinely (see p. 76). The common sites of bleeding due to haemorrhagic disease are the stomach or bowel (haematemesis and/or melaena), the cord stump, and beneath the scalp.

Platelet deficiency may occur as a complication of maternal thrombocytopenia (see p. 12), or due to platelet iso-immunisation, or as a complication of neonatal illnesses such as congenital viral infections, or in marrow hypoplasia.

Disseminated intravascular coagulation (which is also associated with thrombocytopenia) is only likely to occur in babies who are ill with hypothermia, severe hypoxia, severe Rhesus incompatibility or serious infections.

### Investigation

Though treatment of haemorrhage is often urgent, an accurate diagnosis cannot usually be made unless specimens are taken for certain investigations before treatment is started. The following tests should always be done on a baby who is bleeding or has bled:

(a) blood group (and crossmatch);

(b) haemoglobin and haematocrit;

(c) thrombotest;

(d) platelet count.

The flow-chart on the following page suggests a scheme for further investigation and diagnosis of possible bleeding tendencies.

### Swallowed Maternal Blood

When the problem is vomiting of blood in the first 48 hours, the cause is sometimes swallowed maternal blood. Apt's test is worth doing if the vomitus appears to consist of pure undenatured blood.

APT'S TEST TO DISTINGUISH BETWEEN MATERNAL AND FETAL BLOOD

(1) Dissolve the specimen in half a test tube of water in sufficient quantity to match the colour obtained by dissolving two drops of adult blood in a similar quantity of water.

(2) Set up a third tube containing two drops of baby's blood in the same volume of water.

(3) Add enough 1%NaOH to the tubes to increase the volume of each by one-fifth.

207

Within one or two minutes a colour change takes place in the tube containing adult blood; the pink turns yellow-brown as the adult haemoglobin is denatured by the alkali. The tube containing fetal blood remains pinkish, changing only over a much longer time interval. The specimen will show a rapid change, or not, depending on the origin of the blood in it.

*Points to note:*

If the specimen does not change colour, check that it is alkaline, using a universal pH paper. The extra buffering power of the body fluids or initial reaction of acid vomit could prevent the alkaline conditions necessary for the denaturation of adult haemoglobin to take place.

### Estimation of Amount of Blood Lost

The haemoglobin and haematocrit will only be of limited value in cases of acute haemorrhage. Clearly, immediately after an acute bleed, the haemoglobin and haematocrit will be unaltered. However, haemodilution seems to occur rapidly in the newborn. A reasonably accurate estimate of blood loss could only be made were one to

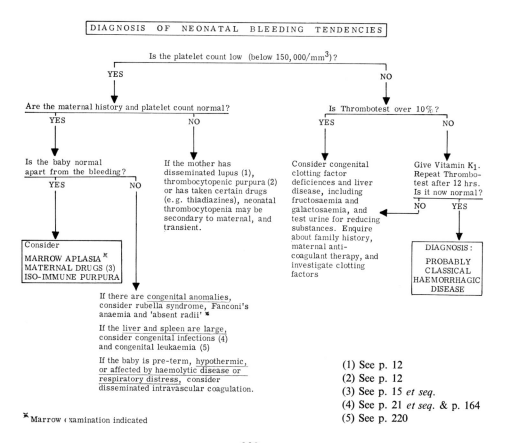

DIAGNOSIS OF NEONATAL BLEEDING TENDENCIES

Is the platelet count low (below 150,000/mm$^3$)?

YES / NO

Are the maternal history and platelet count normal?

YES / NO

Is Thrombotest over 10%?

YES / NO

Is the baby normal apart from the bleeding?

YES / NO

If the mother has disseminated lupus (1), thrombocytopenic purpura (2) or has taken certain drugs (e.g. thiadiazines), neonatal thrombocytopenia may be secondary to maternal, and transient.

Consider congenital clotting factor deficiencies and liver disease, including fructosaemia and galactosaemia, and test urine for reducing substances. Enquire about family history, maternal anti-coagulant therapy, and investigate clotting factors

Give Vitamin K$_1$. Repeat Thrombotest after 12 hrs. Is it now normal?

NO / YES

Consider

MARROW APLASIA *
MATERNAL DRUGS (3)
ISO-IMMUNE PURPURA

DIAGNOSIS:

PROBABLY CLASSICAL HAEMORRHAGIC DISEASE

If there are congenital anomalies, consider rubella syndrome, Fanconi's anaemia and 'absent radii' *

If the liver and spleen are large, consider congenital infections (4) and congenital leukaemia (5)

If the baby is pre-term, hypothermic, or affected by haemolytic disease or respiratory distress, consider disseminated intravascular coagulation.

(1) See p. 12
(2) See p. 12
(3) See p. 15 *et seq.*
(4) See p. 21 *et seq.* & p. 164
(5) See p. 220

* Marrow examination indicated

obtain haemoglobin and/or haematocrit measurements immediately after the first bleed, and to repeat the tests in, say, 24 hours when full haemodilution had taken place.

However, a rough estimate of blood loss can be made by assuming a normal blood volume of 85ml/kg bodyweight, and an initial haemoglobin level of 16g/100ml, from the following formula:

$$\text{Blood loss (ml)} = \text{calculated blood volume} \times \frac{16 - \text{Hb}}{16}$$

where Hb is the haemoglobin level found.

Try, also, to estimate directly by guesswork the amount of blood lost, or by comparing with known amounts of old stored blood spilt on similar material, or by elution of the blood in a measured volume of normal saline and measurement of the haemoglobin content.

When bleeding occurs under the scalp, an approximate estimate of the volume of blood in the subaponeurotic cephalhaematoma (*i.e.* one not confined to the area overlying a single skull bone, see p. 254) can be made from the formula $\dfrac{C^3 - C_{Ex}^3}{12\pi^2}$

where C is the actual and $C_{Ex}$ the previously measured or expected head circumference (see p. 326 and p. 327).

The amount is approximately 38ml for each cm by which the head circumference exceeds expectation.

However, don't waste time on these estimations if the baby obviously needs urgent transfusion.

The clinical signs of blood loss are pallor, rapid and deep respiration, rising pulse rate and, finally, falling blood pressure (see p. 218). If any of these signs is present, the baby has almost certainly lost 10 per cent of his blood volume and probably substantially more.

Note that the blood pH falls in severe haemorrhage.

**Treatment**

In all cases, give phytomenadione 1mg I.V. or I.M. as soon as blood has been taken for the initial investigations. If the baby has any of the clinical signs of blood loss listed above, or if the estimated blood loss is more than 20 per cent of the blood volume, a blood transfusion (see below for blood to be used) should be given immediately. In the absence of a reasonable estimate of blood loss, give 30ml per kg bodyweight for the first transfusion. The first 20-40ml may be given rapidly (in about 10 minutes) when there is air hunger.

If the baby has no signs, or none other than pallor, the situation is less urgent. However, if the haemoglobin level has fallen below 10g/100ml it is probably advisable to give a blood transfusion, (*a*) to forestall collapse in the event of further bleeding, and (*b*) because a baby whose haemoglobin has fallen so low shortly after birth is likely to become seriously anaemic in the next six weeks.

The umbilical vein is the simplest route for transfusion. In cases of acute blood loss, a direct transfusion is given to restore blood volume. It is only in cases of slow bleeding in which the haemoglobin level has fallen very low that an exchange transfusion is indicated to avoid overloading the circulation. Following transfusion, measure pH and correct acidosis with bicarbonate if necessary (see p. 129 for suggested amounts).

If in doubt as to whether transfusion is necessary, re-examine the baby and re-measure pulse, respiration and blood pressure every half hour, remembering that following a severe internal haemorrhage a newborn baby may maintain an adequate circulation for a while and then suddenly deteriorate and be in urgent need of transfusion.

If there is either thrombocytopenia or deficiency of clotting factors, it is best to use fresh blood* for transfusion, but the urgency of the situation may preclude getting fresh blood. In these circumstances use compatible stored blood—even, if necessary, unmatched Group O Rh-negative blood. If possible, this should be treated with heparin, calcium gluconate and THAM, as for exchange transfusion (p. 272), but these measures may be waived in desperate circumstances.

Fresh platelet infusions may be useful when there is thrombocytopenia from any cause, and fresh plasma transfusions when there is a deficiency of clotting factors other than those dependent on vitamin K.

In the case of disseminated intravascular coagulation, the logical treatment would be intravenous heparin, controlling the dose by whole blood clotting time, partial thromboplastin time with kaolin (P.T.T.K.) and plasma heparin level, but we have little experience of this treatment in the newborn.

**Jaundice**

Remember that massive haemorrhage into tissues may lead to serious hyperbilirubinaemia.

*But see p. 272.

# Heart Disease

Some form of heart disease—usually but not invariably a structural malformation—is present in upwards of 1 in 200 newborn babies; thus it constitutes a relatively common problem.

Heart disease may present with:

(1) a cardiac murmur heard on the routine examination of an apparently healthy baby;

(2) (rarely) an abnormality of cardiac rate or rhythm also found on routine examination;

(3) cyanosis;

(4) respiratory distress;

(5) feeding difficulty and failure to thrive.

None of these five findings is necessarily indicative of heart disease, although a combination of two or more increases the likelihood. Thus one finding should make you examine carefully for the other four.

## Cardiac Murmurs

Note the character and localisation of the murmur and examine for other evidence of cardiac disease. Look for cyanosis, thrills, cardiac enlargement, dextrocardia, and femoral pulses (are they palpable and are they synchronous with the radial pulses?). Check blood pressure in arms and legs and look for signs of congestive failure (see below). Examine the obstetric notes for a family history of congenital heart disease and of rubella in pregnancy. (*N.B.* A coloured mother may have had rubella without knowing it.)

If the murmur is very loud, or if there is any evidence of cardiac disease besides the murmur, arrange for chest x-ray and ECG. It is true that even the loudest and most bizarre murmurs may disappear in infancy and are not necessarily associated with cardiac disease, and that the risk to the infant of not investigating an isolated murmur in the neonatal period is small. However, at the risk of causing anxiety to the mother, it is as well to tell her of the existence of the murmur to ensure attendance for follow-up examination.

## Abnormal Rate or Rhythm

In contrast to the finding of murmurs, it is most exceptional to discover an abnormality of cardiac rate or ryhthm on routine examination of an apparently healthy newborn baby. A rate of more than 200/min (*i.e.* uncountable with accuracy) usually means paroxysmal tachycardia, but this condition usually presents with respiratory distress (see below). Note that the heart rate in a normal newborn baby may be nearly 200/min when he is crying lustily.

A heart rate consistently below 80/min suggests congenital heart block. In our experience this condition is diagnosed more often *in utero* than it really occurs.

Expect an asphyxiated baby if fetal 'heart block' is reported to you.

A rapid or irregular heart rate may rarely be due to atrial fibrillation, atrial flutter or incomplete A-V block, in which case there is likely to be, as with genuine heart block, a serious cardiac disorder. Obtain an ECG and chest x-ray and inform the cardiologist immediately.

**Cyanosis**

Distinguishing between a cardiac and a non-cardiac origin is not always simple on initial examination. It is easy in the case of so called 'traumatic asphyxia' because, while there may be deep cyanosis of the head and neck, the trunk is pink. Generalised cyanosis with respiratory distress is nearly always due to respiratory rather than cardiac disease, especially if the cyanosis is relatively mild and if there is marked chest retraction (see below). Severe cerebral disturbances may be associated with cyanosis, possibly due to a reflex increase in pulmonary vascular resistance, which in turn causes right-to-left shunts. But there is usually other clinical evidence of neurological disease. Congenital methaemoglobinaemia is a very rare cause of cyanosis, producing a slaty blue colour. The baby appears to be well, apart from cyanosis, except in a rare variant of the condition associated with severe hypotonia. If you suspect this condition, take blood for spectroscopy and do the simple test described below.* Certain drugs also cause methaemoglobinaemia (see p. 306).

Generalised deep cyanosis without obvious lung disease or with mild signs of respiratory distress is nearly always due to cardiac malformations, even in the absence of cardiac murmurs, and it demands urgent investigation. Remember that a cardiac lesion which one might suppose would inevitably cause cyanosis may not do so for hours or even days after birth.

Do a full clinical examination, looking especially for deepening of cyanosis when the baby cries (this is usually the case in cardiac malformations with right-to-left shunts), for differential cyanosis between the hands and feet and for any signs of cardiac failure. Take a sample of arterial blood for $pO_2$, $pCO_2$ and pH; you will also want to know haemoglobin and platelet levels and blood group and to keep some serum for cross-matching. It is also worthwhile doing a nitrogen washout test (see p. 131) since in cyanotic congenital heart-disease $paO_2$ will rise little in 100% oxygen. Obtain a chest x-ray and ECG and inform the cardiologist.

If there is already a metabolic acidosis, the baby is liable to deteriorate suddenly. Treatment with bicarbonate is worthwhile as a temporising measure while possible surgical treatment is considered. It is also worthwhile raising the environmental oxygen to say 40 per cent, although this is not likely to be of striking benefit. Newborn babies with cyanotic heart-disease are particularly liable to hypothermia; thus their environmental temperature should be kept at the upper end of the neutral range (in

*A useful screening test for methaemoglobinaemia, provided you are not colour-blind, is that described by Harley, J. D. and Celermajer, J. M. (1970) 'Neonatal methaemoglobinaemia and the 'red-brown' screening test.' Lancet, 2, 1223. Allow a drop of capillary blood from the baby and one from a normal control to fall onto a piece of blotting paper or No. 1 filter paper. Wave this gently in the air for about 30 seconds to oxygenate the blood; then compare the colour of the two drops People with normal colour vision have no difficulty in differentiating the brown methaemoglobinaemic blood from the red normal blood, when levels of methaemoglobin exceed 10 per cent.

contrast to babies with left-to-right shunting) and care should be taken to prevent cooling during investigations. Although many such infants have irremedial lesions, a proportion may be saved by curative or palliative surgery (such as balloon a trial septostomy), but before operating a precise diagnosis by angiocardiography and perhaps cardiac catheterisation is necessary. Co-operate closely with the cardiologist in arrangements for investigation, making sure that the baby is kept warm and not kept waiting about in the x-ray department, and that his arterial pH is checked on his return to the neonatal ward. There is some evidence that renal damage may be caused by radio-opaque dyes; the dose should if, possible, be limited to 3ml/kg. After investigation, keep a watch for haematuria. In any case, babies with cyanotic heart-disease are subject to heamorrhagic diatheses (probably disseminated intravascular coagulation, see p. 206), a point to be borne in mind in investigation and surgery. Polycythaemia predisposes to cerebral venous thromboses, and fluid intake should be adequate.

**Respiratory Distress**

A combination of respiratory distress, cyanosis and a cardiac murmur is much more likely to be the result of pulmonary disease (and usually hyaline membrane disease) than cardiac disease, even in full-term infants. In newborn babies with congenital heart lesions producing large right-to-left shunts, severe cyanosis rather than respiratory difficulty is the presenting feature.

In cases of respiratory distress without cyanosis, you should look for signs of cardiac failure (see below), since large left-to-right shunts or myocardial weakness are likely to present in this way.

**Feeding Difficulty and Failure to Thrive**

Slowness with feeds (due to effort dyspnoea) and inadequate weight gain are a characteristic mode of presentation of cardiac failure of relatively gradual onset.

**Signs of Heart Failure**

The clinical signs of cardiac failure in the newborn include:
(1) tachypnoea—often up to 100/min or more, but in mild or early cases only during feeds;
(2) tachycardia;
(3) sweating (otherwise very unusual in the newborn);
(4) unexplained vomiting;
(5) gallop rhythm;
(6) cardiac enlargement (not always detectable);
(7) rise in jugular venous pressure (often difficult to detect in the newborn);
(8) hepatomegaly (the liver is often 2cm below the right costal margin in normal newborn babies, so that a previous measurement is very useful);
(9) splenomegaly;
(10) oedema (which may be generalised and often involves the face);
(11) a sudden increase in body weight (say 100g in one day) or inadequate weight gain;

213

(12) fine moist sounds at the pulmonary bases.

**Causes of Heart Failure**
*Cardiac Malformations*

Some malformations, especially those involving the left side of the heart and/or producing left-to-right shunts, are likely to present with cardiac failure, but even in gross and fatal conditions signs may not appear for several days. These malformations include aortic atresia, truncus arteriosus, coarctation of the aorta, ventricular septal defects, transposition of the great arteries and patent ductus arteriosus. The last condition is encountered relatively commonly in pre-term infants who develop signs of cardiac failure when two or three weeks old and are found to have bounding peripheral pulses (*N.B.* take systolic and diastolic blood pressures), an accentuated pulmonary second sound and a systolic or continuous murmur at the left border of the sternum.

These babies are best treated medically because the ductus may well close spontaneously. Where there is continuous deterioration, or even failure to improve, surgery must be considered. This is often a fiendishly difficult decision to make, since most of these babies do improve on medical treatment, and in the few who do not it is easy to postpone the hazards of investigations until the baby is too ill to undergo them. Angiocardiography and sometimes cardiac catheterization are prerequisites of surgery, since differentiation from other defects, especially ventricular septal defect, cannot be made with certainty on clinical examination.

Patent ductus arteriosus causing cardiac failure in a term infant should be treated surgically, since spontaneous closure is unlikely. Examine for other evidence to suggest the rubella syndrome—especially in coloured babies—and obtain urine for virus culture.

*Paroxysmal Atrial Tachycardia*

In the first four months of life this condition is much commoner in males, is rarely associated with cardiac malformations and has a good ultimate prognosis since it is unlikely to recur after one year. It usually presents with a fairly rapid onset of respiratory distress or vomiting or generalised oedema. The heart rate is over 200 and therefore uncountable. You cannot rely on previous recordings, as nurses find it difficult to believe that the pulse rate may be uncountable. Moist sounds in the lungs may lead to a mistaken diagnosis of pneumonia, and the significance of the very rapid heart-rate may not be appreciated. Get an ECG at once and start digitalisation. Almost all cases respond to digoxin within about 12 hours. If digoxin is ineffective, other drugs such as practolol (see p. 303) should be given. In the rare drug-resistant case, D.C. shock is usually successful.

After normal rhythm is restored, repeat the ECG to exclude the Wolff-Parkinson-White syndrome. Continue digoxin for the first few months to cover the period when recurrences are likely.

*Myocarditis*

Myocarditis presents as unexplained heart failure with a gallop rhythm and usually without murmurs. Get an ECG, which is likely to show low-voltage complexes

214

and T wave abnormalities, and an x-ray which may show cardiac enlargement. Ask the mother if she has had a 'flu-like illness in the previous month and take throat swabs from the baby for Coxsackie B virus culture. Consider also the slender possibilities of toxoplasmosis and bacterial sepsis. Treat for heart failure (see below). Most babies with myocarditis die. Should this happen, ask the virologist what specimens are required to establish the diagnosis.

*Arteriovenous Aneurysms*
An intracranial arteriovenous malformation (see p. 174) or a large benign hepatic vascular tumour may present with cardiac failure, so always auscultate the head and liver.

*Sudden or Severe Anaemia*
The latter is most commonly seen in hydrops fetalis due to Rhesus haemolytic disease.

*Severe Hypertension*
Cardiac failure may be the presenting symptom of coarctation of the aorta, renal disease and the hypertensive form of congenital adrenal hyperplasia.

*Endocardial Fibroelastosis*
This may present at birth with signs similar to those of a mild myocarditis, but with a slowly progressive course. There may be a history of the condition in a sibling.

*Glycogen Storage Disease*
Glycogen storage disease of the heart may also present in the neonatal period, and there may be skeletal muscular hypotonia and a family history.

*Congenital Thyrotoxicosis*
(See p. 10.)

*Intravenous Fluid Overload*
(See p. 99.)

**Treatment of Heart Failure**
*Oxygen Therapy*
Nurse in an oxygen-enriched atmosphere if the arterial $pO_2$ is low or if the baby has signs of respiratory distress. There is little advantage in giving concentrations higher than 40 per cent.

*Digitilisation*
Use digoxin, which may be given orally, by intramuscular injection or by slow intravenous injection. The total digitalising dose is 0.02 to 0.06mg/kg; small preterm infants and seriously affected Rhesus babies require the smaller dose. This total

dose is given in three divided doses over 24 hours; in seriously ill babies, a major fraction (about half) of the digitalising dose is given in the first injection and the total digitalising dose is made up by the subsequent injections. Twelve hours after the last part of the digitalising dose has been given, start maintenance digoxin in two doses daily, each dose being 0.006mg/kg. If there is a bradycardia ($<$ 100 beats per minute), or coupled beats, or ECG signs of intoxication, the next projected dose of digoxin should be withheld.

### Diuretics

Use frusemide 1 to 3mg/kg; it is usually given intramuscularly but can be given I.V. or orally. If possible, weigh the baby before and four hours after the dose. Re-assess the cardiac status, and the urinary output produced by the first dose, before giving more. Usually it need not be given more often than once daily in the acute situation, and much less frequently for maintenance.

### Choice of Milk

Breast-milk has the advantage over cow's milk formulae in that it has a lower sodium content. Very low sodium milks are highly artificial and have become un-necessary since the advent of frusemide.

### Position

The baby should be tipped head-up. Although there are advocates of nursing the child in a near-vertical position using a suitable harness, we have no experience of this procedure.

### Sedation

The best sedation is relief of respiratory distress, and of positioning or gently swaddling the limbs so that he is comfortably supported. For very distressed, hyper-kinetic babies, try chloral hydrate in a single dose of 60mg. On rare occasions, we use morphine 0.1mg/kg/dose, after which the child's breathing must be observed with unusual care.

### Venesection

In hydropic Rhesus babies in whom the venous pressure has been measured and found to be high, and in babies who for some reason have had too much intra-venous fluid, removal of 20 to 40ml of blood can produce remarkable relief. It is, however, not often indicated.

### Environmental Temperature

Babies with acyanotic congenital heart defects and large left-to-right shunts tend to sweat and to have a high metabolic rate. In contrast to blue babies, they should be nursed in an environmental temperature at the lower end of the neutral range.

# TAKING BLOOD PRESSURE IN THE NEWBORN

*Direct Measurement*

If an arterial catheter has been inserted for the measurement of blood gas tensions, we usually take the opportunity of obtaining a direct measurement of blood pressure using a transducer. However, the purpose of this measurement is to compare with the usual indirect measurements, and direct measurement of blood pressure has no particular advantage over indirect measurement in terms of clinical diagnosis.

*Indirect Measurement*

*Cuff size.* Use a 2.5cm wide cuff, the inflatable portion of which is sufficiently long completely to encircle the upper arm. We find the plastic 'Neligan' cuff the most suitable. (In many cloth-covered cuffs, the rubber inflatable cuff is of appropriate width (*i.e.* 2.5cm) but much too short to encircle the arm). We have always found it difficult to measure blood pressure in the lower limbs by auscultation and we therefore use the flush method in comparing blood pressure in the upper arm and calf. Use the same cuff on both the upper and lower limb, and make sure the inflatable part is long enough to overlap in both places.

*State of baby.* Wherever possible, avoid taking readings when the baby is crying or active, or when the baby is having a feed or sucking actively on a dummy. In any of these situations the blood pressure may be 10 to 15mmHg higher than a resting level. It is best to apply the cuff and then wait patiently until the baby is in the right state.

*Method.* Pump the cuff up to above systolic pressure. In most cases 110mmHg will suffice and higher compressions merely disturb the child. Try one of the following means of assessing blood pressure, as the pressure is released *very* slowly.

(*a*) Auscultate over the brachial artery with a small stethoscope (and the popliteal artery if you are not discouraged by our experience). One often can hear the systolic and diastolic endpoints in the arm; if one is successful, this is better than the other methods below.

(*b*) Use the oscillometer: as the pressure is released the point at which the needle begins to flick regularly is the systolic pressure and the point where oscillation is maximal is the diastolic pressure.

(*c*) Palpate a peripheral artery (radial in arm, dorsalis pedis or posterior tibial in leg). This only gives a systolic pressure.

(*d*) Use a pulse monitor. A number of such devices have had a vogue (*e.g.* bead of xylene, photocell, thermistor head) and some personal preference is experienced. In all of them it is difficult to identify and exclude artifact.

(*e*) Use the flush method. Firmly compress the limb in one hand to squeeze the blood out *before* blowing up the cuff to above systolic pressure. Release the pressure 3 or 5mm at a time, holding for five seconds at each step. The end point is when the limb flushes, and is usually obvious. Repeat this two or three times. The flush method gives a systolic reading about 5mmHg less than that obtained by auscultation.

(*f*) We have no personal experience of the use of the Doppler technique for measuring blood pressure but it seems to be a promising recent development.

217

# Unexpected Collapse

It is obvious that collapse is most likely to occur in the course of other illnesses, but below we list some of the situations in which it may come 'out of the blue'.

**Haemorrhage**

If an infant looks extremely pale and collapsed at birth, feto-maternal haemorrhage, or haemorrhage from a torn velamentous cord vessel should be considered. Urgent replacement of blood, and sometimes correction of acidosis, may be necessary (see p. 209).

Massive blood loss after birth may be from one of the following.

(a) The umbilical cord—due to slipped clamp (any time) or associated with haemorrhagic disease (second or third day).

(b) Gastro-intestinal tract—most frequently associated with haemorrhagic disease (see p. 207).

(c) Intracranial haemorrhage (see p. 182), which may be subdural following difficult delivery (first or second day,) intraventricular in the very immature (first, second or third days), or massive intracerebral and subarachnoid in infants with erythroblastosis fetalis associated with disseminated intravascular coagulation.

(d) Ruptured solid abdominal viscus—usually the liver, rarely the spleen (second or third day), usually associated with breech or difficult deliveries, or where there is marked hepatosplenomegaly as in some severe cases of erythroblastosis. Adrenal haemorrhage is described on p. 219.

(e) From any site in addition to intracranial (c) above when disseminated intravascular coagulation is present, commonly with hypothermia, asphyxia and acidosis.

**Pneumothorax**

(See p. 140). This occurs most commonly in severe birth asphyxia, meconium aspiration and RDS.

**Biochemical or Metabolic Disorders**

The most important to exclude immediately is hypoglycaemia (commonest in small-for-dates infants) following severe birth asphyxia, or in severe erythroblastosis fetalis (see p. 147). Some inborn errors of metabolism, which are all rare, may present with profound hypotonia, unresponsiveness and sometimes fits and acidosis (*e.g.* organic acidaemias such as propionicacidaemia and maple syrup urine disease). When you are clearly dealing with an unusual disorder, measure the blood pH, and have the plasma and urine examined for amino-acids and other organic acids (see p. 225).

**Infection**

Septicaemia can occur at any time in the neonatal period, but is commonest after the first 48 hours, in males, and those of low birthweight. Though the majority of severe infections are Gram-negative, the picture of shock within a short time of onset seen in older patients may not be clear-cut in the newborn, and when collapse occurs the infection may already be well established in various systems (see p. 163).

### Adrenal Failure

This may occur in the salt-losing type of congenital adrenal hyperplasia, when hyponatraemia and hyperkalaemia will be present (see p. 61). It is important to realise that the diagnostic clue provided by virilisation in the female does not exist in the male, in whom the disease occurs with the same frequency.

The symptoms of congenital adrenal hypoplasia are similar. Both conditions are inherited as autosomal recessives.

### Adrenal Haemorrhage

Massive unilateral or bilateral adrenal haemorrhage is a rare consequence of breech or difficult deliveries, asphyxia, haemorrhagic diatheses or septicaemia. Shock, sometimes with fits, may suddenly develop within a few days of birth and abdominal distension with large swellings in one or both flanks is usually found. The urine is free from macroscopic blood, thus distinguishing the condition from renal vein thrombosis. Not all cases are fatal and survivors may present later with symptoms of adrenal insufficiency and show adrenal calcification on x-ray.

### Heart Failure

(See p. 213.) This is most common in congenital heart disease, often as the ductus is closing after the first few days of life, but it may occur with paroxysmal tachycardia, myocarditis due to intra-uterine or post-natal viral infection, and even more rarely in association with arteriovenous communication, especially intracranial.

### Airway Obstruction

Once spontaneous respirations are established after birth, the most common causes are inhaled stomach contents, severe degree of Pierre Robin syndrome, and bilateral choanal atresia (see p. 51 and p. 53).

# Congenital Tumours

A large variety of tumours have been recognized as presenting occasionally at birth, and a selection of them is listed in Table XI. Many of these are hamartomas (*i.e.* localized overgrowths of tissue elements normal to the site where they occur) rather than true neoplasms.

The only common lesion is the benign haemangioma of the skin (strawberry mark)—see p. 249 for full description and treatment.

Obtain the advice of a surgeon about other tumours recognised in the neonatal period.

Two points should be remembered.

(1) Internal masses discovered on x-ray or abdominal palpation may represent either an abnormally formed or abnormally sited organ (*e.g.* a low-lying kidney), or a neoplasm.

(2) Malignant tumours presenting in the newborn are mostly embryonic tumours. Their clinical behaviour is not well correlated with their histological structure and they are often adequately treated by simple excision. Some, *e.g.* neuroblastomas, occasionally regress spontaneously.

### Congenital Leukaemia

Acute myelogenous leukaemia presents rarely at birth. The child may be born with haemorrhages or slate-coloured nodular infiltrations in the skin, he usually has an enlarged liver and spleen, and often bleeds from umbilicus, mucous membranes or the gastro-intestinal tract. The platelet count is reduced and there are large numbers of circulating nucleated cells in addition to myelocytes and myeloblasts. Anaemia is not usually a presenting sign, but develops within a few days. The presence of many myeloblasts on blood and marrow smears enables the condition to be differentiated from haemolytic disease of the newborn, congenital thrombocytopenic purpura, haemorrhage due to disseminated intravascular coagulation, or a leukaemoid reaction associated with infection.

Like acute leukaemia in later childhood, congenital leukaemia has an increased incidence in Down's syndrome. Drug treatment in the newborn has so far proved unsatisfactory, and death usually occurs within the first two months of life.

Myeloid metaplasia has been described in the newborn, unassociated with infection or Rh iso-immunisation, and may have been responsible for some reports of congenital leukaemia with spontaneous remission.

TABLE XI
**Tumours and neoplastic disease which may present at birth**

| Site | Benign | Malignant |
|---|---|---|
| Head and neck | Epidermal inclusion cysts, congenital epulis of jaw, melanotic epulis, teratoma. | Retinoblastoma, glioma, teratoma. |
| Skin or subcutaneous tissue (any part of body) | Haemangioma, lymphangioma, neurofibromatosis, multiple lipomas. | Sarcomas of connective tissue and muscle. |
| Visceral and retroperitoneal | Haemangiomas of liver, etc., lymphangioma, cysts of intestine or ovaries, mesenchymal tumours, teratomas. | Neuroblastoma, nephroblastoma*, hepatoblastoma. |
| Sacral region | Teratoma. | |
| Testis | | Orchidoblastoma. |
| Reticulo-endothelial and haemopoietic systems | | Letterer-Siwe disease, congenital leukaemia. |

*It has recently been claimed that all cases of nephroblastoma reported at birth are examples of a different (and benign) tumour.

# The Infant of a Narcotic Addict

We have no direct experience of this problem, but we have kept the following standing instructions for dealing with it if it does arise. For an account based on very extensive experience, see Zelson *et al.* (1971)*.

The baby is likely to be of low birthweight but there will probably not be any knowledge of the mother's dates. Withdrawal signs usually develop within the first 24 hours of life, but may be delayed as long as four to five days, so prolonged and careful observation is necessary in a suspect case.

**Signs of Withdrawal**

*Early:* vigorous sucking with regurgitation of feeds;
increased tone and tendon jerks;
hyperirritability and tremulous movements;
shrill continuous high-pitched cry;
nasal stuffiness, sneezing, yawning, lacrimation, sweating, increased mucus secretion;
hyperventilation with alkalosis and low $paCO_2$.

*Late:* vomiting and diarrhoea;
excitability, convulsions;
fever;
dehydration and electrolyte disorders;
circulatory failure.

If withdrawal symptoms are untreated, the mortality rate may be as high as 90 per cent, death being due to circulatory failure, often with additional infection. With treatment, mortality should be less than 10 per cent.

**Management** (for dosages, see p. 299 *et seq.*)

(1) Await symptoms before introducing therapy, as severity of withdrawal is not predictable.

(2) *Early stage:* (*a*) chloral; (*b*) phenobarbitone.

(3) *Late stage:* (*a*) chlorpromazine; (*b*) i.v. fluids and electrolytes.

(4) Antibiotics as indicated.

**Further Investigations**

If the baby is small for dates, perform appropriate investigations, *e.g.* blood sugar. Check w.r. and hepatitis associated antigen in all cases.

*Follow-up*

If it is felt that the mother is incapable of caring for the child, the Department of Medical Social Work should arrange for the infant to be taken into care.

*Zelson, C., Rubio, E , Wasserman, E. (1971) 'Neonatal narcotic addiction: 10 year observation.' *Pediatrics*, **48**, 178.

222

# Chromosomal Disorders

These may be found in about 1 per cent of live births, and are approximately equally divided between the autosomes and the sex chromosomes. Turner's syndrome apart, abnormalities of sex chromosomes often go undetected in the neonatal period unless a screening programme is in progress, for they are less commonly associated with obvious congenital defect than are autosomal defects.

## Autosomal Disorders

We cannot describe here the clinical features of all the different anomalies recognised so far. Consult Thompson (1965) and Smith (1970)* for helpful catalogues and photographs.

Suspect autosomal anomaly in any infant with low birthweight for gestational age and multiple defects. The external defects may not always be gross, and you should be alert to deviations such as a single transverse palmar crease, clinodactyly and missing interphalangeal crease, a single umbilical artery, low-set or abnormal ears (see Smith for definition), retrognathia, hypertelorism, epicanthic folds, abnormal slant of palpebral fissures, scalp defects, unusual whorling of hair, extra lax skin-folds at the back of the neck, high-arched palate, abnormal finger flexion, in addition to serious lesions such as congenital heart disease, cleft lip and palate, and abnormality of the external genitalia. You should try and record the dermatoglyphic patterns—palm prints will be necessary for a detailed analysis—but it is always helpful to note down the finger-tip patterns and positioning of the palmar triradii; this can be done quite quickly using the light and magnifying lens of an otoscope without the aural speculum attached (see Miller and Giroux (1966) and Penrose (1968)†).

You will diagnose Down's syndrome most commonly. If the mother is over 35, and the baby's features are typical, chromosomal studies might be left undone. However, in most cases, particularly when the parents are young, and in all infants in whom you suspect abnormalities of other autosomes, you should arrange for analysis wherever possible. This is particularly important if early neonatal death seems likely, so do not delay. Though successful cultures have been made on post-mortem material, collection of specimens during life is preferable. A study of two tissues (*e.g.* blood and skin for lymphocyte and fibroblast culture) will help to exclude mosaicism. If an infant proves to have an abnormal karyotype, and particularly if there is a family history of spontaneous abortions, congenital anomalies and/or mental defect, the parents' chromosomes should be examined, again preferably in two tissues, so that they can be given the most informed genetic advice about the future.

*Thompson, H. (1965) 'Abnormalities of the autosomal chromosomes associated with human disease: selected topics and catalogue.' *American Journal of Medical Sciences*, **250**, 718.
Smith, D. W. (1970) *Recognizable Patterns of Human Malformations. Major Problems in Clinical Pediatrics, Vol. VII.* Philadelphia and London: W. B. Saunders.
†Miller, J. R., Giroux, J. (1966) 'Dermatoglyphics in pediatric practice'. *Journal of Pediatrics*, **69**, 302.
Penrose, L. S. (1968) *Memorandum on Dermatoglyphic Nomenclature.* Birth Defects, Original Article Series, Vol. 4, No. 3. New York: National Foundation—March of Dimes.

## Sex Chromosomes

See Insley (1970)* for a helpful review of the various permutations possible. About one-half the live-born cases of Turner's syndrome will show pitting oedema of the dorsum of the feet, sometimes of the hands as well, and extra lax posterior cervical skin-folds. Buccal smear is a helpful preliminary, but normal females may be chromatin negative in the first week of life.

## Collection of Specimens

When possible, contact the laboratory first — they have the special media necessary. If the special medium is not immediately available, put 2cc of the infant's blood into a sterile heparinized container and store at 4°C until the laboratory can deal with it. Cultures can be made quite successfully from a few drops of blood collected in a sterile Pasteur pipette washed out with heparin. This blood must, however, be added to the special media within a very short time, and stored at 4°C until it goes to the lab. Remember that sterile technique during collection is especially important, for infection will prevent successful cultures.

For fibroblast culture, a small pinch of skin should be put straight into the special media.

*Insley, J. (1970) 'Sex chromosome abnormalities in children.' *British Journal of Hospital Medicine*, **4**, 103.

# Inborn Errors of Metabolism

These rare genetically determined disorders, mostly inherited as autosomal recessives, are each due to defective synthesis of a specific enzyme. The wide variety of missing enzymes leads to a great diversity of disease; and disease due to a single inborn error may vary in clinical severity.

An abnormal accumulation of metabolites before the enzyme block, or possibly deficiency of one produced after it, may prove harmful to rapidly growing tissues at this period of life. Brain damage with consequent mental retardation may occur relatively early in life in certain of the disorders. It seems to be well established that avoidance or reduction of brain-damage results if diagnosis is made very early and effective treatment is instituted. In a few cases, the disorders lead to a clinically recognisable illness in the neonatal period; in others the damage is so insidious or the abnormality is so mild that only comprehensive screening programmes will detect them. We do not list the inborn errors and give their clinical features here: we merely give some guidance for their diagnosis. They will probably soon number one hundred. Some useful references are Buist (1968), Cone (1968), O'Brien and Goodman (1970) and Raine (1972)*.

## Screening

The merits and difficulties of screening programmes are under intense discussion at present.

A modification of the Guthrie test, which detects abnormal amounts of methionine and histidine, in addition to phenylalanine, is carried out for us at the Hospital for Sick Children, Great Ormond Street. The test can be performed on blood obtained by heel-prick, and is done on the sixth or seventh day after birth (see p. 84 for details).

If a metabolic disorder is already known to exist in a family, you should of course arrange for the relevant screening procedures to be done when any subsequent child is born.

## Neonatal Illness and Metabolic Disorder
### Protein Metabolism

Certain of the inborn errors of protein metabolism may present with an acute and fulminating illness in the first weeks of life. Suspect metabolic disorder, *particularly* if there is any family history of unexplained neonatal death or mental retardation, in an infant who seems well at birth and who develops any of the following within a few days.

*Buist, N. R. M. (1968) 'Set of simple side-room urine tests for the detection of inborn errors of metabolism.' *British Medical Journal*, **2**, 745.
Cone, T. E. (1968) 'Diagnosis and treatment: some diseases, syndromes and conditions associated with an unusual odor.' *Pediatrics*, **41**, 993.
O'Brien, D., Goodman, S. I. (1970) 'The critically ill child: acute metabolic disease in infancy and early childhood.' *Pediatrics*, **46**, 620.
Raine, N. (1972) 'The management of inherited metabolic disease.' *British Medical Journal*, **2**, 392.

(1) Feeding difficulties—refusal, and vomiting leading to dehydration.

(2) Respiratory difficulties—tachypnoea, apnoea.

(3) Lethargy, progressing to unresponsiveness, with profound hypotonia and areflexia.

(4) Seizures, either tonic fits or myoclonic jerks.

(5) Abnormal smell, either from the baby or his urine.

Final diagnosis will need the help of a specialist laboratory.

(a) Collect blood from the infant, 1-2ml if possible.

Is there a metabolic acidosis? (pH, $pCO_2$, base excess).

Separate plasma; if the laboratory is unable to use specimen at once for amino-acid chromatography, store at $-20°C$.

Store red cells.

(b) Collect all urine passed.

Has it an abnormal smell (such as maple syrup, sweaty feet, tom-cat, oast house)? Test for ketonuria with 'Acetest'.

Test for ketoaciduria with DNP hydrazine test: (add a saturated solution of 2-4 DNP hydrazine in HCl drop by drop to 1 volume of urine until up to $\frac{1}{2}$-volume of reagent added; a precipitate will appear in 3-5 minutes if ketoacids are present). Give some to the laboratory for chromatography—paper, thin layer and column. Store at $-20°C$ if they are unable to use it immediately.

(c) If a metabolic acidosis, ketonuria, ketoaciduria and hyperglycinaemia are present, the infant may have one of the organic acidaemias. Gas chromatography of blood and urine will be necessary for final diagnosis in these cases.

**Initial Treatment**

Until the laboratory are able to reach a precise diagnosis with the specimens you have given them, and if the child is profoundly ill:

withdraw protein (i.e. milk) from the diet;

substitute oral or intravenous glucose;

try to correct metabolic acidosis with alkali;

support respiration if necessary.

In desperate cases, an exchange transfusion or even peritoneal dialysis might be considered.

After diagnosis, a suitable synthetic low-protein preparation will be necessary (remember, complete vitamin supplementation with these is essential). Biotin, $B_{12}$ and thiamine may be of value in the treatment of certain of these disorders.

If death should occur despite these measures before a proper diagnosis has been reached, further help may be obtained at post-mortem. By freezing unfixed autopsy tissues, particularly liver, amino-acids, volatile organic acids and glycogen will be preserved, and further diagnostic tests can be carried out. It is particularly important to try to reach a diagnosis, so that genetic advice to the parents can be as precise as possible.

*Carbohydrate Metabolism*

Two disorders of carbohydrate metabolism may be mentioned here.

(1) *Galactosaemia* may be present with hepatomegaly, jaundice, haemorrhages

due to deficiency of vitamin K dependent factors associated with liver damage, vomiting, failure to thrive, and the development of cataracts.

Test the urine for reducing substances with Fehling's or Benedict's reagents or 'Clinitest'. Strip tests (like 'Clinistix') which react specifically with glucose are not suitable for this purpose. The reducing substances can be identified by sugar chromatography. Test the urine for protein and arrange for animo-acid chromatography, since proteinuria and an abnormal amino-aciduria are also present. Estimation of blood-sugars will show higher levels of total reducing substances than of glucose. The diagnosis is established by demonstration of the enzyme defect (galactose 1-phosphate uridyl transferase) in the red cells, and treatment consists of withdrawal of lactose (*i.e.* milk) from the diet. Give phytomenadione 1mg I.M. and be prepared for blood transfusion if there are any haemorrhagic manifestations.

(2) *Fructose intolerance* may present in a very similar way, and similar initial steps are needed for diagnosis. Fructose, and frequently abnormal amino-acids, will be present in the urine, and estimation of blood sugars will again show higher levels of total reducing substances than of glucose. Final diagnosis will rest on quick clinical improvement when fructose is withdrawn from the diet, and a profound fall in blood glucose if a test dose of fructose is given (proceed with great care in the neonatal period). Give phytomenadione and/or transfusion as above if haemorrhagic manifestations are present.

Several other inborn errors of metabolism have been mentioned elsewhere, *e.g.* congenital adrenal hyperplasia (p. 61), cystic fibrosis (p. 195), disaccharidase deficiency and other disorders of carbohydrate metabolism (p. 202), glucose 6-phosphate dehydrogenase and pyruvate kinase deficiencies (p. 160).

# Polycythaemia

The viscosity of blood increases gradually with increasing haematocrit until the packed cell volume exceeds 70 per cent when viscosity increases abruptly, causing poor flow in small vessels. Polycythaemia of this degree has been described in some neonatal conditions and may cause symptoms and require action.

The baby is usually reported as looking plethoric, and sometimes as having cyanosis. In fact such cyanosis is usually confined to the extremities, but it should be remembered that even relatively mild hypoxaemia in the presence of a very high haematocrit may lead to > 5g/100ml of reduced haemoglobin, and thus true central cyanosis. Gross polycythaemia is also associated with symptoms of cerebral hyper-excitability (including fits) or, alternatively, apathy (see 'Neurological problems', p. 178) and on rare occasions with cerebral thrombosis. Polycythaemic babies sometimes have some degree of respiratory distress and may become severely jaundiced.

Babies in whom polycythaemia is likely to occur are those with delayed clamping of the cord (p. 30), babies who are very small for dates (usually less than 3rd percentile), infants of diabetic mothers, and the recipient twin in the twin transfusion syndrome. This last condition occurs in identical twins where, presumably over a fairly long period of intra-uterine life, one twin has transfused blood into the other through a placental vascular connection (p. 70). At birth there is a gross disparity in Hb concentrations (and colour) between the two twins. The recipient plethoric twin may be in a worse condition than the donor, often with congestive heart failure and the problems associated with polycythaemia. The donor twin will be anaemic, occasionally severely anaemic, is likely to be small for dates and therefore to become hypoglycaemic.

If a baby is unduly plethoric, take *venous* blood for a haematocrit estimation, since heel-prick blood may give unreliable results. In any case of suspected twin transfusion, estimate Hb concentration and haematocrit in both babies. If the venous haematocrit is greater than 70, perform an exchange transfusion with plasma using 20 to 30ml/kg.

# What To Do When A Baby Dies

First inform the consultant paediatrician, the obstetrician and the postnatal ward sister. Between you, decide who shall break the news to the mother. If the father is quickly available by telephone, he may prefer to do it himself.

*Always* inform the general practitioner by telephone.

The consultant paediatrician will see both parents together at a suitable time and will write to them when the full post-mortem results are available. A second interview may then be desirable.

## Post-mortem Examination

It is highly desirable that any baby who dies should be submitted to post-mortem examination by a pathologist experienced in this branch of morbid anatomy. Post-mortem examinations always contribute to good clinical standards, but there are two reasons why they are of special importance in neonatal paediatrics.

(1)  Accurate diagnosis in life is often impossible in the small baby, due to the brief duration of his illness.

(2)  Confirmation of the cause of death is important in order to advise the parents on the prospects for future pregnancies.

## Immediate Post-mortem Sampling

If death is suspected to be due to infection and no blood culture has been set up previously, an immediate post-mortem culture of heart blood is preferable to the culture of specimens taken hours later during routine autopsy. Bladder puncture and collection of CSF may also be done if post-mortem is likely to be delayed.

### Permission for Post-mortem Examination

Written permission for necropsy should be obtained as soon as possible after death, following the standard practice of the hospital. If permission for post-mortem is refused, the consultant should be informed immediately if he has not already seen the relatives, as he may be able to obtain a reversal of this decision.

### Attendance at Post-mortem

The residents should attend post-mortem examinations unless engaged in urgent duties on the wards, and should inform the pathologist of any clinical details which may not readily be ascertained from the notes, *e.g.* a positive blood culture report obtained by telephone after the baby's death.

## Death Certificate*

The death certificate may be completed before or after post-mortem examination.

*These paragraphs refer to the law in England and Wales.

If the certificate is completed after necropsy, the pathologist will advise on the correct diagnosis to include. Often, however, the certificate has to be completed by the resident before necropsy is done.

Neonatal deaths must be reported to the coroner if resulting from or accelerated by negligence or assault, or if occurring within 24 hours of an operation or anaesthetic. If in doubt, telephone the Coroner's Officer and ask for advice.

The precise wording of the death certificate is important. If death is certified as due to septicaemia in a case of generalised infection, the registrar of births and deaths will refer the case to the coroner. The certification of death as due to inflammation of whichever organ is primarily involved, *e.g.* pneumonia or meningitis, is, however, entirely acceptable.

# Section 5: Less Urgent Neonatal Problems

*NOTES*

# Continuing Care of the Low-birthweight Infant

Infants of low birthweight are likely to have a more or less prolonged stay in the neonatal ward. After the first week of life the condition of the majority no longer causes anxiety, and there is a risk that in competition with ill new arrivals they may get less than their share of attention from busy staff.

For feeding, see p. 96; for eye-examination, see p. 241.

**Regular Examination**

This should be made at least once weekly, and the findings recorded. There are three important aspects: (1) detection of illness or abnormality; (2) assessment of physical growth; and (3) assessment of neurological maturation.

(1) Look carefully for any minor abnormalities which may have been missed if the infant was ill in the first days of life. Note particularly the presence of tachypnoea, cardiac murmur, skin lesions, or herniae, and the state of the umbilicus. Look particularly for herniae in the groin. Record the important normal findings, such as a good stream of urine in the male.

(2) Chart head-circumference and weight on percentile charts (see pp. 324-327) once weekly, in order to detect major and continuing deviations from normal. Although the charts are derived of necessity from cross-sectional rather than longitudinal data, they are a helpful guide to progress. Head-circumference percentiles may be crossed in an upwards direction in many very immature babies, and the increased PA and narrower biparietal diameters of these infants may increase the circumference and give a false impression of hydrocephalus. The length of time taken to regain birth weight is usually inversely proportional to gestational age, being longest when this is lowest. With modern feeding methods, most pre-term babies of appropriate birthweight for gestation should be above the tenth percentile on their expected date of delivery, whereas small-for-dates infants who are also pre-term are unlikely to be. A rapid weight gain over a 24 to 48 hour period is most likely to be due to fluid retention, and the commonest causes are congestive cardiac failure, or a change from breast milk to cow's milk. Conversely, a marked weight loss over a 24 to 48 hour period means fluid loss, usually from the gastro-intestinal tract. If weight gain is very slow, check first that the infant is having and retaining an adequate feed, *i.e.* at least 180ml of undiluted breast-milk or full-strength half cream dried milk per kg expected weight. Consider the possibility of late metabolic acidosis and measure pH and bicarbonate in capillary blood. Treat with oral sodium bicarbonate (see p. 303). Static or falling weight is always an indication for further investigation, examination of the urine being one of the most important first steps. Also assure yourself of the normality of the stools.

(3) Record, in the case of infants who are more than three or four weeks pre-term, the various reflexes which are helpful in assessing gestational age (see p. 91). Their appearance at certain intervals after birth may be a further check on the accuracy

233

of your initial assessment. Record when the baby is first able to take a feed from a bottle or the breast. If the baby is awake and alert, see if he will look at you and whether you can make him smile. In any case, ask the nurse about his visual attention and smiling.

### Haemoglobin Estimation, Iron and Folic Acid Therapy
Check the haemoglobin weekly. The majority of very immature infants develop an anaemia which is normocytic at first, with hypoplastic marrow. Later, there is increased marrow activity, a high reticulocyte count, and iron deficiency gradually appears. The prescription of iron as Ferrous sulphate mixture paediatric, B.P.C. (30mg b.d.) from approximately two weeks will lessen but not prevent this*. The continued importance of iron to the infant should be stressed to the parents when he is discharged. Make sure an initial supply is given, and that the family's doctor knows the prescription. We also give folic acid tablets (B.P. 0.1mg once weekly) to infants with birth weights less than 1800g (see also p. 236).

### Vitamin Supplements
We use a proprietary multivitamin preparation and 0.6ml is given once daily from two weeks of age. Again, a supply should be given on discharge, and the family's doctor notified. 0.6ml of the drops contains:-

| | |
|---|---|
| vitamin A 5000 i.u. | vitamin B 1mg |
| vitamin C 50mg | vitamin $B_2$ 0.4mg |
| vitamin D 400 i.u. | vitamin $B_6$ 0.5mg |
| nicotinamide 5mg | |

### Transfer from Incubator to Cot
It is only in writing this book that it has occurred to us that we have left this decision entirely to the nursing staff. Sister Castle normally transfers a low-birthweight baby to a cot when he weighs between 1500 and 1750g. Before doing so, she clothes the baby in the incubator and lowers the incubator temperature to make sure that he is still able to maintain his body temperature. A baby who is feeding from a bottle, or who is very active, may be transferred to a cot at a lower weight. A baby who still has respiratory difficulty or who needs especially close observation will generally be kept in an incubator. This general policy is in keeping with that of other neonatal units, but we think that the whole question of the use of incubators should be reviewed. Incubators have disadvantages in that they may be a source of infection and they may be noisy: they must also be very uncomfortable to lie in.

### Parents
Try to keep the parents informed of their baby's progress, and make sure their

---

*There may be objections to giving iron as early as this since it has been shown that iron may aggravate the early anaemia of pre-term babies by interfering with the absorption of vitamin E (Melhorn and Gross 1971).

Melhorn, D. K., Gross, S. (1971) 'Vitamin E-dependent anemia in the premature infant: effects of large doses of medicinal iron.' *Journal of Pediatrics*, **79**, 569.

questions are answered as far as possible. Except in a very few cases, cheerful optimism about present and future is justifiable. Remember that the mother may feel a tremendous sense of isolation from the infant, particularly if he is nursed in an incubator at first. She should be encouraged to come and see him, touch him when she wants to, and participate in his care, particularly feeding, from an early stage. It is your responsibility to see this is happening, and it may require tactful discussion with the nursing staff.

**Discharge from Hospital**

The families of low-birthweight infants often have more than their share of social and economic problems. The Obstetric Medical Social Worker usually knows about most of them, but if she doesn't, you may need to make gentle enquiries of the parents. In general, a baby will be ready for discharge when he reaches 2250 to 2500g; an even lower weight may be suitable during the summer for babies with the most satisfactory homes. Before he goes, his mother (or foster mother) must be thoroughly conversant with the preparation of his feeds, and feel confident that giving them to him presents her with no problems. She must understand the continued need for iron and vitamin supplements. These explanations are generally given by the nursing staff but the medical staff should make sure they have been understood. They must also assure themselves that the parents are able to keep the infant's bedroom at least at a reasonably steady temperature of about 20°C (70°F) throughout the 24 hours during winter, and that there are no infections in the home. Young siblings with diarrhoea or respiratory infection pose a particular threat. The parents should also be told of the staff's continued interest in the infant's wellbeing, and an appointment should be made for the follow-up clinic after a suitable interval, usually 4 to 8 weeks in the first instance. Ask them to let you know of any change of address. Finally, enquire *how* the parents are going to get the baby home: do not allow an infant who weighed 1000g at birth and who has spent eight weeks in your care to leave for a distant destination by public transport at the rush hour in a snowstorm!

# Anaemia

The commonest situations associated with anaemia in the neonatal period are:

(1) Haemorrhage (see p. 206).

(2) Haemolytic disease of the newborn, which may be associated with anaemia at birth (normally corrected by exchange transfusion), and with a later anaemia usually occurring at two to six weeks of age (see p. 154).

(3) Anaemia of prematurity: pre-term babies may become anaemic in the first few weeks and/or later in the first year. Here we are concerned with the former situation.

**Early Anaemia of Prematurity**

In term newborn babies, the haemoglobin level normally falls during the first two months of life. In infants of low birthweight, the fall is more pronounced and these babies may become markedly anaemic at some time during their stay in the neonatal ward. The age at which the haemoglobin level is lowest is usually between five and nine weeks, and the minimum haemoglobin concentration is usually between 7 and 12g/100ml. Why the marrow cannot keep pace with the rapid increase in blood volume during the period of rapid growth is not known. Iron deficiency is not an important factor, and while folic acid deficiency may sometimes play a part, it is not a major factor either. There are three practical questions to be asked in an infant of low birthweight who becomes anaemic during the first few weeks of life.

*Is Any Further Investigation Indicated?*

If the anaemia follows the expected time course, the haemoglobin level dropping to a minimum at five to nine weeks and then beginning to rise, further investigation is not indicated. The reticulocyte count rises from the age of about one month (earlier in babies of very low birthweight). Check the haemoglobin and reticulocyte count once weekly.

*Should Haematinics be Given?*

In our special care nursery, all low-birthweight babies are given ferrous sulphate mixture 30mg b.d. from the age of two weeks. This does not significantly alter the course of early anaemia, though it lessens the degree of later anaemia. No other haematinics are indicated if the problem appears to be straightforward anaemia of prematurity. Babies below 1800g birthweight are also given folic acid 0.1 mg weekly, because these babies have been shown in several studies to be folic-acid deficient. We do not give vitamin E; the cases of vitamin E deficiency reported in low-birthweight babies have been in infants fed on artificial milk lacking this vitamin, but see p. 234.

*Should the Baby be Transfused?*

Babies with early anaemia of prematurity usually recover spontaneously: transfusion is therefore only indicated if the baby is seriously disturbed by the anaemia when the haemoglobin level is at its lowest. We do not routinely transfuse when the haemoglobin level falls below some arbitrary level, though we would always seriously consider transfusion if the Hb fell below 7g/100ml. We attach greater importance to the presence of symptoms—breathlessness or increasing slowness over feeds—for which there is no other explanation, and in such cases we might transfuse even though the haemoglobin level were above 7g/100ml. We may take further factors into account in deciding on transfusion; for example, if a pre-term baby were ready to go home and had not yet definitely passed the trough, we would usually transfuse rather than delay the baby's going home.

In practice, we find that transfusion is rarely needed in anaemia of prematurity.

If a baby is transfused, special care must be taken to avoid precipitating heart-failure. The blood should be given slowly—over the course of several hours—and the baby should be watched carefully for breathlessness or tachycardia. If in doubt, stop the transfusion at once. If there are signs of incipient heart-failure or pre-existing heart disease, or the baby has been anaemic for a considerable time, intraperitoneal rather than intravenous transfusion may be considered (see p. 274).

Aim to raise the Hb level to about 12g/100ml. A rough calculation of the volume of blood needed (V) based on an expected blood volume in the baby of 85ml/kg can be made from the formula:

$$V = \frac{(12 - Hb)}{12} \times 0.085 \times W$$

where Hb is the baby's present haemoglobin level in g/100ml and W his present weight in grammes. The calculation refers to the volume of donor blood *before* dilution with ACD solution or packing. We like to give fresh heparinized blood, which is partially packed (see p. 272).

### Rarer Causes of Anaemia

If a baby has anaemia which does not fit into any of the above categories, a number of rare conditions must be considered. (See Oski and Naiman 1972.)

Oski, F. A., Naiman, J. L. (1972) *Hematological Problems in the Newborn*. 2nd. Edn. Philadelphia and London: W. B. Saunders.

# Delayed Pulmonary Insufficiency in Pre-term Infants

We recognise the existence of delayed pulmonary insufficiency of pre-term infants (including the Wilson-Mikity syndrome) and always look for it, but must acknowledge that we seldom find a case in our survivors of very low birthweight.

Surviving pre-term infants, especially those of very low birthweight (*i.e.* less than 1.5kg), should be looked at twice weekly for evidence of late respiratory distress while they remain in the special care nursery, or immediately, should the nursing staff report rapid breathing or slowness with feeds.

Whether or not there has been respiratory distress (presumptive hyaline membrane disease) in the early neonatal period, and whether or not recovery from classical respiratory distress has been complete, pre-term infants may insidiously develop signs of respiratory failure in later weeks, manifest by tachypnoea, costal recession, abdominal distension and slowness with feeds; in severe cases cyanosis occurs and, in a very few extreme cases, death.

Immature infants may become breathless during or after feeds, without necessarily being ill. The differential diagnosis of continuous dyspnoea includes severe anaemia, various forms of pneumonia, and some rare malformations of the lungs; however the principal problem is to distinguish heart failure (usually due to patent ductus arteriosus) from delayed pulmonary insufficiency of pre-term infants, and this is sometimes difficult, especially as cardiac murmurs and oedema may occur in the latter condition. We used to see a similar sort of illness in babies following prolonged ventilator treatment (broncho-pulmonary dysplasia) but in recent years it has become an unusual occurrence.

In all cases of late respiratory distress obtain:
(1) a chest x-ray;
(2) electrocardiogram;
(3) radial artery blood for $paO_2$, $paCO_2$ and pH, and bicarbonate;
(4) blood culture;
(5) haemoglobin, PCV and reticulocyte count.

The signs of delayed pulmonary insufficiency of pre-term infants may be continuous with those of early respiratory distress in the immediate neonatal period; more often their onset is delayed—perhaps for several weeks. A gradual deterioration may lead to the death of the baby, but more often is followed by a gradual improvement with a full recovery after several weeks.

The x-ray of an early or mild case may be practically normal, but in later severe cases there are diffuse changes of streaking and mottling, often with over-inflation of both lower lobes and, in the worst cases, the appearance of multiple cysts separated by coarsely thickened strands.

The aetiology is unknown but we favour the suggestion of Burnard *et al.* (1965)*

---

*Burnard, E., Grattan-Smith, P., Picton-Warlow, C. G., Grauaug, A. (1965) 'Pulmonary insufficiency in prematurity.' *Australian Paediatric Journal*, **1**, 12.

that abnormally compliant and collapsible airways lead to patchy over-aeration and atelactasis, with consequent ventilation/perfusion inequalities.

Treatment can only be symptomatic; give oxygen to raise abnormally low $paO_2$ and try to avoid tiring the baby. This may involve continuation of, or reversion to, tube-feeding and not being too obsessional about changing nappies and other forms of disturbance. Attention to adequate warmth is important.

# Insidious Deterioration — The Baby Who 'Goes Off'

The nursing staff or the mother may tell you that they are worried about a term baby who has hitherto been thought to be perfectly normal. Also, it sometimes happens that when a low-birthweight baby has passed the period when the more urgent neonatal problems occur, the nursing staff report that he has 'gone off'—or some other phrase conveying the idea that there has been some ill-defined change for the worse in his behaviour, feeding or general state of well-being. We are not here considering observations of the nursing staff which can be clearly defined, such as lethargic sucking and refusal of feeds, vomiting (see p. 192), diarrhoea (see pp. 201 and 202), and abdominal distension, nor are we considering acute and obvious deterioration where the comment is much more urgent and the problem more obvious (see p. 218).

There is one important rule to follow in these circumstances; take what the nurses or mother say seriously. We have sometimes not done so and regretted it.

A reasonable procedure in these circumstances is as follows.

(1) Ask the nurses or mother to define as clearly as they can what it is about the baby that concerns them, but do not take what they say less seriously if they are unable to do so.

(2) Look carefully through the baby's past and present records. Look at the present pattern of feeding, weight gain, bowel action, temperature, pulse and respiration. Make sure there are no abnormal results of investigations which have been overlooked.

(3) Do a complete medical examination of the baby, looking particularly for evidence of infection (see p. 163), and also measuring the blood pressure and doing at least a limited neurological examination.

It may be that when these things have been done, there will be some definite symptom or sign which requires further investigation or suggests a particular diagnosis to be verified or excluded. The commonest cause of vague symptoms of slow onset is infection, but rarer disorders (e.g. cardiac failure and adrenogenital syndrome, see p. 61) may present in this way. In low-birthweight babies after the second week of life, anaemia is a common cause of vague ill-health.

If, even after these things have been done, there is still no definite evidence of abnormality other than the nurses' complaint, the following investigations should be done as a minimum:

(1) haemoglobin;
(2) white count and differential;
(3) urine culture.

If the complaints persist, or there are other ill-defined grounds for uneasiness, consider blood culture and lumbar puncture. In any case, examine the baby daily till everybody is happy that he is thriving, or a diagnosis has been made.

# The Eyes

## Examination of the Eyes

Visual responses and their value in the neurological examination are described on p. 175. In this section, we are concerned with abnormalities of the eye itself.

The examination of the eye requires considerable skill and practice, and certain parts of it can only satisfactorily be done by an ophthalmologist who is experienced in looking at the eyes of newborn babies.

If the eyes are closed, the baby will often open them if he is lifted into the prone position above your head. However, as this is not a very practicable position in which to carry out further examination, it is usually best to have a nurse with clean hands to hold the eyelids open *gently*. As an alternative, try examining the eyes when the baby is being fed, when he usually keeps his eyes open.

Observe the sclerae, the cornea for size and clarity (see 'Glaucoma', p. 244), and the pupils for size and shape—colobomata often escape notice. Note any obvious cataract. (Less obvious cataract is seen with the ophthalmoscope.)

Ophthalmoscopy requires dilatation of the pupils if much of the fundus is to be seen: use cyclopentolate ('Mydrilate') 0.5%, 1 to 2 drops in each eye. The best view of the retina is obtained with the indirect ophthalmoscope, but it takes a great deal of practice to see anything at all through this instrument, and the paediatrician should be satisfied with the less complete view obtained through the ordinary direct ophthalmo-scope.

### When and Who?

(1) In the routine discharge examination we have suggested that the eyes should be seen open to exclude obvious abnormalities, but ophthalmoscopy should not be attempted.

(2) In the neurological examination we have suggested that the paediatrician should try to see the fundi, but not spend too much time on this part of the examination (see p. 175).

(3) The low-birthweight baby should certainly have a complete ophthalmic examination at regular intervals (every one to two weeks) because of his special risk of developing particular ophthalmic problems—signs of oxygen toxicity or cataract. At Hammersmith these examinations are done by our ophthalmologist who visits the ward routinely.

(4) Any baby who has an actual symptom or problem related to the eyes (other than subconjunctival haemorrhage or straightforward conjunctivitis), should have a full ophthalmic examination, preferably by the ophthalmologist.

(5) The fundi should be examined in cases of suspected embryonic or fetal infection.

**Acknowledgement:** We are very grateful to our colleague Mr. Alan Mushin, F.R.C.S., D.O., for his help in the preparation of this chapter.

## Changes with Gestational Age

There are marked and visible changes in the eye with increasing gestational age. We are not yet certain how valuable these changes (other than the appearance of the pupillary reaction to light, see p. 92) are in assessment of gestational age. However, they are certainly important in that they affect the interpretation of ocular findings in pre-term babies. The following is a rough statement of the sequence of changes seen. The gestational ages are approximate, and we do not know their confidence limits.

*The eyelids* are lightly fused until 26 to 27 weeks gestation.

*The pupil reactions to light* appear between 29 and 31 weeks gestation.

*The pupillary membrane* begins to disappear in the centre at 28 weeks gestation and has largely gone by 32 weeks gestation. It is seen through a +12 lens in the ophthalmoscope as a dense collection of blood vessels in front of and behind the lens. It obscures the view of the retina.

*The vitreous humour* is very hazy until about 32 weeks gestation. This haze gradually clears, from the central region outwards, until the vitreous is clear by 40 weeks gestation.

*The retinal vessels* are first visible about 32 to 33 weeks gestation. At first they only reach to the equator (the macula is the North Pole and you are at the South Pole). By 38 weeks they reach the periphery of the retina.

## Problems

### Retrolental Fibroplasia

The prevention of retrolental fibroplasia (RLF) depends on the control of oxygen therapy (see p. 107). Remember that the more immature the baby ,the greater the risk of RLF and therefore the greater the caution that must be exercised in adding even small amounts of oxygen to the air the baby breathes.

We do not believe that ophthalmoscopy has any place in the control of oxygen therapy; there is therefore no point is disturbing the baby frequently during an acute respiratory illness to look at his eyes. Gross constriction of retinal vessels is not to be regarded as an early sign of oxygen toxicity: we have only seen it in babies who have been given grossly excessive oxygen therapy (Baum and Bulpitt 1970*a*)*. The early changes in the fundi if RLF is developing (usually when the baby is no longer receiving oxygen therapy) are seen in the following order.

(1) Dilatation of the central vessels.

(2) Appearance of retinal haemorrhages which were not previously present. These haemorrhages are usually small dots, placed very peripherally, and therefore not often visible except with the indirect ophthalmoscope.

(3) Capillary proliferation.

(4) Tortuosity of retinal arteries may develop at the same time as (2) and (3).

If signs of RLF do develop, no specific treatment can be given. Do *not* put the baby back in oxygen. He must be followed very carefully from the ophthalmic point of view, and an examination under anaesthetic will probably be necessary at some time. The child's visual capabilities should be assessed as early and as accurately as

*Baum, J. D., Bulpitt, C. J. (1970*a*) 'Renal vasoconstriction in premature infants with increased arterial oxygen tensions.' *Archives of Disease in Childhood*, **45,** 350.

possible, so that a plan for management can be made.

The very few cases of retrolental fibroplasia we have seen in recent years have nearly all been of relatively minor degree, and have not caused severe handicap. Note that myopia is another problem not uncommonly seen at follow-up in babies of low birthweight, and in some cases appears to be related to minor degrees of oxygen toxicity.

*Retinal Haemorrhages*

These are very common in normal newborn babies and appear to have no diagnostic significance, even if they are very large and subhyaloid (Baum and Bulpitt 1970*b*)* except when they first appear after the first week of life in babies at risk for RLF (see above). Retinal haemorrhages usually disappear rapidly—most are gone within one week—but the larger ones take longer to resolve.

*Conjunctival Haemorrhages*

These are harmless but may cause some concern to the mother (see p. 78). They usually take two or three weeks to disappear.

*Cataract*

These are often best detected using a light shining obliquely into the eye. If a baby is seen to have a cataract it is important:

(1) to look for a cause—it may be a sign of an accompanying or underlying disorder;

(2) to obtain ophthalmic advice about further management.

The causes of cataracts include the following.

(*a*) *Hereditary factors.* There are several inherited forms, usually autosomal dominants.

(*b*) *Congenital infections.* Rubella is the commonest infective cause, but toxoplasmosis and syphilis must also be excluded.

(*c*) *Prematurity.* Transient lens opacities have been seen in pre-term infants, but they are only apparent on very careful ophthalmic examination;

(*d*) *Smallness for dates.* In the past, an increased incidence of cataract has been described in small-for-dates babies. However, the significance of this finding is uncertain. Conditions such as intra-uterine rubella infections and certain syndromes predispose to both cataract and smallness for dates. Hypoglycaemia, which used to be common in small-for-dates babies but should now be rare, may have lead to cataract formation. We have not found cataract to be an important problem in small-for-dates babies.

(*e*) *Galactosaemia.* Cataracts do not usually appear till after the age of 10 days in cases of galactosaemia, by which time the diagnosis should already have been suspected because of vomiting, failure to thrive or prolonged jaundice. Nevertheless, the urine should be tested for galactose in all cases of cataract. (See p. 226).

(*f*) *Syndromes.* Cataract is a feature of a large number of syndromes, the common-

*Baum, J. D., Bulpitt, C. J. (1970*b*) 'Retinal and conjunctival haemorrhage in the newborn.' *Archives of Disease in Childhood*, **45**, 344.

est of which is Down's syndrome. The importance of this fact is that the discovery of cataract should lead to a careful search for other congential abnormalities. Other syndromes associated with developing cataract, which is not usually obvious at birth, include Lowe's syndrome, oxycephaly, punctate epiphyseal dysplasia, Marinesco-Sjorgren syndrome, incontinentia pigmentii and a good many others. For syndromes, see Smith (1970)*.

### Glaucoma (Buphthalmos)

Photophobia is usually the first symptom of congenital glaucoma, and it may make the eyes particularly difficult to examine. The affected eyes may look large and the corneal diameter may exceed 11mm (normal newborn 9.5mm). Eyeball tension may be palpably raised (if in doubt compare with another baby). Haziness of the cornea and redness of the conjunctivae are common. If a baby has photophobia, or a large or hazy cornea, call the ophthalmologist at once. The treatment of congenital glaucoma is a matter of urgency.

### Other Congenital Ocular Malformations

A very large number of other ocular malformations has been described (see Brown 1963)†.

### Infection

(See p. 169).

### Blocked Naso-lacrimal Duct

The signs of blockage of the naso-lacrimal duct are persistent wateriness or, more usually, persistent purulent discharge, in which case a drop of mucopus can usually be expressed from the lacrimal sac by pressing the little finger against the side of the baby's nose, just below the inner canthus.

If the eye is merely watery, no immediate treatment is indicated. If there is persistent conjunctivitis, the discharge should be cultured and treatment given with antibiotic drops to which the organism is sensitive, or 10% sulphacetamide eye-drops if there is no growth. The lacrimal sac should be expressed *before* putting in the drops, and they should be given at least four times daily for at least four weeks. The great majority of cases of blocked tear duct will be permanently cured by this treatment, but if wateriness of the eyes or persistent or recurrent infection are still present after six months, the child should be referred to the ophthalmologist for probable probing of the duct.

Occasionally a newborn baby shows visible swelling and redness of the skin overlying the lacrimal sac (*i.e.* just below the inner canthus), sometimes combined with systemic signs of infection. The condition will probably respond to expression of the sac, combined with local and (if appropriate) systemic antibiotics, but the

*Smith, D. W. (1970) *Recognizable Patterns in Human Malformations. Major Problems in Clinical Pediatrics, Vol. VII.* Philadelphia and London: W. B. Saunders.
†Brown, C. A. (1963) 'Abnormalities of the eyes and associated structures.' *In* Norman, A. P. (Ed.) *Congenital Malformations in Infancy.* Oxford: Blackwell. p. 138.

ophthalmologist's advice should be sought.

Marked orbital swelling and inflammation suggest osteomyelitis of the maxilla, particularly if there is a purulent unilateral nasal discharge.

# Abnormalities of the Genitalia

## Male

### Undescended and Ectopic Testes

Descent of the testes into the scrotum is usually complete in a full-term baby, but seldom in a baby born before the 34th week. When one or both testes are undescended, look for other clinical evidence of genital abnormalities, and in the case of bilateral undescent, do a buccal smear. Otherwise no immediate action is required, but follow-up must be arranged. Most undescended testicles will descend in the first few weeks; if they have not descended within one year, later spontaneous descent is unlikely. Ectopic testes are usually found in the superficial inguinal pouch but may be in the perineum; we have rarely detected this condition in a newborn baby, but if we do, we ask for the opinion of our paediatric surgeon.

### Hydrocele and Torsion of the Testis

Hydrocele of the testis is not always obvious at birth but develops within the first few weeks. However large, treatment—by aspiration or surgery—is seldom required. A hydrocele must, of course, be distinguished from an inguinal hernia—this is usually easy, save perhaps in some cases of a communicating hydrocele which, like a hernia, will vary in size. The differential diagnosis also includes testicular tumours and torsion of the testis. The latter condition is not associated with fever and vomiting in the new-born nor, apparently, with pain. It is accompanied by discolouration and induration of the scrotal skin and necessitates immediate operation, since there is a small chance of saving the testis. A confusing differential diagnostic problem is provided by babies who have had fetal blood transfusions into the peritoneum, from which blood may track down into the tunica vaginalis.

### Abnormal Prepuce

The *inaction* to be taken in the case of a hooded prepuce is explained on p. 64. The preputial opening in a normal male newborn is very small and the prepuce cannot and should not be retracted:, we have never seen a case of genuine stenosis or atresia necessitating circumcision. A brief discussion of this topic appears on the next page.

## Female

### Vaginal Discharge

All female infants have mucoid vaginal secretions and some menstruate for a day or two within a few days of birth. This is presumably due to oestrin withdrawal and is not abnormal. If there is a completely unperforated hymen, the normal mucoid or menstrual secretions will be retained and the hydrometrocolpos may be mistaken for a pelvic tumour. Inspection of the genitalia and the appearance of a bulging hymen (and its perforation) will give the show away.

## Ambiguous External Genitalia (see p. 60).

# Circumcision

"The anatomists have not studied the form and the evolution of the preputial orifice.... they do not understand that Nature does not intend it to be stretched or retracted.... what looks like a pin point opening at seven months will become a wide channel of communication at 17.... Nature is a possessive mistress, and whatever mistakes she makes about the structure of the less essential organs such as the brain and stomach, in which she is not much interested, you can be sure that she knows best of the genital organs"—*The late Sir James Spence.*

We have never known this operation be to indicated on medical grounds in the neonatal period. It is certainly not indicated simply because, on inspection, the foreskin seems to have a pinhole meatus. It is contraindicated if the baby has hypospadias (see p. 64), jaundice, a bleeding disorder or a significant family history of bleeding disorder, or a rash in the napkin area.

However, we recognise that the operation is required by some for religious, tribal or social reasons.

The advantages and disadvantages of circumcision in adult life are largely imponderable, and if a father feels strongly that his son should be circumcised it is probably best not to argue with him. If the parents want it for no very good reason ('I thought it was cleaner'), we think it is worth some time and trouble to try to dissuade them.

Although the do-it-yourself 'Plastibell' technique is technically simple, it is not trouble-free and we prefer that a surgeon takes the responsibility for this surgical procedure, especially since a tidying-up operation is occasionally subsequently needed. Before calling the surgeon, however, check that none of the above contraindications is present, and that the baby has definitely had his routine 1mg dose of phytomenadione. If in doubt, repeat the dose.

# Herniae

**Umbilical Herniae**

Herniae *into* the cord are referred to on p. 30. The ordinary type of central umbilical hernia and the less common supra-umbilical hernia are of no importance in the neonatal period and require no treatment. For exomphalos, see p. 54.

**Herniae in the Groin**

These are commoner in the pre-term infant. Unlike the common form of umbilical hernia, they are unlikely to resolve spontaneously. Strangulation is not uncommon in the first few months, and to prevent this, herniotomy is usually advisable within the first few weeks. An inguinal hernia in a girl should make one suspect the testicular feminization syndrome (see p. 61).

# Skin Lesions

Skin lesions are relatively common in newborn babies; most are harmless, but a few indicate serious disease. The following is an account of skin lesions we commonly see, with some that we rarely see but that are of serious import. Even the harmless lesions must be taken seriously, since they may cause concern to a mother.

## Birth Marks

(1) *'Stork bites'*. See p. 78.

(2) *'Port-wine stains'*. These are dense flat capillary haemangiomata which look quite different from the diffuse and sparse stork bites and which, unlike the latter, are permanent. They may appear anywhere on the body and usually have a sharply defined edge. When a port-wine stain is confined to one side of the face and head it suggests association with intra-cranial haemangiomata (the Sturge-Weber syndrome) which may later—although this should not be said to the parents at this time—lead to hemiplegia and fits. It may also be associated with glaucoma (see p. 244) and this should be borne in mind at follow-up examination.

(3) *'Strawberry naevi'*. These capillary cavernous haemangiomata are frequently multiple especially in babies born early and, unlike port-wine stains, grow and become raised above the level of the skin. In fact they are not present at birth, except in the form of small flat capillary haemangiomata which may well escape notice. These lesions continue to grow for several months before beginning to whiten and flatten. They usually disappear before school age and are best left untreated, for the cosmetic result seems best after natural regression. They are said to be likely to become locally malignant if situated on or near mucous surfaces, but in practice this is very exceptional and we have seen lesions on the lips, palate and even the conjunctiva regress spontaneously. However, a rapidly expanding lesion may be arrested by the use of a steroid cream, and parenteral steroid treatment may be necessary if there are very large lesions and, as is sometimes the case, a consumption coagulopathy with thrombocytopenia. Bleeding from a strawberry naevus is usually small and self-limiting, but lesions do rarely become eroded and infected. Ligating the feeding arteries has been reported as a method of treating very large lesions, but we have no personal experience of this treatment.

(4) The *'pigmented naevus'* may grow *pari passu* with the baby; it is a permanent birth mark.

(5) *'Mongolian' blue spots*. This form of pigmentation has nothing to do with Down's syndrome. They are large ill-defined bluish-black patches of pigmentation most commonly seen in the sacral area but also on the limbs. They are usually seen in babies of African or Asiatic ancestry and are entirely harmless. The pigmentation usually becomes less obvious with the passage of time.

(6) *'Café-au-lait' and 'white' spots*. Four of us are unaware of having detected these lesions in the immediate neonatal period, but we believe the fifth (P.A.D.)!

When there are only one or two such spots they are of no particular significance, but when there are several café-au-lait spots there is a possibility of neurofibromatosis and several white spots will suggest tuberous sclerosis.

(7) *Skin lesions over the spine.* A hairy patch over the midline of the back usually indicates an abnormality of the underlying spinal column and sometimes also of the spinal cord. The same significance must be attached to dorsal midline capillary naevi.

### Rashes

(1) *Petechiae.* Petechiae confined to the head and neck are due to 'traumatic cyanosis' and are of no serious consequence (see p. 47). Generalized petechiae must always be taken seriously. The possibilities are thrombocytopenia or infection. Take blood for a platelet count and do the appropriate tests for fetal infection. See p. 165 and p. 208.

(2) *Urticaria of the newborn.* We prefer this term to 'erythema toxicum' which suggests a serious disease. It is a rash which occurs commonly in term babies between the ages of two and ten days and which, when florid, looks alarming. We have rarely seen this rash at birth or in a baby of less than 34 weeks gestation. It is usually most obvious on the trunk, but also occurs on the proximal parts of the limbs and on the face. Individual lesions are rhomboid, red areas up to 1cm across which develop a small central yellow spot often taken for a pustule. One should be able to distinguish this rash from a pustular rash, which is usually concentrated in one area; if in doubt, scrapings from the central spot can be shown to contain numerous eosinophils but not pus cells or organisms. The rash disappears spontaneously in a few days.

(3) *Rash after exchange transfusion.* A blotchy rash, most obvious on the belly and trunk, often occurs after exchange transfusion. There is no petechial element about this rash—pressure blanches it. We have no explanation for the rash, though we always take cultures in case it represents sepsis. It disappears within a day or two.

(4) *Rashes of Gram-negative sepsis.* Several different kinds of rash may occur in association with Gram-negative infection. Sometimes there are individual erythematous lesions about 5mm in diameter with a blanched and occasionally necrotic centre. Sometimes there is a petechial element to the rash, and at other times there are large raised patches of red discolouration.

Any rash in an ill child is supportive evidence of infection, and an indication that you should take blood cultures and start antibiotic treatment at once (see p. 167).

(5) *The rash of congenital syphilis.* This consists of reddish circular maculopapular or vesicular lesions which may be widespread but which tend to be concentrated at mucocutaneous junctions and on the palms of the hands and soles of the feet. For diagnosis, see p. 23.

(6) *Vesicular lesions.* There are a number of rare but serious conditions which can present in the neonatal period with vesicular rashes. In every case, consider the possibility of infection or of an inherited defect of the skin.

(a) *Pemphigus Neonatorum.* This now rare but previously common rash is caused by a staphylococcus or haemolytic streptococcus and usually appears after a few days in a baby who is obviously unwell. Equally rare today is widespread exfoliation of the skin due to staphylococcal infection. Prompt parenteral antibiotic treatment and

250

isolation are necessary.

(*b*) *Virus infections.* Vesicular rashes may be caused by herpes simplex, vaccinia and chicken pox and you should enquire about maternal exposure and maternal disease. For diagnostic measures, see p. 24.

(*c*) *Syphilis.* Characteristically, the lesions are on the palms and soles although they may occur elsewhere on the body. They are highly infectious. For diagnosis see p. 23.

(*d*) *Epidermolysis bullosa.* This condition is genetically determined, but there is more than one variety. Bullae may appear anywhere on the skin, particularly at pressure points, and also in the mouth. In the serious variety, skin will peel off when it is rubbed lightly. Call in the dermatologist and consult him about steroid therapy, which is said to be effective when large doses are given. Avoid unnecessary handling.

(*e*) *Incontinentia pigmenti* (Bloch-Sulzberger syndrome). This is an inborn defect of the skin and central nervous system which is much commoner in girls. The skin lesions follow the lines of peripheral nerves.

(*f*) *Urticaria pigmentosa* (mast cell infiltration of the skin). This condition may produce urticaria or blisters in the newborn baby. We have never seen a case—or at least recognized one—in the newborn.

### Other Lesions

(1) *Milia*, which are almost a normal part of the newborn, are fine white sebaceous concretions, most dense on the nose but also seen on the forehead and cheeks. They disappear.

(2) *Pustules and paronychia.* These may be, but usually are not, outward evidence of a systemic infection. Take skin swabs; if a lesion is intact but superficial, prick it first. Paint with a local antiseptic, *e.g.* gentian violet. If the lesions are extensive or the baby appears ill, treat for systemic infection (see p. 167).

(3) *Nappy rashes.* See p. 252.

(4) *Acne of the newborn.* This is very rare: the individual lesions and their distribution are similar to those of adolescent acne. They gradually disappear but it may take some months for them to do so.

(5) *Subcutaneous fat necrosis.* In this rare condition there is patchy hardening and swelling of subcutaneous tissues, most commonly in the scapular region and buttocks. (In contrast, sclerema is diffuse hardening which does not raise the skin.) Subcutaneous fat necrosis resolves spontaneously unless it becomes secondarily infected, in which case antibiotic treatment will be required. Hypercalcaemia may be present and subcutaneous calcification may occur. Temporary hardening of subcutaneous tissues (small firm nodules) may occur under the line of application of forceps.

# Rash in the Napkin Area

**Perianal Excoriation**

The commonest variety of sore bottom seen in the neonatal period is perianal excoriation. The skin is red and raw in an area on both buttocks, usually not actually contiguous with the anus but a little displaced from it—at the point where the buttocks meet if the thighs are adducted.

The main factor causing perianal excoriation is contact of faeces with the skin. It is commoner in babies fed on cow's milk than in breast-fed babies, but low-birth-weight babies fed on expressed breast-milk are also subject to it. Loose stools from whatever cause are another factor. Once perianal excoriation has arisen, it is aggravated by contact with wet napkins, and probably even by contact with dry ones. The most effective treatment is to expose the buttocks. The room should be at a temperature of at least 25°C (75°F) if this is be to done. If exposure is impracticable, the napkins must be changed as soon as they are wet or dirty.

Local applications are probably not of much help in this condition. Barrier creams, and zinc and castor oil ointment are of more value in protecting unaffected skin than in treating the excoriation when it has arisen. We were astonished to learn that Sister Castle sometimes applies fresh egg-white to the buttocks in severe cases and even finds it helpful.

If the lesions look infected, or are very slow to heal, take a swab for bacterial and fungal culture; in practice, we have seldom had to use antibiotics and thrush does not usually cause a rash limited to the distribution described.

**Thrush**

Thrush infection sometimes occurs in the napkin area in low-birthweight babies, especially if they have been on antibiotics. The groin is the site most often affected, and the rash goes down into the creases—unlike ammoniacal dermatitis. At the edges of the rash there are small, red, ulcerated satellite lesions. Sometimes there is slight sogginess of the affected skin, accompanied by what look like small broken blisters.

If skin thrush is suspected, take a culture for *C. albicans*, and apply gentian violet (Crystal violet paint 0.5%). If recovery does not begin in two or three days, and *C. albicans* is cultured, use nystatin ointment. We have no reason to suppose that nystatin is more effective, and as it is much more expensive it should not be used as the drug of first choice. Expose the affected area if possible. Give nystatin by mouth, too, if the rash is prolonged.

**Ammoniacal Dermatitis**

Although we do not see this condition in hospital in newborn babies, it is so common in later infancy that it deserves a mention. It is caused by splitting of urea (in the urine) to ammonia by faecal organisms: the ammonia then causes blistering of the area with which it is in contact. The rash therefore involves those areas which come into direct contact with wet napkins, and spares the creases. The skin becomes red, blistered and excoriated.

Treatment is very similar to that described for perianal excoriation, the most effective treatment being exposure. When the baby wears washable, rather than disposable, napkins, it is helpful to complete the washing process with a rinse in diluted vinegar (1 oz in 1 gallon water, *i.e.* approx. 1 in 100) or benzalkonium chloride (1 in 8,000).

# Cephalhaematoma

This is an effusion of blood under the scalp, and it may occur in one of two tissue planes.

(1) *Subperiosteal*. The bleeding is under the periosteum of one or more vault bones of the skull. The bleeding and the swelling are therefore confined to the area over a vault bone—usually a parietal bone—and are bounded by the sutures. More than one subperiosteal cephalhaematoma may be present, but each will be distinct from the other. The swelling is not present at birth, but appears within the first two or three days. The amount of blood loss is comparatively small and, apart from the occasional aggravation of jaundice, the condition is harmless. No treatment is indicated; the blood should not be aspirated. Warn the mother that the swelling will take several weeks or even months to disappear. The edge may sometimes, misleadingly, feel like a depressed fracture.

(2) *Subaponeurotic*. The bleeding is between the epicranial aponeurosis (*galea aponeurotica*) and the periosteum. Bleeding may be much more severe than in the ordinary subperiosteal type of cephalhaematoma (see p. 209).

# Oedema

Oedema is a relatively common finding in the newborn, especially the pre-term baby, and does not necessarily mean serious trouble. Oedema may be recognised either because it is visible and palpable, or because there is a sudden increase in weight (say, over 100g in one day). Oedema is not necessarily confined to dependent parts in the newborn. There may be a generalised puffiness, including the face, or localised swelling and pitting, especially shins, scalp and dorsa of hands and feet, as well as the back. Even in normal babies, very firm pressure may leave a little pitting.

**Localised Oedema**

Strictly localised oedema clearly calls for a local explanation, *e.g.* trauma or infection. The commonest example is caput succedaneum. Oedema of the dorsa of the hands and feet is common in newborn infants with Turner's syndrome. Do a buccal smear for Barr bodies and take blood for chromosome analysis.

**Generalised Oedema**

Hydrops fetalis is discussed on p. 67. The following causes should be considered in the baby who develops oedema after birth.

(1) *Increased sodium load.* Pre-term babies in particular are liable to become oedematous when first given cow's milk, which has a much higher sodium content than breast milk. Check the feeding regime and weight chart. Probably no action is needed, for the baby will become able to excrete the load, but make sure he is not being given an excessive amount of salt by mistake. If the oedema is persistent and trouble-some, it may be necessary to dilute the feeds temporarily or change to breast milk or other milk with a lower sodium content. However, you should also consider the possibilities listed below.

(2) *Heart-failure* (see p. 213). The first sign of right heart-failure may be generalised oedema, not obviously of dependent parts.

(3) *Urinary protein loss, e.g.* congenital nephrotic syndrome or renal vein throm-bosis. Measure urinary albumin.

(4) *Oedema in babies on positive pressure ventilation.* This often occurs. Reduce the inflating pressure if possible.

**Scleroedema (Sclerema)**

We apply these terms interchangeably to a hardening of subcutaneous tissue, principally in babies who take a long time to die, although it is not invariably a fatal complication. This is quite different from subcutaneous fat necrosis (see p. 251). It is often associated with hypothermia and Gram-negative sepsis. The treatment is that of the causative disease. Although some advocate treatment with high doses of steroids, we are unimpressed that this is helpful.

255

# Circumoral Cyanosis

We find it difficult to think of anything sensible to say about this common and curious condition. Many babies become blue about the mouth during or shortly after feeds. There is no accompanying sign of central cyanosis. The condition often seems to be associated with wind, and to be relieved by burping. It is harmless and should not cause concern. We do not understand it.

# Harlequin Colour Change

This condition bears no resemblance to the harlequin fetus (a severe form of congenital ichthyosis) and neither bears the slighest resemblance to the parti-coloured costume of Columbine's consort.

The harlequin colour change is sometimes seen in a newborn baby lying naked on his side; the dependent half of the body is red and the upper half pale; the two colours are sharply demarcated by a line which bisects the body from head to feet. This colour change usually disappears spontaneously in a few minutes, or may be made to disappear by lying the baby supine, or to reverse by lying him on the other side. It is said to be commonest in low-birthweight babies in the first week of life, but this may only be because these are the circumstances in which the newborn baby is most often seen naked. Its causation and significance are unknown and we seem to have seen it less often in recent years. Murmur something about autonomic imbalance and 'retire in dignity and optimism'.*

*A remark we have misappropriated from the late Dr. Bronson Crothers.

# Skeletal and Connective Tissue Disorders

Certain of these may be recognisable in the neonatal period. Here we are only concerned with conditions likely to require active intervention in the first weeks of life. (We again recommend you to refer to Smith (1970)* for a helpful catalogue with photographs.) Many of these conditions are genetically determined and you should look up the mode of inheritance. For references, see p. 6. Some of the disorders, such as congenital dislocation of the hip (see p. 84), talipes (see p. 57) and fracture associated with birth trauma (see p. 47) have been described elsewhere.

**Osteochondrodystrophies**

By far the commonest type is achondroplasia, but the condition is seldom recognised at birth, possibly because all newborn babies have relatively short limbs and large heads. When this diagnosis is made in the neonatal period it is quite likely to be mistaken, the baby having one of several more severe forms. Many such babies may be stillborn or die shortly after birth; others may present with illness in the neonatal period. We have seen one or more examples of the following four conditions.

*Thanatophoric Dwarfism*

These infants have marked shortening of the extremities, a very narrow thorax, a relatively large head, and a more-or-less normal trunk length. They rarely survive more than a few hours, due to the associated respiratory distress. Radiology of the skeleton shows very short, bowed, tubular bones, flared irregular metaphyses, wide iliac bones, and poorly developed vertebral bodies.

*Lymphopenic (Swiss-type) Agammaglobulinaemia with Short-limbed Dwarfism*

Infants with this hereditary syndrome may have low birthweight for their gestational age, short upper and lower limbs, and prominent foreheads. The radiological features are similar to but not identical with those of achondroplasia (see Gatti *et al.* 1969)†. The diagnosis would be suggested in such a child by the finding of lymphopenia, poor lymphoblast transformation with phytohaemagglutinin, agammaglobulinaemia, and absence of palpable lymph glands. Be on the look-out for severe infection. Avoid wholeblood transfusion, as it has been reported to be followed by graft-versus-host disease, and death.

*Asphyxiating Thoracic Dystrophy*

In this condition, inherited as an autosomal recessive, the thorax is extremely small due to shortness of the ribs, with irregularity of the costochondral junction.

*Smith, D. W. (1970) *Recognizable Patterns of Human Malformations. Major Problems in Clinical Pediatrics, Vol. VII.* Philadelphia and London: W. B. Saunders.
†Gatti, R. A., Platt, N., Pomerance, H. H., Hong, R., Langer, L. O., Kay, H. E. M., Good, R. A. (1969) 'Hereditary lymphopenic agammaglobulinemia associated with a distinctive form of short-limbed dwarfism and ectodermal dysplasia.' *Journal of Pediatrics*, **75**, 675.

The limbs are also somewhat short, and x-ray shows metaphyseal flaring. Respiratory failure occurs very early in the more severe forms, for the lungs are hypoplastic with a reduced number of alveoli and alveolar ducts. Surgery to increase the size of the thoracic cage offers the only hope for survival in these children.

*Hypophosphatasia*

In the most severe form of this recessively inherited disorder, the limbs appear deformed with bowing of the legs. The ribs are short and the thoracic cage small. x-ray appearances of the skeleton are diagnostic and show incomplete mineralisation of the metaphyses and hypoplastic bones; rickets may be present. Respiratory failure will occur early in severe cases.

**Osteopetrosis (Albers-Schönberg Disease)**

Severe recessively inherited forms present soon after birth. There may be a haemorrhagic tendency with bruising: pancytopenia results from marrow encroachment. Hepatosplenomegaly is frequently present. The diagnosis should be suspected if x-rays reveal abnormally dense bones. A slowly deteriorating course may be expected in many cases, though dietary calcium restriction and cellulose phosphate aimed at producing a negative calcium balance has been reported to have some success in reducing new bone density (Yu *et al.* 1971)*.

**Connective Tissue Disorders**

*Ehlers-Danlos Syndrome*

Many of these infants are born pre-term following premature rupture of membranes. The condition is inherited as an autosomal dominant. The usual complications of immaturity, depending on gestational age, should be anticipated (see p. 90). Hyperelasticity of the skin may be obvious in the neonatal period, but we have not seen the more serious manifestations (widespread arterial disease, herniae, mediastinal emphysema or pneumothorax, to mention some of them) presenting at this age.

*Osteogenesis Imperfecta*

In the most severe forms, the infant is born with limb deformities due to multiple fractures. x-ray of the skeleton will nearly always reveal fractures of ribs as well in these cases, and skull bones are excessively thin, with large fontanelles and Wormian bones. We have seen one infant present at birth with bilateral femoral fractures only, one of them already surrounded by dense callus formation, having occurred *in utero*. Prognosis is poor for the most severe forms. Involve the orthopaedic surgeons in care of the fractures from the beginning.

**Miscellaneous**

*Vertebral Anomalies*

Infants are occasionally born with bizarre anomalies of the thoracic vertebrae which result in much distortion of the thoracic cage. The trunk looks abnormally

*Yu, J. S., Oates, R. K., Walsh, K. H., Stuckey, S. J. (1971) 'Osteopetrosis.' *Archives of Disease in Childhood*, **46**, 257.

short, and the postero-anterior diameter of the chest may be increased. Respiratory distress may be present from birth in the severe cases, necessitating ventilation.

### Arthrogryposis Multiplex Congenita and Congenital Amputations

These babies will not be ill, but you should involve the orthopaedic surgeons in plans for their long-term care from the beginning, and be prepared to give the parents much support.

### Abnormalities of the Radius and Thrombocytopenia

Marked hypoplasia or even complete absence of the radius, sometimes with malformations of the lower limbs such as talipes equinovarus, has been described in association with thrombocytopenia in more than one member of a family. Haemorrhage may occur within a few weeks of birth, thus differentiating the condition from Fanconi's syndrome, in which the haematological manifestations are not usually seen in babies. The risk of haemorrhage is greatest in early infancy and appears to be uninfluenced by steroids.

# Section 6: Procedures

Some of the procedures described in this section, like lumbar puncture, are essentially the same as those done on older patients, but the technique may be modified in detail to allow for the baby's smaller size or different anatomy. Other procedures, like umbilical artery catheterization, are only performed on the newborn baby.

For procedures not covered in this Section, see the Index, p. 337.

*NOTES*

# Sterile Precautions

All the procedures described, except arterial puncture, venepuncture and capillary blood sampling, should be done with full sterile precautions. This means:

(1) wear a mask;
(2) wash hands thoroughly (we no longer use scrubbing brushes);
(3) wear a sterile gown and gloves;
(4) clean the relevant areas of the baby's skin with 70% isopropyl alcohol, and let it dry;
(5) cover the rest of the baby with sterile towels;
(6) observe no-touch technique wherever possible.

These precautions will not be repeated as each procedure is described.

For arterial puncture, venepuncture and capillary puncture, wash your hands, clean the baby's skin with isopropyl alcohol, and observe no-touch technique.

# Umbilical Catheterization

The initial procedure is the same whether the artery or vein or both are to be catheterized. Umbilical catheters are transparent flexible polyvinyl infant-feeding tubes with a rounded blind distal end and sidehole, and a female Luer fitting (with stopper) at the proximal end. We use No. 5 (French gauge) for the umbilical artery and No. 8 for the vein.

### Preparation of Catheters and Cord

Add heparin to sterile saline to make a solution containing 1000 units heparin per 100ml.

Attach each catheter to be used to a 10ml syringe of heparinized saline, and fill the catheter, leaving it attached to the syringe.

Inspect the legs for discoloration or bruising before starting arterial catheterization, so that these are not subsequently attributed to the catheter.

Place a loose tape ligature around the base of the cord, and cut the cord cleanly with a scalpel about 1cm from its base.

Identify the umbilical vessels. The vein is usually superior and central, and looks like a slit. The two arteries usually stand out as small whitish protrusions, the lumen not always being obvious.

### Umbilical Artery

*Holding the Vessel.* In a fresh cord, the vessels are best held by gripping the entire stump with a gauze swab. Alternatively, hold the artery with fine-toothed forceps. A useful arterial retractor can be made by jabbing a No. 1 needle against a sterile metal surface; the barb may then be used to hold the edge of the artery.

*Dilatation of the artery.* With an umbilical arterial dilator (see p. 287), gently tease open the lumen of the artery and insert the dilator to about ½cm. It is worthwhile taking a little time to get the mouth of the artery well open.

*Inserting the catheter.* Remove the metal dilator from the artery and insert the catheter tip. Push the catheter in until blood flows freely—usually when it has passed in about 8cm. Not infrequently, one encounters resistance at about 2cm, which may be overcome by steady pressure. Try elevating the cord stump and pushing the catheter in the line of the umbilical artery, *i.e.* caudally. If it is impossible to introduce the catheter, fiddle with it but remember that it is quite easy to make a false passage into the rectus sheath or peritoneal cavity. If it still does not go in, try redilating the vessel, if necessary retrimming it first, or try the other artery.

*Tighten the cord ligature.* Stitch the catheter in place. Spray the area with polybactrin.

Ensure the catheter is filled with heparinized saline and the rubber stopper pushed home and held with a piece of adhesive tape. Label the catheter with a piece of sterile red 'Sellotape'.

Inspect the legs for discoloration and feel for the dorsalis pedis pulses. If a leg goes white or blue and pulseless, the catheter must be removed.

### Umbilical Vein

Hold the cord stump with a gauze swab, or on its upper aspect with a pair of toothed forceps. In a fresh cord soon after birth, the vein is usually easy to identify. The closed point of a small artery forceps makes a good probe for venous catheterization. In older cords, or when the vein has been used previously, carefully remove any clot or debris with forceps: sometimes the mouth of the vein cannot be seen clearly but it can nonetheless be entered at the depth of the funnel-shaped depression in the centre of the cord left by picking away clot. Usually the catheter slips into the vein easily: do not push hard. If it sticks at 1cm, especially if there has been any appreciable amount of clot at the mouth, insert an open-ended catheter, apply suction on the syringe and withdraw to suck out loose clot. Repeat several times if necessary.

The catheter should only be advanced until a free flow of blood is obtained. Do not insert too far—it may traverse the ductus venosus, I.V.C. and enter the coronary sinus or left atrium. In a baby of, say, 1500g, the right atrium is only about 1cm from the ductus venosus.

Whenever it is intended to leave a catheter *in situ*, arrange for an x-ray to show where it has gone (chest x-ray, PA and lateral). If left in, it should be labelled with dark blue 'Sellotape'. NEVER leave a venous catheter open to air: there is a serious danger of air embolism. (Measurement of venous pressure via the umbilical vein is of doubtful value, unless one is certain of the exact position of the tip of the catheter).

### Maintenance of Catheters

Volumes of catheters: Arterial (No. 5 F.G.) = 0.2ml; venous (No. 8 F.G.) = 0.65ml.

When filling with heparinized saline after use, inject $1\frac{1}{2}$ times the dead space volume (*i.e.* 0.3ml U.A.C., 1.0ml U.V.C.). Pinch off, insert stopper and fix it with adhesive. It is important to remember that each such injection involves giving the baby a few units of heparin. Ensure that the labelling of catheters is with the appropriate coloured 'Sellotape'. Except in emergency, the arterial catheter should only be used for sampling or for injections of physiological fluids (normal saline or blood).

Strap free ends of catheters to the abdominal wall, well away from the perineum. Blocked venous catheters, which cannot be cleared by suction, should be removed and not replaced unless the indications for catheterization are still very strong.

### Removal of Catheters

The risks of prolonged catheterization include thrombosis and infection. Catheters should be removed as soon as the clinical situation will allow. In general, umbilical venous catheters, if left in, should be removed after not more than 24 hours. We aim to remove umbilical arterial catheters by 48 hours, but see p. 130.

*Procedure*

Observe sterile precautions.

Insert a purse-string suture and have forceps ready.

Dissect away any horny inspissated Wharton's jelly.

The venous catheter usually slides out easily and any bleeding can be controlled by pressure and/or pulling tight the purse-string.

The arterial catheter should be removed in two stages. Draw the catheter out until only 1 to 2cm remain in the artery as a plug. Wait about a minute—the part of the umbjlical artery from which the catheter has been removed may contract down during this time. Then finally remove the catheter. Should bleeding occur, control it at once by: (*a*) artery forceps on the end of the vessel (not always possible); (*b*) pressure on the line of the umbilical vessel just below and to the side of the umbilicus, together with direct pressure on the bleeding point; (*c*) purse-string suture.

All catheters removed (except for those needed for short periods, *e.g.* exchanges) should be cultured by cutting off the tip. In laboratory hours, the tip should be put in a sterile universal tube and sent to the laboratory at once. At night, cut the tip off into a blood culture bottle and send it to the laboratory in the morning.

# Radial Artery Catheterization

**Procedure**

Use a No. 2 F.G. polyvinyl intravenous catheter (of external diameter 0.63mm). Prepare heparinized saline 10 units/ml, and fill the catheter with it.

Place the cuff around the upper arm and connect to the sphygmomanometer. Splint arm firmly above and below the wrist, leaving the wrist free.

Locate the radial artery at the wrist carefully. It is in the centre of the lateral third of the flexor aspect of the wrist.

Cut down over the artery with a longitudinal skin incision. Incise the skin carefully and locate the artery by blunt dissection. Isolate a length of the vessel from the surrounding tissue with care, keeping the skin edges apart with a butterfly self-retaining retractor.

Under-run the vessel with two lengths of fine silk tie and separate them as far as possible. Allow the proximal tie to lie free and tie a loose knot in the distal tie that can be tightened if necessary.

Keeping the artery taut, by pulling gently on the distal ligature, make a small longitudinal nick in the artery. Take great care that the incision does not go through to the opposite side of the vessel as well. Use the sphygmomanometer to control the flow of blood from the cut. (The nurse can do this.)

Dilate the vessel *very carefully* with the radial artery dilator and then insert the catheter about 1cm, previously filled with heparinized saline (10 units/ml), *but not* attached to the syringe. If necessary bevel the end of the catheter, but try to leave as blunt a point on it as possible or the catheter will cut out of the artery when pushed in.

Tie the catheter in with 3.0 plain catgut, after removing both silk stay ties. Flush the catheter frequently with heparinized saline while closing the wound with 3.0 chromic catgut.

*Either:* (*a*) flush the syringe every half-hour with 0.5ml of heparinized solution; or *preferably* (*b*) connect the catheter to a constant infusion pump delivering 0.5 ml of heparinized solution per hour.

# Blood Sampling Other Than From Indwelling Catheters

If the umbilical or radial artery catheters are in place, blood required for any analytical purpose other than blood culture can be obtained from them. Blood for culture should not be taken from catheters since the specimen so obtained may be contaminated with bacteria which are not present in other parts of the blood-stream.

The other possible routes for obtaining blood are arterial, venous or capillary, *Always* state in the notes where blood was taken from, and how much.

*Arterial blood* is suitable for any analytical purpose, and for blood culture.

*Venous blood* is suitable for blood cultures and for analytical purposes other than pH, $pCO_2$ and $pO_2$. (These can, of course, be measured accurately in venous blood, but it is the arterial value in which we are interested.)

*Capillary blood* is unsuitable for blood cultures. It can be used for pH determination—there is little difference between arterial and capillary pH—but not for $pO_2$ or $pCO_2$ estimations, since even arterialized capillary values correlate poorly with arterial values. Capillary blood can be used for all other biochemical estimations, but if a great deal of squeezing is necessary the values obtained for serum potassium or calcium may be falsely high. Blood which has become haemolysed cannot be used, for example, for bilirubin or potassium estimation.

Unless there is an indwelling catheter, it is difficult to obtain more than 2 to 3ml of blood by any of these routes without puncturing a deep vein which is, in general, best avoided. If larger quantities of blood are called for, (*a*) ask yourself how high a priority you give to obtaining the information which the test(s) would provide; and (*b*) ask the laboratory if they *really* need as much blood as they say. Remember that 10ml of blood taken from a 3kg baby is equivalent to about 200ml taken from an adult, and that many of the babies whom you treat are smaller than 3kg. (Our pathologists would never ask for this amount, and indeed do most of the tests on a few drops of blood.)

## Arterial Puncture*

### Radial Artery Puncture

The radial artery is the vessel we have most commonly used for obtaining arterial blood by puncture. We have followed the technique described by Shaw (1968)† and have encountered few technical problems and no complications.

Using a 1ml syringe, wedge a 23 gauge needle on tightly, bevel upwards, aligned with the markings of the syringe. Fill the dead space with heparinized saline. Do not extend the wrist—keep it in line with the forearm. The radial artery may be visible as a

---

*We have evidence from the use of the intra-arterial electrode that $paO_2$ may fall during painful procedures. Results of arterial puncture must therefore be interpreted with caution.

†Shaw, J. C. L. (1968) 'Arterial sampling from the radial artery in premature and full-term infants.' *Lancet*, **ii**, 389.

blue streak in a very small baby; it lies in the centre of the lateral third of the flexor aspect of the wrist, just lateral to the tendon of the flexor carpi radialis. Palpation may not help. The syringe is held by the plunger. Introduce the needle at an angle of 45°, bevel upwards, just proximal to the proximal skin crease, aiming to transfix the artery and just to touch the bone. Apply gentle suction and withdraw the needle slowly until blood flows into the syringe. If the artery is missed, the needle can be pushed to one side or the other without withdrawing it from the skin. After a sample has been obtained, ask a nurse to apply firm pressure for five minutes to secure haemostasis. If correctly performed, this sampling procedure can be repeated as frequently as four-hourly from the same vessel.

*Brachial Artery Puncture*

A similar technique to that used for the radial artery can be applied to the brachial artery. The vessel is located at the elbow by palpation.

*Temporal Artery Puncture*

The temporal artery runs vertically just in front of the tragus of the ear. It can be located by palpation, or by seeing the pulsations after the hair has been shaved just in front of the ear. The artery can be punctured with a scalp-vein needle directed against the flow of blood in the artery (*i.e.* directed from the vertex to the jaw). Blood is allowed to fill the scalp-vein needle tubing and then drawn into a 1 or 2ml syringe in which the dead space has been filled with heparin.

**Venepuncture**

Venous blood can be obtained from superficial veins in the antecubital fossa, the scalp, the back of the wrist, or the foot. The main difficulty is not in entering the vein, but in obtaining much blood having done so. We would make three suggestions.

(1) Try to become expert at sampling from one or two chosen sites. We would favour the antecubital fossa as the first choice. Scalp veins are often quite large and easy to puncture, but it will be necessary to shave some of the scalp to do so, and the baby's mother may think this much more of a mutilation than you do. Do not use a scalp vein without good reason, but use it without hesitation rather than expose the baby to the slightest risk by using some less safe procedure.

(2) Use a reasonably large needle—the largest you think can enter the vein. This both makes it easier to enter rather than transfix the vein and also makes it easier to get blood out.

(3) Be patient over withdrawing blood. Do not apply excessive suction, which often seems to stop the flow altogether.

We are deliberately not giving instructions for femoral, external or internal jugular vein or sagittal sinus puncture, because we believe they are very rarely justified or needed in the newborn, and each has its own particular dangers. If forced to do one of them, we prefer external jugular puncture.

**Capillary Puncture**

In the newborn, capillary blood is most easily obtained from the heel. Some warming of the heel may be helpful, but it must be done with great care to avoid burning the skin, and is probably unnecessary if the baby has been lying under bed-clothes or in a sufficiently warm incubator. If warming must be done, soak a large pledget of cotton-wool in water at 40°C (not hotter) and hold it around the heel for about five minutes.

Correct holding of the leg and foot is the key to successful capillary puncture. If the baby is not in an incubator, have him held on someone else's lap with his legs hanging free. With the left hand grasp the leg with the foot dorsiflexed in such a way that your thumb and fingers surround the heel, which protrudes through the circle made by them. When the heel is held in this way the heel pulp stands out and looks engorged with blood. Clean it with isopropyl alcohol and allow it to dry. Then stab the edge of the heel with the special lancet (*e.g.* 'Sterilette').

Experience is needed to know exactly how to make the stab. The sharp part of the lancet should be pushed in to a depth of about 2mm. If it is withdrawn exactly in the line in which it was inserted, it may be difficult to obtain more than about 0.5ml of blood. If more blood than this is needed, a very small cut should be made in the skin as the lancet is withdrawn. But don't make too big a cut: we have seen some nasty scars on baby's heels subsequently, and inclusion dermoids are a possible complication.

When the stab has been made, wipe away the first drop of blood with a piece of sterile cotton-wool. Then milk blood out of the heel by alternately squeezing and releasing with the four fingers around the calf. Let the drops of blood form freely and drop straight into a container (or onto the paper in the case of the Guthrie test). Do not scrape the skin with a container—this is likely to cause haemolysis of the specimen. Be as un-messy as possible. Only the skin within a few mm of the stab should be wet with blood and the drops should form and detach themselves in this area. If blood gets spread all over the heel it will flow off in the wrong directions and be more difficult to collect—wipe the heel dry if this happens.

After the collection is finished, release the foot, press on the puncture site to stop oozing and apply a piece of plaster.

# Intravenous Infusion: Drips

Drips can normally be given by percutaneous puncture rather than cut-down, however small the baby. However, when the baby is going to the operating theatre, it is safest to do a cut-down. In the exceptional case of babies requiring long-term total parenteral nutrition, it is possible to manage for some days by percutaneous needling of peripheral veins, the drip site being changed every 12 or 24 hours. When this is no longer possible, it is best to have a superior vena caval catheter inserted by a surgeon. We prefer not to use the umbilical vein for intravenous infusions (particularly of glucose-containing solutions), though we would do so if other routes were technically impossible, knowing that our treatment of the umbilicus keeps it sterile in the majority of cases (see p. 111). We have also rarely used the umbilical artery for giving infusions; this can be done provided an infusion pump is used, but because of the slight risks to the arterial circulation to the legs, we prefer to use a small vein if possible.

For percutaneous intravenous infusion we use a scalp-vein set. The scalp veins are usually the best and easiest to use for drips. They are numerous, easily seen and comparatively large, and needles can be very easily fixed against the skull. First, shave the scalp in the frontal region. If the veins do not stand out well enough, ask the nurse to press on them proximally, or put a rubber band around the scalp in the occipito-frontal circumference, or, as a last resort, make the baby cry, for instance by flicking his feet. When the needle is in the vein, secure it with small strips of 'Micropore' or plaster of paris.

If the scalp veins prove impossible or have been used up, try the saphenous veins at the ankle, which usually stand out well. After this, use any visible superficial vein, *e.g.* those on the back of the hand or dorsum of the foot. For instructions on what fluid to give and how much, see p. 99. Once the drip has been set up, the main technical problem is that of giving very small quantities of fluid very accurately. With gravity drips it is essential to have a burette in the system so that the volume given can be recorded accurately. It is difficult to maintain even flow-rates without very frequent adjustments of the clamp, and the drip has to be watched virtually continuously to prevent it stopping, or the baby being flooded. Many of these problems can be avoided by using a continuous infusion pump, and we do this increasingly often.

# Blood Transfusion

**Cross-matching**

We have sometimes given uncrossmatched blood of the same ABO and Rh groups as the baby, or group O Rh-negative blood. In an emergency, this is most unlikely to cause trouble, for haemolytic transfusion reactions are almost unknown in the newborn period. However, blood used for transfusion in newborn infants should normally be cross-matched. We follow the procedure recommended by Dr. P. L. Mollison (1961)[†], which we have summarized on the flow-sheet.

The essence of these rather complicated instructions is as follows. Provided the infant's red cells are compatible with the mother's serum, the mother's serum should be used for cross-matching, as any blood group antibodies present in the infant's serum will be present in the mother's serum in at least equal titre. If the infant's red cells are incompatible with the mother's serum, serum from the infant must be used for cross-matching if blood of the same ABO group as the infant is to be transfused. An Rh-negative infant, or an infant with haemolytic disease of the newborn due to Rh, must be given Rh-negative blood at any transfusion. In the case of exchange transfusions, the blood used for the first exchange should be cross-matched in this way. Blood used for subsequent exchanges should be cross-matched against a sample of the baby's serum obtained since the last exchange. If group O blood was used for the first exchange, it should be used for subsequent ones, even if the baby is not group O.

When the baby is more than four weeks old, or has had a previous blood transfusion, use his own serum for cross-matching.

In case of doubt, consult the blood transfusion department.

**Blood Transfusion Other Than Exchange**

(See 'Haemorrhage', p. 206 and 'Anaemia', p. 236).

**Site of Infusion**

The instructions for intravenous infusion apply, but in the first few days there is no objection to using the umbilical vein, provided the umbilicus is not thought to be infected. For intra-peritoneal transfusion, see below, p. 274.

**Type of Blood**

We have a slight preference for fresh heparinized rather than stored ACD blood under any circumstances, because of the tendency of ACD blood to produce hypocalcaemia, hyperkalaemia and metabolic acidosis.* When the transfusion to be given

---

*Note: We realise that this policy may have to be abandoned unless, in the future, blood donors are screened at regular intervals for hepatitis-associated antigen (HAA, Australia antigen).

†Mollison, P. L. (1961) *Blood Transfusion in Clinical Medicine* (3rd Edn.). Oxford: Blackwell. p. 426.

1. Find the ABO and Rh groups of mother and baby

2. Has the baby had previous transfusions (including fetal intraperitoneal transfusions)?

          **YES**                                  **NO**

**YES branch:** Was the blood used before of the same ABO group as the baby?

**NO branch:** Is he more than four weeks old?

---

**(YES → NO):** Use blood of same ABO group as before (probably O), cross-matched against baby's serum *

**(YES → YES):** Use blood of same ABO group as baby, cross-matched against baby's serum *

**(NO → YES):** → (points to "Use blood of same ABO group as baby, cross-matched against baby's serum *")

**(NO → NO):** What are the ABO groups of mother and baby?

| Mother and baby have same ABO group, or mother is AB, or the combination is one of: | | The combination is one of: | |
|---|---|---|---|
| Mother | Baby | Mother | Baby |
| A | O | O | A, B or AB |
| B | O | A | B or AB |
| | | B | A or AB |

**(left table →):** Use blood of same ABO group as baby, cross-matched against mother's serum *

**(right table →):** Use blood of same ABO group as baby, cross-matched against baby's serum *

---

* GENERAL RULE : NEVER GIVE Rh-POSITIVE BLOOD TO AN Rh-NEGATIVE BABY OR TO A BABY WITH HAEMOLYTIC DISEASE OF THE NEWBORN DUE TO Rh

---

is small, these drawbacks are less important, but it is a pity to use a 500ml unit of ACD blood to give a 50ml transfusion. In these circumstances we prefer to use blood drawn directly from one of us. (A list of blood groups of all HAA-negative members of staff is kept on the neonatal ward, but blood must be cross-matched before use; see below). If ACD blood is used for transfusions of more than 100ml, 1500 units of heparin and 5ml calcium gluconate should be added to a 500ml unit, and the cells partially packed.

If the purpose of the blood transfusion is to replace acute blood loss, whole blood should be given and it may be given rapidly. If it is to correct anaemia, partially packed cells are more appropriate, but do not have the cells packed to such an extent that the blood is too viscous to flow readily through a scalp-vein set (*i.e.* when the haematocrit exceeds 70 per cent).

A transfusion to correct anaemia must also be given slowly for fear of over-loading the circulation and inducing right-sided heart failure, which may supervene with disconcerting suddenness. Give the blood as slowly as is compatible with the drip continuing to flow. A careful watch must be kept for a rising respiratory or heart rate, cyanosis and enlarging liver and spleen. If these signs develop, stop the trans-fusion, and if the baby is in serious heart-failure, remove, say, 20ml of blood and give digitalis and frusemide.

Because of the risk of cardiac failure in cases of severe anaemia in the first few days of life, exchange transfusion may be best.

**Intra-peritoneal Blood Transfusion**

Blood given into the peritoneal cavity is largely absorbed intact into the circulation over the next few days. At one time we used this route for transfusing anaemic babies.

The advantages of intraperitoneal transfusion are:
(1) the blood is absorbed slowly, so there is far less risk of overloading the circulation than with intravenous infusion;
(2) the technique is very easy, as it does not involve entering a vein.

The disadvantages are:
(1) the method is not suitable if the transfusion is to repair acute blood loss;
(2) absorption is not complete, so the baby's haemoglobin level is only raised by two-thirds of the amount expected from the volume given;
(3) this method must not be used if there is intra-abdominal pathology;
(4) there *might* be some risk of peritoneal adhesions, or of tubal blockages in females, though the evidence we have is that the procedure does not cause peritoneal adhesions.

Because of the small possibility of this long-term risk, we now very rarely use this procedure, but we would do so if we thought a baby who required transfusion for anaemia was at particular risk of developing heart-failure, or if there was particular difficulty in entering a vein. In units which are short of staff, there is much to be said for intraperitoneal transfusion.

*Technique*

Use a medium-sized 'Angiocath'. The size is not critical, provided the needle or catheter is big enough for the blood to flow readily. Insert the needle in the left iliac fossa, feeling carefully for any viscera or masses before doing so—especially an enlarged liver or bladder. The blood can be run in from a bag or a bottle, or injected from a large syringe, and the total amount can safely be given in 10 to 15 minutes. We use about one-third more than the total amount of blood which would be given intravenously to correct the anaemia, but the total volume given at one transfusion should not exceed 90ml. For preference, use heparinized blood, partially packed. Blood in which the anticoagulant is acid-citrate dextrose sometimes seems to hurt the baby.

**Exchange Transfusion**

(1) Exchange transfusions are best performed in the neonatal ward.
(2) Warmth. Except in unusual emergency, the baby should be warmed to a

normal body temperature *before* starting the exchange. The exchange is carried out in the incubator. It is quite possible to do this and maintain sterile precautions. There is no need to fasten the baby on a crucifix, but his arms need some restraining. Fresh donor blood is usually used unwarmed. Blood fresh from a refrigerator at 4°C should be warmed by immersing in water at 37°C or by leading the inflow through a sterile heating coil in a bath at 37°C. (*Never heat blood under a hot tap.*) Refrigerated blood can represent a considerable cold stress to a baby, but it is even more important to ensure that the baby himself is properly warmed before and during the procedure.

(3) Attach the ECG oscilloscope. Prepare the exchange transfusion (IN/OUT) record forms.

(4) Specimens to be collected.
- (*a*) Umbilical swab for bacteriology at beginning.
- (*b*) Umbilical blood at beginning for —(i) Hb., PCV, Kleihauer
  - (ii) Bilirubin
  - (iii) Glucose
  - (iv) For serology if required, *e.g.* hepatitis-associated antigen, cytomegalovirus.
- (*c*) Donor blood at beginning for —(i) Hb., PCV
  - (ii) For serology if required as above.
  - If stored blood, also for (iii) Potassium
  - (iv) pH
- (*d*) Umbilical blood at end for —(i) Hb and PCV
  - (ii) Bilirubin
  - (iii) Glucose
- (*e*) Donor blood at end for — Hb, PCV
- (*f*) Catheter tip at the end for bacteriology.
- (*g*) Samples for special current interests.
- (*h*) In addition, we collect all the effluent blood for bilirubin estimation to calculate the total removed.

(5) Use full aseptic precautions. Take a swab of the umbilicus and paint the skin of the abdominal wall and the umbilicus with 70% isopropyl alcohol. Place a loose ligature around the base of the cord to control any excessive bleeding which occurs when the cord is cut. Lift the distal end of the cord with a Spencer Wells, cut the cord about 1cm from the umbilicus and discard the cut end, and do not use the dirty Spencer Wells again. Cover the abdomen with a circum ision towel with the umbilicus protruding. Complete towelling up.

(6) Introduction of the catheter. Details are given under 'Techniques', p. 264. We normally use the umbilical vein, but have occasionally used the artery when the catheter is already in.

(7) Connect the two three-way taps so that leads are connected to the umbilical catheter, the syringe, the donor blood and a sterile bag for the waste. At no time should the umbilical catheter be open to air because of the danger of air embolism.

(8) Take the pre-transfusion specimen of baby and donor blood.

(9) The order of procedure is (*a*) withdraw blood from the baby, and (*b*) inject donor blood. Normally the exchange transfusion will be carried out with 20ml aliquots. In the case of very small or ill babies, 10ml aliquots are safer. Blood can be withdrawn quickly, but only light pressure should be exerted in withdrawing the plunger.

If the flow of blood ceases, pause for a few seconds before continuing withdrawal —it is frequently the case that blood flows intermittently rather than continuously. If the blood-flow ceases altogether, the position of the catheter should be altered by slight further insertion or withdrawal. The cause of the difficulty in withdrawing is often the use of excessive negative pressure in the syringe. It may, however, be due to a clot in the tap or to the plunger sticking in the barrel. If all your fiddling is in vain, withdraw the catheter and examine it for clots. A new catheter should be inserted.

Whenever there is a pause in the exchange—for changing taps or syringes, or for collecting blood specimens—the catheter should be filled with donor blood to prevent clotting.

(10) Injection of donor blood. When the syringe has been filled, the plunger should be held upwards, nozzle down and the barrel should be sharply tapped to displace any bubbles upwards. There should not normally be bubbles in the syringe; if there are, the tap junctions must be tightened. When injecting the blood, the cannula must be watched very carefully and continually to detect the passage of any bubble.

AT LEAST TWO MINUTES SHOULD BE TAKEN TO INJECT 20ml OF BLOOD INTO THE BABY. With faster injection rates, cardiac failure may be precipitated.

It is of great importance that the bottle of donor blood should be gently agitated from time to time to keep the cells and plasma mixed.

The amount of blood injected and withdrawn at each phase of the operation *must* be noted exactly, as potentially serious changes in blood volume can occur with even a small constant error of measurement in withdrawal or injection.

(11) Note keeping. Following each phase of the procedure, the operator must call out the number of ml injected or withdrawn. The nurse then enters this figure in the appropriate cell on the chart, noting the exact time, and repeats the figures aloud, totting them up as the transfusion proceeds. Also to be noted on the chart are the baby's name, the date, the number of the donor-blood bottle and details of the donor blood (*i.e.* fresh heparinized or stored citrated, and the date of collection), and whether an arterial or venous catheter is used. The nurse must record the heart rate (preferably from the oscilloscope) and respiration rate, every quarter of an hour. The feet should be observed frequently when an arterial catheter is used, and if possible the pulses should be felt.

(12) Volume to be changed. The usual total volume to be exchanged is 180ml/kg bodyweight up to a total of 500ml. *There should be no hesitation in stopping the exchange for a period, or altogether, if any untoward signs appear.* A smaller total volume is used for the first exchange in hydropic or very anaemic babies (see p. 65). Remember that much more is achieved in the first 100ml than subsequently.

(13) Warnings of impending cardiac failure. Restlessness, distressed respiration, or a heart rate above 150 or below 110, grunting, soft heart sounds, or deterioration in the colour of the cord venous blood (this is normally almost as red as arterial blood) should be taken as an early warning sign of cardiac failure and the procedure should be

interrupted until the baby has recovered. Sometimes cardiac failure is precipitated by insertion of a venous catheter too far into the left atrium via the ductus venosus and the foramen ovale. This is very easily done.

(14) End of the transfusion. Take samples of donor and baby blood (para 4).

The vein must be closed by purse-string suture of catgut. The catheter is then removed before the ligature is tied tightly. The cut end of the stump should be sprayed with Polybactrin. A light dressing should be placed over the umbilicus so that any bleeding may be rapidly detected.

When you have finished the exchange, go and see the mother.

### Exchange Transfusion by Other Routes

If it is not possible to insert a catheter into the umbilical vein, first try the artery (see p. 264). Should this fail, a cut-down should be performed. Make an incision through the skin of the umbilicus on the cephalic side; the umbilical vein lies in a surprisingly deep trough, and the catheter can be inserted directly into it. It is very seldom impossible to carry out an exchange transfusion via the umbilical vein. When it is impossible, the saphenous vein is the best alternative.

The saphenous vein is located as follows. A line is drawn at right angles to the mid-point of the line joining the anterior superior iliac spine to the pubic tubercle. The incision is made at right angles to and medially from the first mentioned line, parallel to the second mentioned line and 1½cm from it. The incision should be 1 to 2cm long and should be about ½cm below the inguinal fold. The saphenous vein is *very small indeed* and lies just above the deep fascia.

Sometimes after cutting down on a small vein in a small baby, blood can be injected but none withdrawn. If no adequate means of withdrawing blood can be established, cut down on the radial artery (see p. 267) and insert a catheter, withdraw blood with a syringe, or allow it to drip into a measuring cylinder. Replace the blood by injecting into the existing cut-down vein, and thus perform an exchange. At the end of the procedure, a very firm dressing on the radial artery will control the haemorrhage.

CONSENT FOR BLOOD TRANSFUSION

It is not usual to obtain formal consent for blood transfusion, though the reason why transfusion is necessary should be explained to the parents beforehand.

If the parents have religious or other objections to blood transfusion, follow the advice of the Department of Health and Social Security of 14th April 1967. Briefly, this is as follows.

(1) Legal procedures, such as an application to a juvenile court to obtain a fit person order should *not* be used as this may cause a serious delay and it is doubtful if it confers any added protection on the doctor.

(2) The consultant should take personal responsibility for deciding whether transfusion is necessary. He should explain his decision to the parents. If they withold

consent he should:

(*a*) obtain a written supporting opinion from a colleague (presumably another consultant would be most appropriate) that the child's life is in danger if transfusion is withheld;

(*b*) obtain an acknowledgement, preferably in writing, from the parent or guardian that, despite the explanation of the danger, they refuse consent; and

(*c*) write his own opinion, and what he has said to the parents in the notes and sign it.

(*d*) Although this is not stated in the Department of Health's circular, it is wise to inform the Hospital Secretary, and the Secretary of the appropriate medical defence organization, of what has happened as soon as it is convenient.

(*e*) Go ahead with the transfusion.

# Neurological Procedures

**Lumbar Puncture**

There are no specific contraindications to lumbar puncture, but the handling required and the flexion of the trunk may provoke apnoeic attacks in babies who are prone to them.

(1) The needle. A conventional L.P. needle with a stilette has the advantage that it will not become blocked by tissue during insertion. Select the shortest L.P. needle available. If pressure measurement is required and an ordinary L.P. needle is being used, take a plastic feeding tube and cut off the connection at the end so that the new cut end will just fit snugly into the wide end of the L.P. needle. The tube is used as a manometer. Some of our residents prefer to use a scalp vein needle: this has the advantage that it is directly connected to a piece of fine tubing which can be used as a manometer.

(2) Position the baby. The best method is probably to sit the baby up with the dorsal and lumbar spine flexed as much as possible. Alternatively, the baby may be lain on his side with the spine flexed as much as possible, parallel with the ground, and not rotated. In the case of very small and sickly babies, too much flexion may hinder respiration.

(3) Identify the spine of the fourth lumbar vertebra, which usually lies on a line joining the two iliac crests.

(4) Infiltrate the skin over the space between L.4 and L.5 (but not the deeper structures) with not more than 0.4ml of 0.5% plain lignocaine hydrochloride injection. We usually do this, but we are not sure if it is worthwhile.

(5) Insert the needle between the L.4 and L.5 spines, precisely in the midline and precisely in the antero-posterior plane.

(6) Do not go too far. The depth to which the needle has to be inserted is usually less than 1cm and the sensation of penetrating the ligamentum flavum is often absent. The stilette should therefore be withdrawn frequently as the needle is advanced. Inserting the needle too deeply results in a blood-stained tap. Slight rotation of the needle may help the CSF to come out.

(7) Measure pressure, using the tubing as a manometer, alongside a ruler.

(8) If no fluid is obtained, repeat in space L3/4. But do not go higher than this because of the risk of damage to the spinal cord (in the newborn the cord comes down to L. 3).

(9) Dry taps will sometimes be obtained despite adequate technique. Consider whether examination of the CSF is important enough to justify cisternal puncture. If the CSF is bloodstained, it may be difficult to decide whether this is due to a traumatic tap, or to the presence of blood in the CSF. The following points may help the decision. (a) Note whether the puncture seemed clean and straightforward, or whether there was difficulty in entering the theca. (b) Collect CSF in numbered bottles and see whether the blood-staining is uniform.

279

(c) Have the CSF centrifuged and see if the supernatant is xanthochromic: this suggests that blood has been present in the CSF for some time, *provided* the baby is not jaundiced. However, if the baby is significantly jaundiced, the CSF will be xanthochromic anyway. (d) Have the red and white cell count and culture done on the CSF, however blood-stained it is. Ask the haematologists if there are any macrophages on the film: their presence suggests that the CSF has been blood-stained for at least a few hours.

**Cisternal Puncture**

*N.B.* Cisternal puncture is contraindicated in babies with myelomeningocele (who are likely to have the Arnold-Chiari malformation) and in any case where cerebellar malformation is suspected.

*Procedure*

(1) Shave hair from the occipital bone and back of the neck and measure the circumference of the neck.

(2) Select an L.P. needle of medium length (4-5cm).

(3) Arrange for the baby to be securely held, lying on its side. The neck should be flexed as much as possible, and the entire spine should form a straight line as viewed from behind. A little padding may be needed under the baby's left cheek and ear to obliterate any lateral flexion of the cervical spine.

(4) Identify the landmarks. Feeling in the midline posteriorly at the junction of the head and neck, a small depression is palpable. Its upper edge (in relation to the baby) is formed by the base of the occipital bone, which is the lowest palpable portion of the skull. The lower edge of the depression is formed by the spine of the axis (C. 2), which is the highest palpable portion of the cervical spine. The lateral borders of the depression are formed by the posterior nuchal muscles on each side. The needle will be inserted into the centre of this depression.

(5) Infiltrate the skin between the base of the occipital bone and the spine of the axis with a small quantity (about 0.5ml) of local anaesthetic such as 0.5% plain ligno-caine. Do not infiltrate the deeper structures and avoid using a larger quantity, since this obscures the landmarks.

(6) Take the L.P. needle and penetrate the skin precisely in the midline between the base of the occipital bone and the spine of the axis. Keeping the needle horizontal, aim it towards a point on the forehead just above the glabella and push it in to a depth of about 1cm. Withdraw the stilette. If no fluid is obtained, push the needle in a further few mm and again withdraw the stilette. Continue until either the needle hits the occipital bone or the cistern is entered. Usually the needle will hit the occipital bone. In this case, partly withdraw the needle and re-insert it, aiming at a slightly lower point on the forehead) *i.e.* aiming just to avoid the base of the occipital bone rather than to hit it). Repeat the procedure as before. Usually the moment of entering the cistern will be obvious from a distinct 'pop', but this should not be relied on, and the stilette should be withdrawn frequently as the needle is advanced.

The usual depth to which the needle needs to be inserted is about 1.5cm in a term baby; this is about one-eighth of the circumference of the neck.

(7) We do not normally measure pressure when cisternal puncture is done, since

we prefer not to manipulate the needle if this can be avoided.

**Subdural Tap**

This is rarely indicated in the neonatal period (see p. 184).

(1) Shave the entire anterior part of the head to well behind the posterior angle of the anterior fontanelle.

(2) Select two subdural tap needles. These are very short and of much wider bore than an L.P. needle.

(3) Identify the landmarks—the lateral angles of the anterior fontanelle and the coronal sutures.

(4) Position the baby on a locker-top, with a wrapper round the whole body keeping the arms firmly in place and with the top of the baby's head on the edge of the locker, towards the doctor.

(5) Infiltrate the skin with a small quantity (about 0.5ml) of 0.5% plain lignocaine at the proposed sites of insertion of the needles in the coronal suture lines, just lateral to the lateral angles of the fontanelle.

(6) Insert the subdural tap needle through the skin at the site described, on one side of the head. Keep it perpendicular to the scalp surface. As soon as the skin and suture are penetrated, withdraw the stilette. Wait for at least a half-minute. Subdural fluid is often viscid. If no fluid comes out, push in further to a maximum depth of 1.5cm, withdrawing the stilette frequently. If no fluid is obtained, withdraw slowly, rotating the needle. After complete withdrawal of the needle from the skin, it is usual and normal for a drop of CSF to ooze out.

(7) IN NO CIRCUMSTANCES SHOULD SUCTION BE APPLIED BY A SYRINGE ATTACHED TO A NEEDLE IN THE HEAD.

(8) If there is strong reason (*e.g.* from transillumination) to suspect that subdural fluid is present and no fluid is obtained by the procedure described, taps may be repeated at sites further lateral in the coronal suture line.

**Ventricular Tap**

We rarely do ventricular taps. They may occasionally be required in hydro-cephalus, when they should only be done after consultation with the neurosurgeon, and in meningitis (see p. 168).

(1) Shave the head, position the baby, identify the landmarks and infiltrate the skin in exactly the same way as for subdural taps.

(2) The right ventricle should be tapped unless there is some over-riding reason to choose the left one.

(3) Select a fine L.P. needle at least 5cm long and prepare a manometer as for lumbar puncture.

(4) Push in the needle cautiously in the coronal plane, slightly inwards to a depth of up to 4 to 5cm in a term baby, withdrawing the stilette frequently. Generally speaking, ventricular taps will only be done on babies who are thought to have en-larged ventricles, in which case the ventricle will usually be encountered without difficulty at a depth of not more than 2.5cm—often much less. The depth should be measured while the needle is being inserted—not while it is being withdrawn, which

often gives a misleading measure of cerebral mantle thickness.

(5) If no fluid is obtained after two attempts, inserting the needle to a depth of 4.5cm, it is unlikely that the doctor will reap any information (or the baby any benefit) from persisting with the procedure.

(6) IN NO CIRCUMSTANCES SHOULD SUCTION BE APPLIED TO A SYRINGE ATTACHED TO A NEEDLE IN THE HEAD.

(7) After removal of the needle, ventricular fluid may continue to ooze out. Sit the baby up 'and apply local pressure till it stops.

## Air Ventriculography

(1) Sedation with chloral is helpful.

(2) Tap the ventricle as described above.

(3) Carefully measure the quantity of CSF removed by comparison with a universal container containing a measured 10ml of water.

(4) After removal of 10ml of fluid, inject 10ml of air which has been drawn into a syringe through a sterile filter of gauze. DO NOT SUCK ON THE SYRINGE.

(5) Repeat removal of 10ml aliquots of fluid and injection of equal amounts of air until enough air has been injected. In a baby with normal-sized ventricles, 10ml of air would be sufficient, but ventriculography is not done under such circumstances. In a baby with hydrocephalus, up to 25-30ml of air should be enough.

(6) Keep the baby in the brow-up position from the moment the air is inserted until he reaches the table in the x-ray department. This is not difficult, and generally easier than doing the whole procedure in the x-ray department.

# Urine Collection

Meticulous attention to detail is essential when collecting urine for bacteriology.

(1) Urine collecting bags, sterile or unsterile, give a falsely high number of significant ($10^5$ organisms/ml) cultures, and cell counts are significantly raised in the female. A clean catch method of collection should be used if possible.

(2) However carefully any collection is made, the results will be invalidated by increase in bacterial number if the urine is kept at room temperature for more than one hour without being plated out; if there is to be delay beyond that time, refrigeration at 4°C will prevent such multiplication for up to 48 hours.


**Methods**

*Mid-stream Clean Catch*

This gives the most reliable results without hazard to the baby. If you cannot collect it yourself, explain to the nurses exactly what to do.

(1) Clean buttocks and perineum with soap and water.

(2) Dry with sterile swabs.

(3) Support infant with thighs abducted, separating the labia in females but not retracting the foreskin in males.

Collect, after the first few drops are passed, into a sterile container which must not touch the infant's skin. Tricks to ensure the immediate passage of urine (and there are many described) usually give 100 per cent success in everybody's hands except your own.


*Urine Collecting Bag*

Wash perineum with soap and water before putting it on, and remove for examination as soon as urine is passed, snipping the lower corner of the bag and allowing the urine to drain into a sterile Universal container.


*Bladder Puncture*

This should be reserved for (*a*) ill infants in whom a urine culture is a matter of extreme urgency and (*b*) infants from whom equivocal results have been obtained on more than one occasion using the above methods. It has a failure rate of about 10 per cent. If possible, do the puncture an hour or so after urine has been passed, when a dull percussion note above the symphysis pubis suggests a full bladder.

With the infant lying supine, and legs held in the frog position, clean the suprapubic area thoroughly with 70% isopropyl alcohol. Using a 20cc syringe with No. 21 (3.8cm) needle, and holding it vertically 1.5 to 2.0cm above the symphysis pubis in the mid-line, pierce the abdominal wall and bladder in one rapid movement. The bladder will usually be entered at a depth of 1.0 to 2.0cm or occasionally 2.5cm. Aspirate urine, withdraw needle, remove from the syringe, seal the syringe with a cap, and arrange for immediate examination and plating. Transient haematuria may occur following the procedure, and should be recorded.

### Cell Count

You should do this yourself on all urgent specimens. Place one drop of Trypan blue on either side of the recessed areas and cover slip of a white cell counting chamber, and allow to dry. Mix urine with Trypan blue before allowing it to flow under the cover slip—this helps to distinguish pus from renal tubular cells and red cells by the appearance of the nucleus. Normal urines contain fewer than 10 white cells/mm$^3$ in both sexes NOTE: Cells disappear very rapidly in an alkaline urine, so always record the pH.

### Interpretation of Results

In urines collected by the mid-stream catch technique, as described, or by bladder puncture, bacterial counts of 10$^5$/ml and white cell counts above 10/mm$^3$ should be regarded as significant. If the bacterial count is raised, but the cell count is normal (or vice versa), it is advisable to examine further specimens of urine before starting treatment, unless the baby is obviously ill. Ideally, in all cases, two consecutive positives should be obtained before starting treatment.

If a collecting bag has been used, falsely high cell-counts may be found in a proportion of females due to perineal contamination: false positive cultures may occur to a lesser extent in both sexes. Remember that a normal specimen means that the urine was normal *at the time of collection*, and if real suspicion of urinary infection exists, repeated examinations must be made, as bacteriuria may be intermittent.

# Section 7: Equipment

We would have liked to include in this section a full list of equipment for the special care nursery, and to have included a 'best buy' table. Such a section, however, is impracticable because of the rapid advances in the field, because of individual preferences of nurses and paediatricians, and because the price of various pieces of equipment changes so rapidly. However, much of the equipment we use is not commercially available or is rather expensive if purchased and has, therefore, been made for us in the workshop of the Royal Postgraduate Medical School by Messrs. Ken Lanning, Tony Becket and Peter Goddard. The electronic equipment was devised by Mr. Peter Rolfe, B.Sc. This section, therefore, gives some details of home-made equipment that we have found useful and sometimes invaluable. We are grateful to Mr. Peter Clark, medical artist, and Mr. Bill Hinks, photographer, both of the department of medical illustration of the Royal Postgraduate Medical School, for the drawings and photographs in this book.

*NOTES*

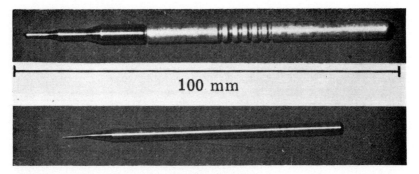

**Fig. 10. Umbilical Artery and Radial Artery Dilators**
These smooth-tipped metal dilators are extremely helpful in opening the arteries before insertion of the catheter. The diameters of the successive steps of the umbilical artery dilator (upper in photograph) are 1.45mm, 2.70mm and 4.70mm. (See p. 264.)


**Fig. 11. Pressure-limiting 'Blow-off' Valve**
The spring-loaded 'blow-off' valve limits the maximum pressure achieved. The desired limit can be varied from 10-70cmH$_2$O by turning the bevelled screw top. It is light, easily sterilised and functions in any position. We incorporate one in any air line which leads from a pressure source (*e.g.* O$_2$ supply) to the baby's airway. Vickers Medical are now producing such valves. Details of the construction have been published (Goddard, P., Becket, A. J. (1971) 'A simple safety valve for infant resuscitator and ventilator gas circuits.' *Lancet*, **ii**, 584).

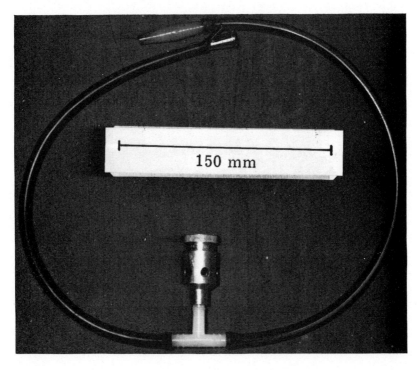

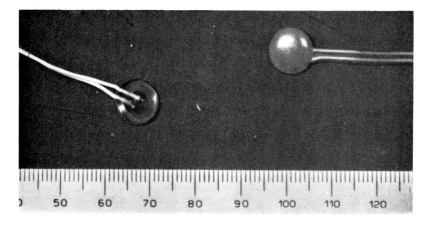

**Fig. 12. Skin Thermistor Probes**
Temperature probes that attach to the skin should be properly designed. The temperature-sensitive element is applied to the skin surface and embedded in a 'button' of plastic for security. (See p. 106.)

**Fig. 13. Clock Which Displays Baby's Age**
This clock is made cheaply from an electric clock motor, two gear wheels and a simple plastic case. The clock is set to the baby's age and then started. The time of investigations, observations, X-rays, etc., can then be read off directly. (See 'Neonatal record keeping', p. 311.)

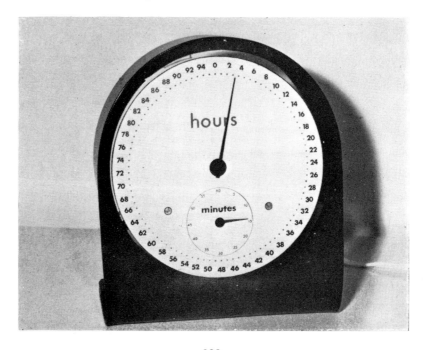

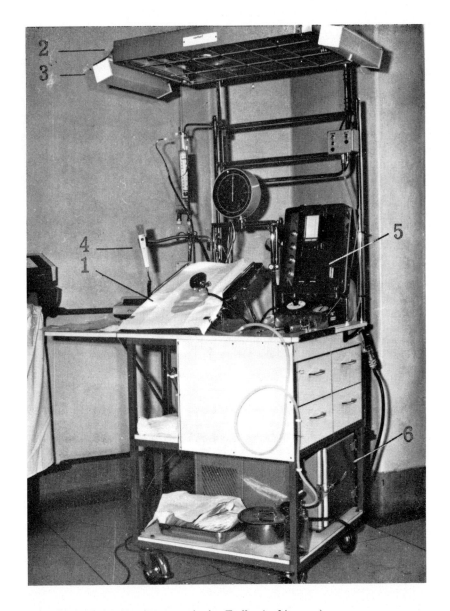

**Fig. 14. The Hammersmith Hospital Resuscitation Trolley** (p. 34 *et seq.*)
The inclination of the baby-shelf (1) is adjustable and the shelf can itself be 'broken' to allow a baby's head to be extended for intubation, which obviates hanging the baby over the edge. Overhead (2) is a home-made radiant heat panel (four electric-fire elements wired *in series* so that the output is limited). The flanking lights (3) are easily turned off to prevent glare when using the laryngoscope. To the left of the baby-shelf is a microphone (4) for the tape recorder; to the right is an ECG machine (5). The supply of 40 per cent oxygen passes through an aneroid pressure-limiting system before reaching the baby's airway. Suction is by a Venturi operated sucker. Beneath the drawers is a refrigerator (6) in which heparin, etc., is kept and in which samples can be stored for analysis. It is very helpful to have some table-top space both to the right and to the left of the baby-shelf.

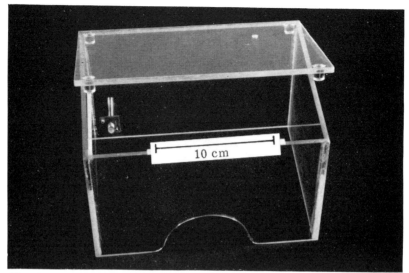

**Fig. 15. The 'Gairdner' Head-box** (p. 132)

Such a plastic head-box has a removable lid for access to the face, an inlet for oxygen-air mixtures, and a sampling hole for analysis. It is easy to make and much cheaper than its commercial equivalent. It is essential if very high ambient $O_2$ concentrations are needed around the face and, incidentally, it reduces the amount of oxygen used.

**Fig. 16. Perspex Heat Shield**

The function and importance of the heat shield **are** described on p. 103. It is essential if meaningful interpretations of 'environmental' temperature are to be made from readings of the air thermometer in an incubator. Such a shield may be made cheaply by cutting two hemicylinders from a tube of perspex, or by allowing a sheet of perspex to settle to the shape (below) over a heated mould.

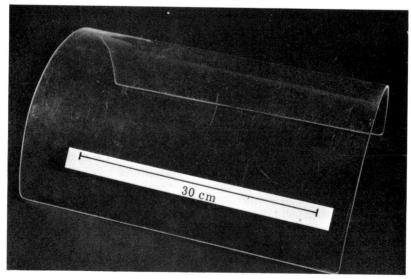

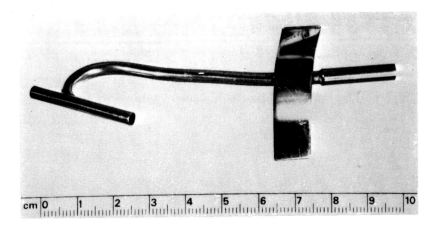

**Fig. 17a. 'Harness' for Securing a Nasotracheal Tube** (p. 134)

We use this easily sterilised harness for securing a nasotracheal tube. The baby is given a bonnet of tubegauze to cover head and forehead. The butterfly wings of the harness are strapped to the bonnet on the forehead and the nasotracheal tube is also secured at the nostril. The opening in line with the nasotracheal tube is used for the humidification infusion and for suction of the tube. This harness enables the U loop of the ventilator (p. 133) or CPAP (p. 128) to pass above the head and the child can easily be turned from side to side, thus obviating his having to lie flat on his back. Dr. A. D. Milner pointed out to us that the internal bore of the metal tube had to be at least 3.8mm to ensure minimal airways resistance. On the other hand, it should not be much bigger than this or there will be an undesirably large dead space.

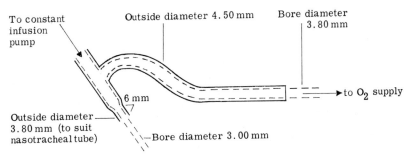

**Fig. 17b.** Dimensions of harness.

Figs. 18-21. The Hammersmith Hospital Ventilator (p. 133)

**Fig. 18.** The ventilator and infusion pump in use. This constant infusion pump is made from an electric-clock motor. The rate of infusion is varied by the bore of the disposable syringe used. Commercial constant infusion pumps are rather expensive.

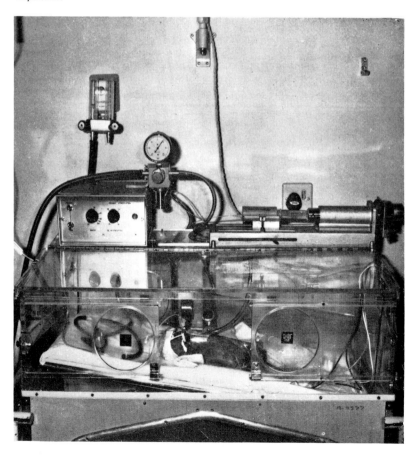

**Fig. 19.** Close-up view of the ventilator. (Modified from Grausz, J. P., Watt, N. L., Becket, A. J. (1967) 'A new positive-pressure respirator for new-borns.' *Lancet,* **ii,** 499.)

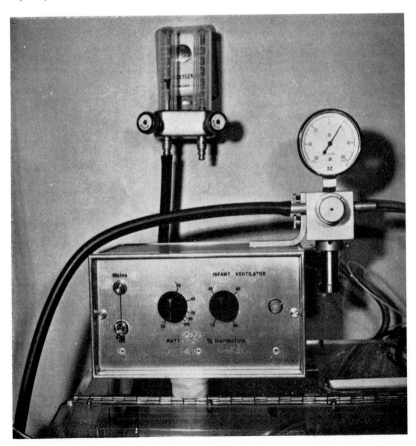

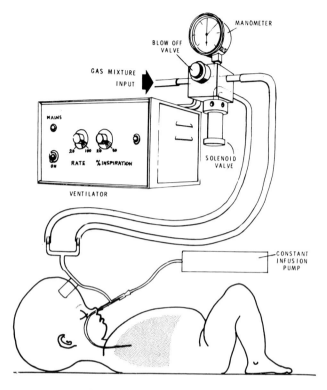

**Fig. 20.** Diagram of the ventilator.

**Fig. 21.** The mode of action.

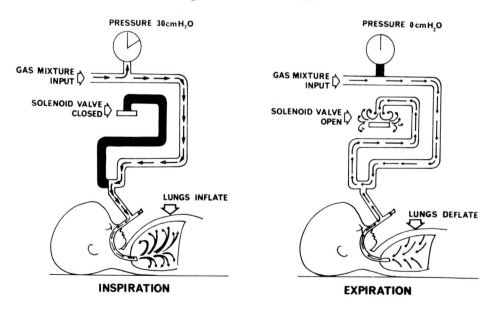

PRESSURE 30cmH₂O

GAS MIXTURE INPUT

SOLENOID VALVE CLOSED

LUNGS INFLATE

**INSPIRATION**

PRESSURE 0cmH₂O

GAS MIXTURE INPUT

SOLENOID VALVE OPEN

LUNGS DEFLATE

**EXPIRATION**

# Section 8: Drugs and Dosage

*NOTES*

# General Considerations

The ability of the newborn to deal with drugs depends on the maturity of specific enzyme systems and on renal function. Because maternal drug metabolism is altered in pregnancy, it has been suggested that an abnormal neonatal response may in part be due to maternally derived hormones. Besides this there are many other factors which have a special influence on the metabolism and excretion of drugs in the neonatal period.

The practical points to remember are that dosage schemes calculated on weight, surface area or a percentage of the adult dose are not applicable to the newborn. There is a multitude of reports of drug toxicity in the newborn which appeared before these facts were generally realised, and which mainly involved the antibacterials. Suitable dosage for most antibacterial drugs has now been established following estimations of blood levels. Unfortunately, this is not true of other categories of drugs, and the suggested doses given below should thus be accepted with caution. Prescribe parsimoniously and unadventurously in the neonatal period, and be constantly on the alert for unusual reactions. We do not wish to imply that drugs are of little value at this time: they may on occasions be life-saving.

## Practical Points in Prescribing and Administration
### Prescribing
Drugs, and the form they may be prescribed in, are listed in Table XII under their approved (British National Formulary, 1971) names. Some proprietary names are also given, but you should become familiar with and use the former. An appropriate strength (*not* always the only one available) is given under the approved name for your guidance, but the exact dosage of a drug in milligrams (mg), rather than the volume of the solution in millilitres (ml), should always be written to avoid accidents. Do not use fixed dosage drug combinations.

Because we are uncertain about rates of absorption from the gastro-intestinal tract in ill babies in the first week of life, we have usually recommended the intramuscular route and given the appropriate dose. But when oral drugs can be effectively substituted, use them. In a few cases, oral drugs are only supplied as tablets. If the tablet strength is appropriate, it can be crushed and given in milk. In other cases the pharmacy will be able to make up a suitable solution or suspension.

### Administration
Drugs should not be injected into the buttock in the newborn, because of the risk of sciatic nerve damage. The anterior or lateral thigh should be used, but care must be taken to rotate sites of injection. We have seen two cases of late contraction of the quadriceps following I.M. injections; avoid unnecessary frequency of injection, and watch carefully for excessive induration at injection sites. Most intramuscular doses

should be well under 1ml, though there are a very few exceptions. For accuracy of administration, it is essential to use syringes graded in 1/10's and 1/100's of 1ml (*e.g.* 'Gillette Scimitar' 1ml syringe). For intravenous medication, see p. 101.

*Never discharge home an infant still having drugs without informing his general practitioner.*

## TABLE XII

**Drugs and dosage. (For antimicrobial drugs, see pp. 170-172.)**

| Drug — Approved name and form | Proprietary name | Route | Single dose | Frequency | Comment | Page in text |
|---|---|---|---|---|---|---|
| Acetazolamide Tablets B.P. (250mg) | Diamox | Oral | 15 - 35mg/kg. | 8-hourly | Consider its use in cases of hydrocephalus. | 179 |
| Aldosterone injection (0.5mg/ml) | Aldocorten | I.M. or I.V. | 1mg. | Give once, repeat in 12 hours if necessary | Salt-losing adrenal crisis. Replaces desoxycorti-costerone acetate (DOCA), now unavailable | 64 |
| Calcium Gluconate Injection, B.P. (10%) Calcium Gluconate | | I.M. or I.V. Oral | 20mg/kg. (0.2ml/kg 10% soln.) 100mg/kg. | Give once, *slowly* if I.V. 6-hourly | Hypocalcaemia | 190 |
| Carbimazole Tablets, B.P. (5mg) | Neo-Mercazole | Oral | 2.5mg. | 8-hourly, gradually reduce once symptoms controlled | Congenital thyrotoxicosis | 11 |
| Chloral Elixir Paediatric, B.P.C. (200mg/5ml) | | Oral | 7.5mg/kg. | 6-hourly | Sedative, anticonvulsant | 190 |
| Chloroquine Sulphate Injection, B.P. (200mg base in 5ml) | Nivaquine | I.M. | 10mg base. | Once daily | Congenital malaria | 171 |
| Chlorpromazine Injection, B.P. (25mg/ml) | Largactil | I.M. | 0.5mg/kg. | 6-hourly | Withdrawal symptoms of maternal drug addiction | 222 |
| Chlorpromazine Hydrochloride Syrup (25mg/5ml) | | Oral | 0.5mg/kg. | 4-hourly | | |

(*continued*)

299

**Table XII (cont.)**

| Drug | | | | | | |
|---|---|---|---|---|---|---|
| *Approved name and form* | *Proprietary name* | *Route* | *Single dose* | *Frequency* | *Comment* | *Page in text* |
| Cortisone Injection, B.P. (25mg/ml) | | I.M. or I.V. | 25mg. | Once daily, or 12-hourly if symptoms very severe | Salt-losing adrenal crisis | 64 |
| Cortisone Tablets, B.P. (5mg; 25mg) | | Oral | 5mg. | 8-hourly (more may be necessary in individual cases) | Maintenance for congenital adrenal hyperplasia | 64 |
| Cyclopentolate Eye-drops, B.P.C. (0.5%) | Mydrilate | Local instillation | 1 to 2 drops each eye | Give once 30-60 minutes before examination | Mydriatic | 241 |
| Dexamethasone Injection (4mg/ml) | Decadron | I.M. | 1mg. | 12-hourly | Cerebral oedema—proof of efficacy in the neonatal situation lacking | 184 |
| Diamorphine Injection, B.P. 5mg; powder/vial | (Heroin) | I.M. | 0.05mg/kg. | 12-hourly | Analgesic; beware of respiratory depression | 197 |
| Diazepam Injection, B.P.(10mg/2ml) | Valium | I.M. or I.V. | 0.25mg/kg. | 8-hourly | Anticonvulsant—do not use if infant jaundiced | 190 |
| Diazepam Elixir (2mg/5ml) | | Oral | 0.25mg/kg. | 6-hourly | | |
| Digoxin Injection B.P. (0.25mg/ml) | Lanoxin | I.M. or I.V. | 0.006mg/kg. For rapid digitalisation give twice stated dose at once, then stated dose 8-hourly for 2 injections | 12-hourly (maintenance) | Congestive cardiac failure | 214, 215 |

| | | | | | | |
|---|---|---|---|---|---|---|
| Digoxin Elixir Paediatric, B.P.C. (0.25mg/5ml) | | Oral | As above | | | |
| Edrophonium Injection, B.P. (10mg/ml) | Tensilon | I.M. or I.V. | 1mg. | Once, give *slowly* if I.V. | In diagnosis of temporary involvement in infants of mothers with myasthenia gravis | 13 |
| Ephedrine Nasal Drops, B.P.C. (0.5%) | | Local instillation | 1 drop each nostril | Give 20 minutes before a feed, but not more frequently than 12-hourly | Nasal congestion. Use for short period only; CNS excitation has occurred from overdose | 17 |
| Ferrous Sulphate Mixture Paediatric, B.P.C. (60mg/5ml) | | Oral | 30mg. | Twice daily | Anaemia of prematurity | 234, 236 |
| Folic Acid Tablets, B.P. (0.1mg) | | Oral | 0.1mg. | Once weekly | Anaemia of prematurity Severe rhesus incompatibility | 154, 234, 236 |
| Frusemide Injection (20mg/2ml) | Lasix | I.M. | <2mg/kg. | Once or twice daily | Diuretic | 216 |
| Hydrocortisone Sodium Succinate Injection, B.P. (100mg powder to be dissolved immediately before use.) | Efcortelan soluble | I.M. or I.V. | 2.5mg/kg. | 6-hourly | Laryngeal oedema | 145 |
| Lignocaine Hydro-chloride Injection, B.P. (0.5%) | | Local infiltration | | | Local anaesthesia before lumbar puncture, etc. | 279 *et seq.* |

*(continued)*

**TABLE XII (cont.)**

| Drug<br>Approved name and form | Proprietary name | Route | Single dose | Frequency | Comment | Page in text |
|---|---|---|---|---|---|---|
| Magnesium Chloride Injection (2.5mEq Mg$^{++}$ and Cl$^-$/ml) | | I.V. or I.M. | 0.3mEq/kg (=15mg/kg.) | Once, give *slowly* if I.V. | Hypocalcaemia, hypomagnesaemia | 190 |
| Morphine Sulphate Injection, B.P. (10mg/ml) | | I.M. | 0.1mg/kg. | 12-hourly | Analgesic. Beware respiratory depression | 197 |
| Nalorphine Injection, B.P. (5mg/5ml) | Lethidrone | I.M. or I.V. | 0.2mg/kg. | Once | Morphine (and analogues) antagonist—birth asphyxia | 36 |
| Neostigmine Injection B.P. (0.5mg/ml) | Prostigmin | I.M. or I.V. | 0.05mg/kg. | Once | Infants of mothers with myasthenia gravis | 13 |
| Neostigmine Tablets, B.P. (15mg) | Prostigmin | Oral | 1mg. | 8-hourly | | |
| Paraldehyde Injection, B.P.C. (2ml) | | I.M. | 0.1ml/kg. | 12-hourly | Anticonvulsant | 190 |
| Pancreatin Powder, Strong (Tryptic activity 5 times that of Pancreatin, B.P.) | Pancrex V Powder | Oral | 25mg/kg. | 6-hourly | Cystic fibrosis | 195 |
| Pethidine Injection, B.P. (50mg/ml) | | I.M. | 1mg/kg. | 12-hourly | Analgesic | 197 |
| Phenobarbitone Injection, B.P. (20% W/V) | | I.M. or I.V. | 2mg/kg. | 8- or 12-hourly | Anticonvulsant, sedative, enzyme inducer | 190 |
| Phenobarbitone Elixir, B.P.C. (15mg/5ml) | | Oral | 1.25mg/kg. | 6-hourly | | |

| Preparation | Proprietary name | Route | Dose | Frequency | Indication | Page |
|---|---|---|---|---|---|---|
| Phenytoin Injection, B.P.C. (250mg powder /vial, dissolved immediately before use) | Epanutin | I.M. or I.V. | 2mg/kg. | Twice daily | Anticonvulsant | 190 |
| Phenytoin Mixture, B.P.C. (30mg/5ml) | | Oral | 1mg/kg. | 6-hourly | | |
| Phytomenadione Injection, B.P. (1mg/0.5ml) | Konakion (Vitamin $K_1$) | I.M. | 1mg. | Once | Prophylaxis for haemorrhagic disease of the newborn | 76, 196, 207 |
| Phytomenadione Oral Solution (1mg/ml) | | Oral | 1mg. | Once | | |
| Potassium Iodide Tablets, B.P.C. (60mg) | | Oral | 5mg. | 8-hourly Reduce gradually once symptoms controlled | Congenital thyrotoxicosis | 11 |
| Practolol Tablets (100mg) | Eraldin | I.V. | 0.1mg/kg. | Once, *slowly*; repeat if necessary | Paroxysmal atrial tachycardia | 214 |
| Protamine Sulphate Injection, B.P. (50mg/5ml) | | I.V. | 1mg for each 100 units of Heparin (max. 50mg) | | Anticoagulant antagonist—treatment of heparin overdosage | 307 |
| Pyridostigmine Tablets, B.P. (60mg) | Mestinon | Oral | 10mg. | 8-hourly | Short-term treatment for infants of myasthenic mothers | 13 |
| Pyrimethamine Elixir (6.25mg/ml) | Daraprim | Oral | 0.5mg/kg. for 3 days 0.25mg/kg for one month | 12-hourly 12-hourly | Congenital toxoplasmosis Given with sulphadiazine | 172 |
| Sodium Bicarbonate (8.4% solution, approx. 1mEq $Na^+$/ml) | | I.V. | Dependent on pH: 1ml/mEq base deficit/kg. | 8-hourly | Acidosis | 35, 129 |

*(continued)*

**TABLE XII (cont.)**

| Drug | Proprietary name | Route | Single dose | Frequency | Comment | Page in text |
|---|---|---|---|---|---|---|
| Approved name and form | | | | | | |
| Sodium Bicarbonate (8.4% solution approx. 1mEq Na$^+$/ml) | | Oral | 1-2mEq per feed, depending on base deficit | | Late metabolic acidosis of immaturity Check base deficit daily | 233 |
| Thyroxine Tablets, B.P. (0.05mg) | | Oral | 0.025mg. | Once daily | Cretinism; temporary hypothyroidism | 17 |
| Tris (Hydroxymethyl) Amino-Methane (3.6% and 7.0%) | THAM | I V. | See pp. 35 and 38 | | In terminal asphyxia | 35, 130 |

# Hazards in Prescribing Drugs

THE FOLLOWING INCOMPLETE HISTORY OF REACTIONS TO
DRUGS GIVEN TO THE NEWBORN IS INTENDED AS A WARNING TO THE
ENTHUSIASTIC PRESCRIBER OF NEW DRUGS

### Drugs; Their Effects, with Reported Total Daily Dose

*Antibacterials*

*Chloramphenicol.* Ineffective conjugation to inactive metabolites, rising blood levels of active drug giving circulatory collapse and death ('grey syndrome'). 100mg/kg.

*Colistin.* Presence of renal tubular epithelial cells and protein in urine, raised blood urea during therapy, disappearing when stopped. 2.5-5.0mg/kg.

*Colistin, kanamycin, neomycin, polymixin, streptomycin.* Muscle end-plate blockers. May cause respiratory paralysis if applied locally and absorbed from large raw areas, or if instilled into peritoneal cavity.

*Sulphonamides* (*sulphafurazole*). Kernikterus—due to displacement of bilirubin from protein-binding sites by drug. Heinz body anaemia. 150mg/kg in babies >1kg b.w.; 100mg/kg in babies <1kg b.w.

*Nalidixic acid.* Reversal of normal low serum/high urinary levels, with resultant metabolic acidosis. 60mg/kg.

*Novobiocin.* Hyperbilirubinaemia due to inhibition of glucuronyl transferase. 150mg/kg.

*Streptomycin* (*and dihydrostreptomycin*). Deafness and vestibular damage. 20mg/kg.

*Tetracyclines.* Permanent yellow-brown staining of primary dentition, extent depending on gestational age at time of administration. Temporary retardation of bone growth. (Molecule chelates with calcium, deposited along with it in tissues undergoing mineralization, *e.g.* tooth buds, bone.) 100mg/kg.

*Digitalis*

As at all ages, but ECG only reliable guide to intoxication in newborn. 0.075mg/kg (digitalising dose).

*Oxygen*

Pulmonary fibroplasia. Retrolental fibroplasia. Safe concentrations of ambient oxygen in respect of lung damage, and safe arterial oxygen tensions in respect of eye damage are not known.

*THAM*

Apnoea. 3.6 and 7% solutions.

305

*Vitamin K Analogues*

*Menadiol sodium diphosphate ('Synkavit') and menadione sodium bisulphite ('Hykinone').* Large doses of water-soluble preparations cause hyperbilirubinaemia (probably due to haemolysis), and kernikterus. 10-30mg. NOTE: Similar reactions have not been seen with naturally occurring $K_1$ or synthetic derivatives.

*Absorption From Intact Skin*

*Aniline dye.* Methaemoglobinaemia. (Usually from marking-ink on napkins. Will not occur if these are laundered after marking.)

*Hexachlorophane.* If allowed to dry on, has caused diarrhoea, dehydration and shock, neuromuscular disturbances.

*Naphthalene.* Haemolytic anaemia (napkins stored in moth-balls).

*Pentachlorophenol.* Excessive sweating, tachycardia, tachypnoea, hepatic enlargement (fatty infiltration liver), renal tubular damage, metabolic acidosis, death. (Disinfectant wrongly used in laundering napkins and bed linen.)

*Ointments containing resorcinol.* Methaemoglobinaemia.

*Absorption From Broken Skin*

*Boric acid (undiluted).* Diarrhoea and vomiting, generalised rash, liver necrosis, renal damage and death.

*Certain antibiotic sprays containing muscle end-plate blockers.* See p. 305.

(*Neomycin.* Deafness has been reported in older patients—not so far in the new-born.)

*Accidental Oral Ingestion of Harmful Substances in the Neonatal Period*

Opportunities are greater in the artificially fed, but have occurred in the breast-fed. The first three occurred in hospital nurseries.

*Hexachlorophane.* Symptoms as in skin absorption (see above).

*Boric acid or Salt (NaCl and even KCl!), used instead of sugar.* Boric acid: symptoms as in skin absorption (see above). Salt: hypernatraemia or hyperkalaemia and death.

*Hexachlorobenzene* (excreted in breast milk of women eating seed-wheat treated with this substance). Generalised skin lesions, gastro-intestinal symptoms, death.

*Lead acetate ointment on maternal nipples, lead nipple-shields.* Lead poisoning.

**Rapid Changes of Osmolality**

The intravenous injection, especially if repeated, of solutions with a high osmolality must be guarded against. Angiographic contrast material (sodium iothalamate) has resulted in metabolic acidosis, haematuria, renal medullary necrosis and severe proximal tubular vacuolization due to production of an osmotic diuresis and renal ischaemia.

Repeated injections of sodium bicarbonate, very high concentrations of dextrose, or THAM might present a danger if brain cells lose water quickly to the extracellular fluid.

**Accidental Overdosage**

This problem is not, of course, peculiar to the neonatal period, but opportunities for overdosage are greater, for instance when the same drugs, dispensed in different strengths, are being used for mother and infant in the same place—*i.e.* delivery rooms and lying-in wards. The following illustrate the hazards.

(1) Accidental heparinisation of the infant has occurred when syringes were rinsed with solutions containing 10,000 units/ml of heparin instead of 1000 units/ml before giving fresh blood transfusions.

(2) Gross streptomycin toxicity has been reported following the use of fixed penicillin-streptomycin combinations used for adults. The appropriate (or at least not grossly harmful) penicillin dose was accompanied by much too high a dose of streptomycin.

(3) Respiratory stimulants such as nalorphine, and water-soluble vitamin K analogues, have been given to the infant in delivery rooms in the past in dangerous amounts when the vial intended for the mother has been used by mistake.

*NOTES*

# Section 9: Neonatal Record Keeping

*NOTES*

The keeping of notes by the resident is an important aspect of neonatal care and, like medical record keeping in general, one that tends to be carried out badly. Several aspects of note keeping are peculiar to neonatal paediatrics.

(1) The mother's obstetric history—both of the present and previous pregnancies —may be very significant and must be accurately obtained and recorded, although this can be difficult if the baby is transferred from another hospital. (See p. 113 and p. 316).

(2) The true course of illness in the neonatal period is often so rapid that observations must be repeated frequently and the changes with time clearly recorded.

(3) The age of any patient is likely to be of significance in the interpretation of illness, but in the newborn baby, so much of life is compressed into the first few days of extra-uterine existence because of the rapid and profound physiological adjustments then taking place, that one must measure and record age in hours or even minutes. The exact time at which an event occurred or an observation was made may greatly alter the interpretation placed upon it. For instance, respiratory distress increasing in the first 12 hours of life is a completely different problem from respiratory distress developing for the first time at 12 hours. If the date alone is recorded, this information will be lost.

(4) The baby's birthweight and gestational age are of great importance in the interpretation of signs of disease.

(5) Frequent and accurate records of therapy (*e.g.* $O_2$ level maintained in incubator) may assume as great importance in relation to subsequent progress as records of changes in the baby's condition.

### The Problem-orientated Approach

These requirements are best met, and the case records are rendered most informative, by adopting the problem-orientated approach coupled with the use of flow-sheets for data recording. The reader is strongly advised to consult the paper by Weed (1968)* on this subject.

A problem list is made out for each baby when first seen—at birth or on admission to the Special Care Nursery—after writing the conventional chronological history. Problems listed and numbered include signs and symptoms (*e.g.* birth asphyxia or fits), and the treatment given (*e.g.* oxygen therapy or artificial ventilation). Further problems can be added to the list as they may develop later, and separate problems found to have a common basis amalgamated; *e.g.* fits and hypoglycaemia could be amalgamated as 'symptomatic hypoglycaemia' when this was established.

### Flow-sheets

The recording of multiple items of data in an orderly, logical and readily retrievable manner during the rapidly changing course of a neonatal illness is only achieved by the use of suitably designed flow-sheets. Items such as incubator $O_2$ concentration, blood gas tensions, serum bilirubin and incidence of fits and apnoeic attacks are conveniently recorded in this way.

*Weed, L. L. (1968) 'Medical records that guide and teach.' *New England Journal of Medicine*. **278.** 593 and 652.

## SAMPLE CASE SUMMARY

Male Infant M....

Born at Hammersmith Hospital 6.9.71. B.W. 1190g (10th-50th centile). Gestation 30 weeks. OFC 26.5 cm (25th-50th centile). Discharged 2.11.71. Weight 2620g.
Mother. Aged 20. Unmarried, English, primigravida. Gp B, Rh positive, WR negative.

Baby problems

(1) Pre-term. Pre-term vaginal birth after spontaneous rupture of membranes. Neurological and morphological assessment consistent with gestational age of 30 weeks. Birthweight 1190g (between 10-50 centiles).

(2) Birth Asphyxia (probably primary). At one minute, limp, apnoeic, heart rate 80. Intubated and given IPPV, he gasped and HR accelerated before going pink. Regular resps. at 5 minutes.

(3) Respiratory distress (? hyaline membrane disease). Grunting and recession present at 1/2 hour, respiratory rate rose to 80/min. Chest X-ray consistent with HMD. During $N_2$ washout at 4 hours $paO_2$ 94, $pCO_2$ 51, pH 7.18. Respiratory distress persisted for 4 days and was treated with alkali, oxygen therapy and CPAP.

(4) Alkali therapy. He was given 4mEq $NaHCO_2$ at $4\frac{1}{2}$ hours; pH rose to 7.3. At the time of starting CPAP, pH had again fallen to 7.2 and he was given a second 4mEq. Thereafter pH rose to 7.34 and no further alkali was given.

(5) Oxygen therapy and CPAP. Umbilical arterial and venous catheters were inserted at 4 hours for monitoring. At 8 hours he was intubated and CPAP 12cmH₂0 applied via an endotracheal tube (indications - inspired $O_2$ > 60% and irregular respirations). $PaO_2$ then maintained between 55 and 90 using CPAP and inspired oxygen, at first 50% reducing by 36 hours to 25%. Weaned off CPAP at 48 hours. Catheters removed at 48 hours. Oxygen therapy 25% continued to 72 hours, monitored by radial artery stabs. Max. $pO_2$ 94mmHg, min 35. The optic fundi were at all times normal.

(6) Apnoeic episodes. Respirations were irregular with apnoeic episodes at 8 hours when CPAP was introduced. Thereafter the baby had a number of short-lived apnoeic episodes until aged 6 days, all of which responded to tactile stimulation.

(7) Low blood sugar (asymptomatic). Blood glucose was less than 20mg at 4 hours but thereafter was always > 20mg.

(8) Jaundice. Total bilirubin levels rose to a maximum of 14mg% at $3\frac{1}{2}$ days, but thereafter fell.

(9) Growth and feeding. He was fed at first by nasogastric tube and regained his birth weight at 15 days. Bottles were taken from 5 weeks.

(10) Cardiac murmur. At 4 days a systolic murmur, loudest under the (L) clavicle, was noted. Pulses full. BP 60/30. No cardiac failure. Probably a persistent ductus arteriosus which we expect to close spontaneously. For follow-up.

(11) Anaemia. Hb fell to a minimum of 8.2g/100 ml (retics 5.8%) at 7 weeks. Hb on discharge 8.5g. Given ferrous sulphate 30mg b.d. and folic acid 0.1mg weekly from age 3 weeks.

(12) Capillary cavernous haemangioma (strawberry) developed on R knee.

(13) Hydrocele. A small R hydrocele was present. No hernia detected.

Conclusion:

A small pre-term baby who suffered moderately severe RDS together with a number of neonatal problems but who did well. The prognosis is good, but at follow-up the cardiac murmur, Hb and minor problems 12 and 13 will be checked. The mother has since married the baby's father and they have all moved to Greenford, but will attend here for follow-up.

The date and time (preferably the 24-hour clock system) must be recorded immediately when observations are made, when samples or x-rays are taken and when any treatment is given or altered. It is helpful also to record the baby's age in hours (up to say four days old), but as doing so involves the possibility of miscalculation, the date and time must not be omitted from the record. The clock shown on p. 288 is useful.

The site of blood sampling must also be recorded.

A series of printed flow-sheets may be used, or more conveniently a universal flow-sheet grid into which the measurements appropriate to a particular baby can be entered according to the timing of observations or procedures. For charts of weight and head-circumference, see pp. 324-327.

### Progress Notes

These should be numbered according to the problem being considered, and the problem list should be consulted regularly to ensure that no outstanding problems are neglected. Research investigations must always be entered in the notes, and if serial studies are performed they should appear on a flow-sheet.

### Discharge Summaries

The purpose of the discharge summary is twofold: (*a*) to provide some background information for the general practitioner and the Infant Welfare Clinic and (*b*) to provide essential details for later hospital use; *e.g.* to refresh the memory of the doctor seeing the child in out-patients follow-up. These requirements are met by recording the major details such as date of birth, birthweight, gestation and head-circumference and then listing the problems, as in the main record, with a few lines on the development and outcome of each one. There is a final brief comment on the prognosis and any special features of the case. A sample case summary is shown on the facing page.

### Flow-charts (pp. 314-315)

Flow-charts for data on babies with respiratory distress and/or ventilator therapy have been referred to above. The frequency of the observations depends on the condition of the baby and is discussed in the text. Our nursing staff prefer to graph (as well as record) the baby's temperature, heart rate, and respiratory rate. Continuation sheets with the vertical and horizontal lines marked are necessary for a baby whose illness is protracted; they can be lined up with and affixed to the original chart, but another addressograph label must be affixed and the date of starting each continuation sheet entered.

# FLOW-CHART FOR CASES OF RESPIRATORY DISTRESS

Affix addressograph sticker

Name and sex

Case number

Date of birth                    Hour of birth

| | Date:../../.. Time (24-hour clock) | | | | |
|---|---|---|---|---|---|
| | Respiratory rate<br>Heart rate<br>Temperature of baby (Rectal = R,<br>    Axilla = A) | | | | |
| (*Usually completed<br>by nurse*) | Temperature of incubator<br>Oxygen flow rate (litres/min)<br>Oxygen inspired concentration<br>    (percentage)<br>Passed urine since last observation?<br>    (0 or +)<br>Bowels open since last observation?<br>    (0 or +) | | | | |
| (*Completed by<br>doctor as 4-hour<br>summary or when a<br>major change<br>occurs*) | Costal retractions (0, +, + +)*<br>Grunting (0, +, + +)*<br>Peripheral pulses palpable (0, +)*<br>Blood pressure*<br>Activity (0, +, + +)*<br>Response to handling (0, +, + +)*<br>Has baby cried in last 4 hours?<br>    (0 or +)<br>CPA pressure (cms H$_2$O)<br>Inspired oxygen % (range last<br>    4 hours)<br>Inspired oxygen % (at blood<br>    gas determination)<br>paO$_2$<br>paCO$_2$<br>pH<br>Drugs and comments | | | | |

*(Space for comment)*

| | Posture (on R or L side)<br>Physiotherapy of the chest given<br>    (0 or +)<br>Tracheal aspirate (0, +, + +)<br>Pharynx aspirated (0 or +) | | | | |
|---|---|---|---|---|---|

*See p.131 for definitions.                    (*continued*)

314

*(Also completed if baby is on ventilator; this is a separate sheet of same size which can be lined up with and stuck to the flow-sheet on the previous page)*

Does chest move with ventilator?
    (0 or +)
Ventilator controls
    Rate (counted)
    Blow-off valve pressure setting
    Manometer (max reading)
    Flow rate (total of $O_2$ plus air)
    Insp:Exp ratio
    Sigh given (0 or +)
    Added dead space (ml)
Constant infusion syringe
    reading (ml)

Comments

# BASIC DATA COLLECTED ON BABIES
# ADMITTED TO THE SPECIAL CARE NURSERY

*Note*: This form is completed by the neonatal resident or nurse on transfer of a baby to the special care nursery (see pages 45 and 113). The use of the form ensures that a minimum of basic data is recorded, but it is not a substitute for a good history).

HAMMERSMITH HOSPITAL                    BABY TRANSFER FORM

### DETAILS OF MOTHER

Name:............................     Age: ............  Case No: ......

Address:  .........................     Marital Status:   M   S   W   D

          .........................     Religion:  .........................

Tel. No:  .........................     Race of Mother: ....................

Where delivered: .....................  Race of Father: ....................

Hospital or Clinic providing antenatal care:  ................................

Consultant Obstetrician or Paediatrician
   requesting transfer of baby:           ....................................

FAMILY DOCTOR:  ................     MIDWIFE: ......................

Address:  .........................     Address:  .........................

          .........................               .........................

Tel. No.  .........................     Tel. No.  .........................

PREVIOUS PREGNANCIES:

Year        Sex        Gest.       Birthweight        Remarks (*e.g.* NND)



PRESENT PREGNANCY:        LMP   ...........   E.D.D.  .................

                          Blood Group  ......   Rhesus  ......   W.R. ....

                          Gestation  ..........   Antibodies .... at  .... wks

PRESENT LABOUR:           Spontaneous    Induction    Medical    Surgical

Rupture of Membranes—     Date  .............   Time ...................

Liquor—Amount:            Normal   Excessive   Little   Colour   ........

1st Stage  .................   hrs ........ mins   Fetal distress:    Yes/No

2nd Stage  .................   hrs ........ mins   Episiotomy:    Yes/No

Mode of Delivery  .............................   Date ........ Time ......

Presentation:  ..............................................................

DRUGS given within 12 hours of birth       DOSE    TIME    ROUTE

Remarks:

## DETAILS OF BABY

Surname: ......................... Sex: ............ Case No: ......

Baptised:....Yes/No Names: .........................

Birthweight: ..................... Multiple Birth: Yes/No

Placenta: (weight) .................. Cord: (no. of arteries) ..............

    (condition) ................. Abnormalities: (i.e. around neck) ....

..................................... .....................................

CONDITION OF BABY AT....... MINUTE(S) AFTER BIRTH (at 1 minute whenever possible)

Apex beat by auscultation: Inaudible Rate if present ............... /min

Respiration: Absent Gasping or irregular Regular or rhythmical

Onset of regular respiration .................... minutes after birth

Did the baby gasp or cry before 1 minute— Yes/No

Muscle tone and movement: Limp    Normal muscle tone
          No movement  Spontaneous movement of limbs

Response to nasal or pharyngeal catheter None Grimace Cough

Colour of trunk    Grey or white Blue Pink

RESUSCITATION:  (Details of aspiration ? blood ? meconium, intubation, drugs, etc.)

BIRTH INJURY:

MALFORMATIONS:

SUBSEQUENT PROGRESS - before admission to neonatal ward (including drugs and intravenous fluids)

Meconium first passed hours after birth.  Urine first passed hours after birth.

FEEDS: Nature, quantity and time given

ABNORMAL SIGNS: (Including the time when first observed) such as:—
      Jaundice, fits, jitteriness, abnormal cry, refusal to suck,
      excessively sleepy or wakeful, excessive mucus, haemorrhage
      and site, apnoeic attacks, signs of respiratory distress
      (tachypnoea, grunting, recession).

T.P.R. at time of transfer .............................................

RESULTS OF ANY LABORATORY TESTS CARRIED OUT:

317

*NOTES*

# Section 10: Morphological, Biochemical and Haematological Standards

*NOTES*

The selection of appropriate standards to include in a book of this type is a difficult task.

Even the simplest morphological data, such as birthweight for gestation, vary with sex, race, parental height and parity so that one might give many different standards or a number of complex correction factors to apply in different circumstances We have compromised in this instance by giving the birthweight data from Thomson et al. (1968)* for singleton boys and girls, uncorrected for parity, with the addition of 10th, 50th and 90th centile lines for 28-31 weeks gestation derived from the data of Babson et al. (1970)†.

Biochemical data which will be of widespread application are even more difficult to select, as the normal values may vary with gestation, often change from day to day over the first week of life, and may vary considerably according to the technique used in a particular laboratory. The resident must learn the sampling techniques and normal range of results appropriate to his own hospital for the more frequently performed tests.

If proposing to carry out some specialized investigation, for instance measurement of urinary 11-oxygenation index, it is essential to contact the laboratory beforehand to find out the type of specimen required, minimum quantity needed and details of container and preservative, or special requirements for transport to the laboratory. It can often be helpful to discuss the case at this stage with the biochemist or other senior members of the laboratory staff who will be performing the relevant test. Let them know what the likelihood of finding an abnormality is on clinical grounds. This may save the laboratory unnecessary work re-checking an abnormal result in what you had already diagnosed as a classical case.

We have not included all biochemical and haematological tests that can be performed in the newborn and have, in the main, confined ourselves to the more frequently used tests and those that we have found useful.

Normal ranges or means are not given for some frequently performed biochemical tests such as glucose and bilirubin estimations, as the significance of variations in the level of these substances is more appropriately discussed under the headings of jaundice and hypoglycaemia.

Where there are complex variations with age and other factors, we have put in appropriate references and have also given references to the methods by which the figures quoted were obtained.

*Thomson, A. M., Billewicz, W. Z., Hytten, F. E. (1968) 'The assessment of fetal growth.' *Journal of Obstetrics and Gynaecology of the British Commonwealth*, **75**, 903.

†Babson, S. G., Behrman, R. E., Lessel, R. (1970) 'Fetal growth. Liveborn birth weights for gestational age of white middle class infants.' *Pediatrics*, **45**, 937.

*NOTES*

# Birthweight / Gestational Age Charts

Percentile curves for birthweight of singleton boys/girls in relation to gestation. Curves for 28-31 weeks are derived from the data of Babson *et al.* (1970), uncorrected for sex or parity: curves for 32-42 weeks are derived from the data of Thomson *et al.* (1968), corrected for sex only.

### Tenth percentile birthweight figures

| Gestation (*weeks*) | Birthweight (*kg*) | |
| :---: | :---: | :---: |
| | Boys | Girls |
| 28 | 0.70 | 0.70 |
| 29 | 0.85 | 0.85 |
| 30 | 1.03 | 1.03 |
| 31 | 1.18 | 1.18 |
| 32 | 1.36 | 1.27 |
| 33 | 1.66 | 1.57 |
| 34 | 1.93 | 1.83 |
| 35 | 2.17 | 2.07 |
| 36 | 2.38 | 2.27 |
| 37 | 2.56 | 2.44 |
| 38 | 2.71 | 2.59 |
| 39 | 2.83 | 2.70 |
| 40 | 2.92 | 2.78 |
| 41 | 2.98 | 2.83 |
| 42 | 3.01 | 2.85 |

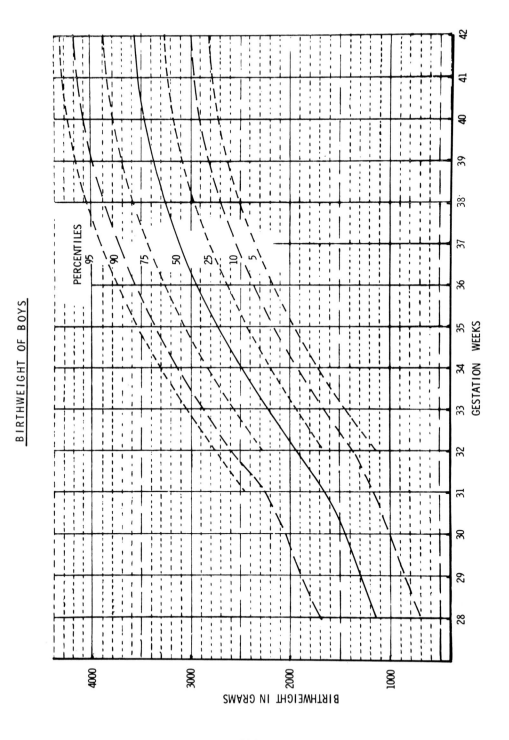

BIRTHWEIGHT OF BOYS

PERCENTILES
95
90
75
50
25
10
5

BIRTHWEIGHT IN GRAMS

GESTATION WEEKS

324

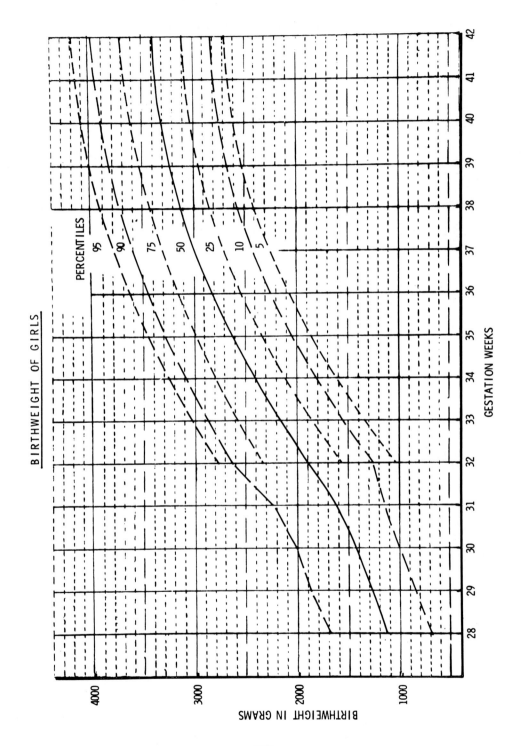

BIRTHWEIGHT OF GIRLS

PERCENTILES

95
90
75
50
25
10
5

GESTATION WEEKS

BIRTHWEIGHT IN GRAMS

4000
3000
2000
1000

28 29 30 31 32 33 34 35 36 37 38 39 40 41 42

# Head Circumference / Gestational Age Charts

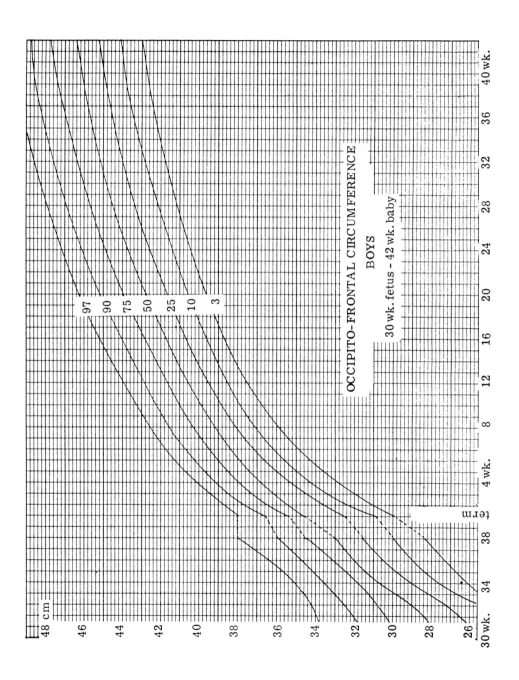

OCCIPITO-FRONTAL CIRCUMFERENCE
BOYS
30 wk. fetus – 42 wk. baby

97
90
75
50
25
10
3

These charts, which have been used by us for some years, are not our data. We cannot discover their origin. We offer free copies of the book to the first reader to enlighten us and, with our apologies, to the original author of the charts.

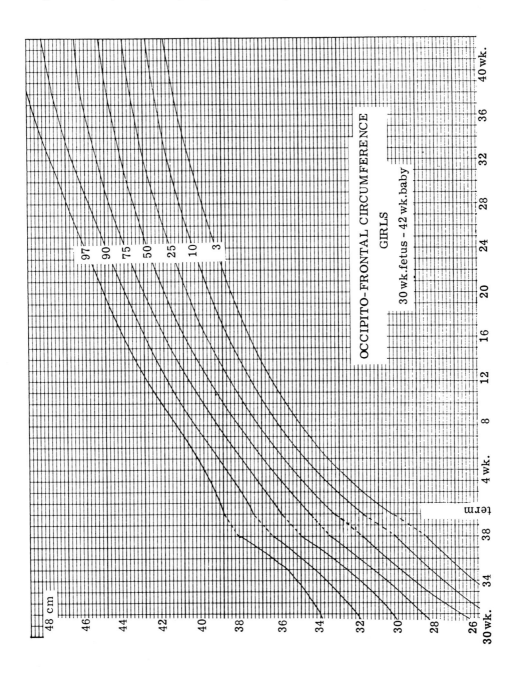

OCCIPITO-FRONTAL CIRCUMFERENCE

GIRLS

30 wk. fetus – 42 wk. baby

## TABLE XIII
### Biochemical standards (Blood)

| TEST | SAMPLE | MINIMUM | NOTES ON SAMPLE | NORMAL RANGE* OR MEAN (For healthy term infants in first 48 hours unless otherwise stated.) | ADDITIONAL INFORMATION AND REFERENCES (See p. 332 for references.) |
|---|---|---|---|---|---|
| Acid base balance | Heparinized arterial blood (see p. 124) | 0.25-0.35ml for a set of measurements | Ensure no air-bubble in sample and preferably analyse immediately. If > 20 mins delay inevitable, store sealed on ice but re-warm in hand before analysis | | |
| pH | | | | 7.3-7.4 | |
| $paCO_2$ | | | | 40mmHg | |
| $paO_2$ | | | | 60-90mmHg | |
| Standard bicarbonate | | | Results derived from pH, $paCO_2$, $pO_2$ and Hb values —see Siggaard-Andersen nomogram | 21 | |
| Base excess | | | | -4 | |
| Bicarbonate | plasma** | ultramicro† | | 21-25mEq/l | Using the Natelson micro-gasometer, one measures total $CO_2$, i.e. bicarbonate plus free $CO_2$. |
| Amino-acids | plasma | ultramicro | Separate and freeze plasma | | See Dickinson et al. (1965), Scriver et al. (1971). |

328

| | | | | |
|---|---|---|---|---|
| Amino-transferases | | | | |
| alanine | plasma | ultramicro | 5.0 i.u./l cord blood | Gautier *et al.* (1962). |
| aspartate | plasma | ultramicro | 21.2 i.u./l cord blood | |
| Amino nitrogen | plasma | ultramicro | 4–9mg/100ml | Stevens (1965). |
| Ammonia | plasma | 0.5ml | 40–100µg/100ml | Rubaltelli *et al.* (1970). |
| Bilirubin | plasma/serum | ultramicro | See 'Jaundice', p. 156 | Analyse at once or keep in dark |
| Calcium | plasma | ultramicro | 7.6mg/100ml on day 2 | Variation with age and feeding. *See* Harvey *et al.* (1970). |
| Cholesterol | plasma | 0.2ml | 78mg/100ml cord blood, S.D. 23mg; 155mg/100ml at 1 week, S.D. 31mg | Darmady *et al.* (1972). |
| Cortisol | plasma | ultramicro | 5–25µg/100ml | Stevens (1970). |
| Creatinine | serum | 0.2ml | 6.4–17.2mg/l cord blood | Josephson *et al.* (1962). |
| Creatinine phosphokinase | plasma/serum | 0.1ml | 5–170 Sigma units | Varies with age at sampling in first week of life. *See* Wharton *et al.* (1971). |
| Electrolytes sodium potassium chloride | plasma in lithium-heparin | ultramicro | 140–150mEq/l 4.5–6.0mEq/l 98–105mEq/l | Separate within half an hour and store on ice Stevens (1965). |

*(continued)*

NOTES

*The validity of the term 'normal range' varies from test to test. It is seldom that data are available in terms of means and standard deviations.

**Heparinized blood is satisfactory for all tests requiring plasma except where indicated.

†By 'ultramicro' we mean methods requiring 50µl plasma or less.

**TABLE XIII (cont.)**

| TEST | SAMPLE | MINIMUM | NOTES ON SAMPLE | NORMAL RANGE* OR MEAN (For healthy term infants in first 48 hours unless otherwise stated). | ADDITIONAL INFORMATION AND REFERENCES (See p. 332 for references.) |
|---|---|---|---|---|---|
| Free fatty acids | plasma | 0.2ml | | 0-0.7mEq/l | Stevens (1965). |
| Folate | serum whole blood | 0.5ml | | 6.2-30ng/ml 230-1250ng/ml | Roberts et al. (1969). |
| Galactose 1-phosphate uridyl transferase | whole blood | 0.5ml | | 14-25μmole UDP glucose metabolised/hour/g. Hb cord blood | Ellis and Goldberg (1969). |
| Glucose | plasma in fluoride oxalate | 0.1ml | proportions of blood: fluoride are important | See 'Hypoglycaemia' p. 147 | |
| Immunoglobulins IgA IgM IgG | plasma | ultramicro | | <2mg/100ml <20mg/100ml‡ 650-1200mg/100ml cord blood | Lower values in pre-term infants. See Hobbs and Davis (1967). |
| Isocitric dehydrogenase | plasma/serum | 0.2ml | | mean 3.7 i.u./l cord blood | Pehrson (1964). |
| Lactate | whole blood | 0.2ml | put into perchloric acid immediately (Boehringer's kit) | <20mg/100ml from 5 hours age | Koch and Wendel (1968). |
| Lactic dehydrogenase | plasma/serum | 0.1ml | | mean 306 i.u./l cord blood | Gautier et al. (1962). |
| Magnesium | plasma | ultramicro | | 1.2mg/100ml on day 2 | For variations with age and feeding, see Harvey et al. (1970). |

330

| | | | | | |
|---|---|---|---|---|---|
| Osmolality | plasma | 0.3ml | 280-310mOsmol/l | | Davis *et al.* (1966). |
| Phosphatase-alkaline | plasma | ultramicro | 35-105 i.u./l | | Thalme (1964), King (1965). |
| Phosphatase-acid | plasma | ultramicro | 3-6 i.u./l | | King (1965). |
| Phosphate—inorganic | plasma | ultramicro | 4.5-6.0mg/100ml | | Stevens (1965). |
| Protein | | | | | |
| total | plasma | ultramicro | 5-7g/100ml | | Stevens (1965). |
| albumin | plasma | ultramicro | 3-4g/100ml | | |
| globulin | plasma | ultramicro | 1-2.5g/100ml | | |
| Protein bound iodine | serum | 0.2ml | 67-92µg/l cord blood | Iodine free tube | Dowling *et al.* (1956). If the laboratory can measure serum thyroxine this is preferable (see below). |
| Thyroxine | serum | 0.2ml | 8.7-14µg/100ml cord blood | | Personal communication from Professor B. E. Clayton. Method is modification of that reported by Maclagan and Howorth (1969). |
| Urea | plasma | ultramicro | 20-50mg/100ml | | Stevens (1965). |
| Uric acid | plasma | ultramicro | 5-9mg/100ml in first 24 hours; 2.5-5.0mg/100ml from 3 days | | *See* Wharton *et al.* (1971). |
| Volatile organic acids | plasma | 0.1ml | | Freeze plasma for gas chromatography | |
| W.R. | serum | 0.4ml | | | |

NOTES

*The validity of the term 'normal range' varies from test to test. It is seldom that data are available in terms of means and standard deviations.

**Heparinized blood is satisfactory for all tests requiring plasma except where indicated.

†By 'ultramicro' we mean methods requiring 50µl plasma or less.

‡Mean values increase from 13.2mg/100ml in first 5 days to 26.8mg/100ml between 20 and 25 days (Blankenship *et al.* 1969).

We are grateful to our senior biochemist, Dr. Elizabeth Hughes, for her help in preparing this Table and Table XV.

# REFERENCES CITED IN TABLE XIII

Blankenship, W. J., Cassady, G., Schaefer, J., Straumfjord, J. V., Alford, C. A. (1969) 'Serum gamma-M globulin responses in acute neonatal infections and their diagnostic significance.' *Pediatrics*, **75,** 1271.

Darmady, J. M., Fosbrooke, A. S., Lloyd, J. K. (1972) 'Prospective study of serum cholesterol levels during the first year of life.' *British Medical Journal*, **2,** 685.

Davis, J. A., Harvey, D. R., Stevens, J. F. (1966) 'Osmolality as a measure of dehydration in the neonatal period.' *Archives of Disease in Childhood*, **41,** 448.

Dickinson, J. C., Rosenblum, H., Hamilton, N. P. B. ((1965) 'Ion exchange chromatography of the free amino acids in the plasma of the newborn infant.' *Pediatrics*, **36,** 2.

Dowling, J. T., Freinkel, N., Ingbar, S. H. (1956) 'Thyroxine-binding by sera of pregnant women, newborn infants and women with spontaneous abortion.' *Journal of Clinical Investigation*, **35,** 1263.

Ellis, G., Goldberg, D. M. (1969) 'The enzymological diagnosis of galactosemia.' *Annals of Clinical Biochemistry*, **6,** 70.

Gautier, E., Gautier, R., Richterich, R. (1962) 'Valeur diagnostique d'anomaliés d'activités enzymatiques du sérum en pédiatrie. I. Valuers normales et influence des corticostéroïdes.' *Helvetica Paediatrica Acta*, **17,** 415.

Harvey, D. R., Cooper, L. V., Stevens, J. F. (1970) 'Plasma calcium and magnesium in newborn babies.' *Archives of Disease in Childhood*, **45,** 506.

Hobbs, J. R., Davis, J. A. (1967) 'Serum γ-globulin levels and gestational age in premature infants.' *Lancet*, **i,** 757.

Josephson, B., Fürst, P., Järnmark, O. (1962) 'Age variation in the concentration of nonprotein nitrogen, creatinine and urea in blood of infants and children.' *Acta Paediatrica (Uppsala)*, **51,** Suppl. 135.

King, J. (1965) *Practical Clinical Enzymology*. London: van Nostrand. p. 202.

Koch, G., Wendel, H. (1968) 'Adjustment of arterial blood gases and acid base balance in the normal newborn infant during the first week of life.' *Biologia Neonatorum*, **12,** 136.

Maclagan, N. F. R., Howorth, P. J. (1969) 'Thyroid function studies using resin uptake of radioactive thyronines from serum and total free thyroxine index.' *Clinical Science*, **37,** 45.

Pehrson, S. L. (1964) 'Serum isocitric dehydrogenase activity in pregnant women and newborn infants.' *Acta Obstetrica et Gynecologia Scandinavica*, **43,** 69.

Roberts, P. M., Arrowsmith, D. E., Rau, S. M., Monk-Jones, M. E. (1969) 'Folate state of premature infants.' *Archives of Disease in Childhood*, **44,** 637.

Rubaltelli, F. F., Formentin, P. A., Tatô, L. (1965) 'Ammonia nitrogen, urea and uric acid blood levels in normal and hypodystrophic newborns.' *Biologia Neonatorum*, **15,** 129.

Scriver, C. R., Clow, C. L., Lamm, P. (1971) 'Plasma amino acids: screening quantitation and interpretation.' *American Journal of Clinical Nutrition*, **24,** 876.

Stevens, J. F. (1965) 'Biochemical changes in the blood of the newborn.' *Journal of Medical Laboratory Technology*, **22,** 47.

Stevens, J. F. (1970) 'Plasma cortisol levels in the neonatal period.' *Archives of Disease in Childhood*, **45,** 592.

Thalme, B. (1964) 'Microliter determination of total and direct bilirubin, alkaline phosphatase, potassium, sodium and urea nitrogen in blood plasma during the early neonatal period.' *Acta Obstetrica et Gynecologia Scandinavica*, **43,** 78.

Wharton, B. A., Bassi, U., Gough, G., Williams, A. (1971) 'Clinical value of plasma creatine kinase and uric acid levels during first week of life.' *Archives of Disease in Childhood*, **46,** 356.

**TABLE XIV**

**Haematological standards**

A blood sample 0.5-1.0ml taken into sequestrene is appropriate for all the standard haematological tests but not for coagulation studies. Venous or arterial samples are preferable.

| TEST | NORMAL RANGE | COMMENTS AND REFERENCES |
|---|---|---|
| Hb (g/100ml) | 16 - 20 | *See* Oski and Naiman (1972) |
| Haematocrit (%) | 52 - 58 | |
| M.C.V. ($\mu^3$) | 96 - 108 | |
| M.C.H. ($\mu\mu$g) | 33.5 - 41.4 | |
| M.C.H.C. (%) | 30 - 35 | |
| Reticulocytes (%) | 3 - 7 (day 1). Drops to 0 - 1 by end of first week. | |
| White cells<br>Total white cells (/mm³) | 9 - 30,000 in first 24 hours | *See* Oski and Naiman (1972) |

|  | *Birth* | *12 hours* | *4 days+* | |
|---|---|---|---|---|
| Neutrophils (/mm³) | 4,500 - 13,000 | 9,000 - 18,000 | 1,500 - 7,000 | |
| Eosinophils (/mm³) | 100 - 2,500 | | | |
| Metamyelocytes (/mm³) | 200 - 2,000 | fall in | | |
| Myelocytes (/mm³) | 100 - 750 | first 3 | | For further details and references, *see* Xanthou (1970) |
| Lymphocytes (/mm³) | 3,500 - 8,500 | days | | |

| TEST | NORMAL RANGE | COMMENTS AND REFERENCES |
|---|---|---|
| Coagulation tests<br>(citrated venous or arterial blood samples) | | |
| Platelets (10³/mm³) | 155 - 373 | Chessells (1970) |
| Fibrinogen (mg/100ml) | 98 - 391 | |
| Thrombin ratio | 1.1 - 2.0 | |
| Thrombotest (%) | 6 - 56 | |
| Thromboplastin generation screening test (secs) | 9 - 20 | |
| Bleeding time } seldom performed on newborn<br>Clotting time } | | |
| Glucose 6-phosphate dehydrogenase screening test (0.5ml in sequestrene) | | Motulsky and Campbell-Kraut (1961) |

333

## TABLE XV

### Urine for biochemical studies

Check requirements with the laboratory before collecting specimens for any of these tests.

| TEST | SPECIMEN | PRECAUTIONS | RESULTS | REFERENCES |
|---|---|---|---|---|
| Amino-acids | 24-hour collection or random sample (2ml) in chloroform or merthiolate | | Some increase in amino-acid excretion is common in pre-term infants. Always collect plasma for quantitative amino-acid chromatography if an inborn error of metabolism is suspected. | O'Brien et al. (1968) |
| Steroids | 24-hour collection in chloroform. For 11 - oxygenation index, random samples can be used | | 11-oxygenation index <1.1 17-hydroxycorticosteroids <1.0mg/24 hours 17-oxosteroids 0.5-2.5mg/24 hours (drops to <1.0mg/24 hours after first few weeks) | Edwards et al. (1964), Visser (1966) |
| Sugars | 6ml in merthiolate | Keep frozen until test | Glucose <25mg/100ml  Galactose <25mg/100ml  Fructose <70mg/100ml  Lactose <120mg/100ml } in first week | Bickel (1961) |
| Catecholamines inc. Vanillyl mandelic acid | 24-hour collection in concentrated HCl | | | Hakulinen (1971) |

CSF Composition, see p. 183.

Faeces - albumin, see p. 195.

334

## REFERENCES CITED IN TABLES XIV AND XV

Bickel, H. (1961) 'Mellituria: a paper chromatographic study.' *Journal of Pediatrics*, **59**, 641.

Chessells, J. M. (1970) 'The significance of fibrin degradation products in the blood in normal infants.' *Biologia Neonatorum*, **17**, 219.

Edwards, R. W. H., Makin, H. L. J., Barratt, T. M. (1964) 'The steroid 11-oxygenation index: a rapid method for use in the diagnosis of congenital virilising hyperplasia.' *Journal of Endocrinology*, **30**, 181.

Hakulinen, A, (1971) 'Urinary excretion of vanilmandelic acid in children in normal and certain pathological conditions.' *Acta Paediatrica Scandinavica*, Suppl. 212.

Motulsky, A. G., Campbell-Kraut, J. M. (1961) 'Population genetics of glucose-6-phosphate dehydrogenase deficiency of the red cell.' *In* Blumberg, B. S. (Ed.) *Proceedings of the Congress on Genetic and Geographic Variations in Disease*. New York: Grune & Stratton. p. 159.

O'Brien, D., Ibbott, F. A., Rogerison, D. O. (1968) 'Chromatography of urine amino acids.' *in Laboratory Manual of Pediatric Micro-Biochemical Techniques* (4th Edn.). New York: Harper & Row.

Oski, F. A., Naiman, J. L. (1972) *Haematologic Problems in the Newborn*. (2nd Edn.). Philadelphia and London: W. B. Saunders.

Visser, H. K. A. (1966) 'The adrenal cortex in childhood. Part I: physiological aspects. Part II: pathological aspects.' *Archives of Disease in Childhood*, **41**, 2 and 113.

Xanthou, M. (1970) 'Leucocyte blood picture in healthy full-term and premature babies during neonatal period.' *Archives of Disease in Childhood*, **45**, 242.

# Subject Index

## NOTES ON THE USE OF THE INDEX

To some extent we have tried to make this a synthetic as well as an analytic index, thus providing what we hope will be some useful lists. However for the sake of comprehensiveness we have sometimes included items about which little or no more information can be gleaned by reference to the text than by reading the index. For instance of Crigler-Najjar disease we can only say that we have never seen a case. To save the reader's time these page references have been bracketed.

Antimicrobial and other drugs and micro-organisms are not separately listed and should be sought under these headings.

*Page numbers in plain type refer to use or preparation of drug; in bold type to dosage and in italics to toxic effects.

339

277.
— necrotizing enterocolitis: 202.
— rashes following: 250.
— fetal intraperitoneal: (7).
— feto-fetal: 228.
— for haemorrhage: 209.
— intraperitoneal: 274.
— parental consent: 277.
— 'top-up': 155.
'Blow-off' valve: 287.
Bone disorders (see Skeletal disorders).
Boric Acid
— toxicity: 306.
Brachial plexus palsy: 48.
— with spinal cord transection: 181.
Bradycardia
— congenital heart block: 211.
— digitalis overdose: 216.
— fetal distress: 212.
— maternal local anaesthesia: 15.
Brain (see Central nervous system).
Breasts
— engorgement in babies: 79.
— size as guide to gestational age: 94.
BREAST FEEDING
— attitudes to: 76.
— contraindicated in maternal medication
with radioactive iodine: 14.
— jaundice: 160.
— low-birthweight babies: 43.
— problems: 79.
Breech delivery
— brachial plexus palsy: 48.
— spinal cord injury: 48.
— visceral injury: 218.
Bronchomalacia: 122.
Bruising (see also Haemorrhage).
— due to birth injury: 47.
— jaundice following: 159.
Buccal smear (see Sex, chromatin).
Buphthalmos: 244.

C
Caesarean section
— hyaline membrane disease: 119.
— not an indication for transfer to Special
Care Nursery: 46.
Café-au-lait spots: 249.
Calcium, blood
— hypocalcaemia: **190.**
— normal standards: 329.
Candidiasis
— maternal: 22.
— neonatal: 164, 165, 171, 252.

— rashes: 252.
— treatment: 171.
Cardiac (see Heart).
Cataracts: **243-244.**
— galactosaemia: 226, 243.
— prenatal infection: 164.
Catheterisation (see Procedures).
CENTRAL NERVOUS SYSTEM (see also
Neurological disorders).
— depression: 178, 185.
— as cause of respiratory distress: 118.
— disorders: **179-191.**
— examination: **173-178.**
— hyperexcitability: 178, 228.
— infection causing abnormal signs: 164.
Cephalhaematoma: 78, **254.**
Cerebral (see Central nervous system).
Cerebrospinal fluid: 166, **183.**
Chicken pox
— maternal: 24.
Chloride-losing diarrhoea: 203.
Chlorpropamide
— maternal medication: 17, 149.
Choanal atresia: (37), 53.
Choking
— in oesophageal atresia: 49.
Cholesterol, plasma
— normal values: 329.
Chorioamnionitis: (29), 71.
Chorionepithelioma: 12.
Choroido-retinitis
— infective causes: 164.
Chromosomes
— abnormal: **223-224.**
— collection of specimens for culture: 4, 223,
224.
— in cases of ambiguous sex: 61, 62.
— karyotyping: 223, 224.
— in fetus: 4.
— placenta in Trisomy 17/18: 71.
Circumcision: 247.
— contraindicated in cases of hooded
prepuce, WARNING: 64.
Circumoral cyanosis: 256.
Cisternal tap (see Procedures).
Clavicle—fracture: 47.
Cleft palate (central): 59.
— in Pierre Robin syndrome: 51.
Cleft palate and hare lip: **59.**
— do not transfer to Special Care Nursery:
46.
— talking to parents: 41.
CLINICAL EXAMINATION
— as guide to gestational age: **91-95.**

*Page numbers by named drugs in bold type refer to dosage (or method of application), in plain type to use or preparation, and in italics to toxic effects.

343

345

Hyponatraemia
— due to maternal intravenous infusions: 18.
Hypophosphatasia: 259.
Hypoplasia (see under appropriate adjective).
Hypospadias: 64.
— deceptive appearance in pseudoherm-
aphroditism: 60.
— talking to parents: 42.
Hypothermia
— cyanotic heart disease: 212.
— disseminated intravascular coagulation:
207.
— infective illness: 165.
— prevention: 102, 114.
Hypothyroidism
— jaundice: 158.
— maternal medication: 17, 18.
HYPOTONIA: **186-187.**
— abdominal distension: 198, 199.
— 'benign congenital': (187).
— cerebral depression: 178.
— glycogen storage disease: 215.
— hyponatraemia: 18.
— kernikterus: 186.
— maternal magnesium sulphate: 19.
— maternal myasthenia gravis: 13, 17.
— metabolic disease: 226.
— methaemoglobinaemia: 212.
— spinal cord transection: 181.
Hypoxaemia
— as guide to oxygen therapy: 124, 126.
— as guide to ventilator therapy: 133.
— during artificial ventilation: 135.
— disseminated intravascular coagulation:
207.

I

Ichthyosis: (257).
Ileus, functional: 197.
Ileus, paralytic: 17.
Immunoglobulins
— agammaglobulinaemia with dwarfism:
258.
— diagnosis of postnatal infection: 166.
— levels as guide to prenatal infection: 162.
— normal standards: 330.
INBORN ERRORS OF METABOLISM:
**225-227.**
Incontinentia pigmenti: (244), 251.
Incubator
— Gram negative infections: 111, 163.
— temperature control: 103.
— transfer to cot: 234.
INFECTIONS (see also Micro-organisms,

Antimicrobial drugs): **162-172.**
— bacterial: 110, **162-172.**
— candidiasis: 22, 162, 164, 165, 171, 252.
— chorioamnionitis: (29), 71.
— cross-infection (see prevention).
— detection: 82, 163, 165, 166.
— listeriosis: 159, 168.
— malaria: 23, 164, 171.
— maternal: **20-26,** 111.
— meningitis: 168, 188.
— pneumonia: 117, 119, 238.
— poliomyelitis: 25, 164, 187.
— prenatal, diagnosis: 20-26, 162.
— prevention: 30, 75, 76, 101, **110-112,** 114,
263.
— rubella: 25, 162, 163, 164, 165, 243.
— signs
— apnoeic attacks: 142.
— diarrhoea: 201-202.
— failure to thrive: 240.
— fits: 188.
— haemorrhage: 207.
— heart failure (myocarditis): 214.
— jaundice: 157, 159.
— rashes: 250, 251.
— respiratory distress: 130.
— shock: 218.
— skin lesions: 82, 250, 251.
— vomiting: 192.
— syphilis: 23, 159, 163, 164, 165, 172.
— toxoplasmosis: 23, 163, 164, 165, 172, 215.
— transfer to Special Care Nursery: 45.
— transmission to fetus: **20-26.**
— treatment: **167-172.**
— tuberculosis: 21, 164, 171.
— urinary: 60, 169, 284.
— viral (see also Micro-organisms): 166.
Inguinal hernia: 61, 248.
Intensive Care Nursery: ii.
Intersex (see Genitalia).
INTESTINAL OBSTRUCTION: **192-200.**
— atresia, duodenal: 192, 194.
— small gut: 194.
— diaphragmatic hernia: 50.
— differential diagnosis from congenital
adrenal hyperplasia: 61, 192.
— Hirschsprung's disease: 192, 194, 195, 198.
— ileus: 17, 197.
— investigation: **194-195,** 200.
— malrotation with volvulus: 192, 194, 196.
— management: **196-197,** 200.
— meconium ileus: 194, 192, 204.
— necrotizing enterocolitis: 192, 194, 199,
**202.**

348

— pyloric stenosis: 192, 193.
— signs
   — abdominal distension: **197-200.**
   — abnormal meconium: 193.
   — maternal polyhydramnios: 7, 192.
   — melaena: 194, 207.
   — visible peristalsis: 193.
   — vomiting: **192-197.**
Intracranial haemorrhage: 182-183.
Intracranial pressure, raised: 184.
Intraperitoneal blood transfusion: 274.
Intrauterine infection: 20-26.
Intrauterine growth failure (see Small-for-dates babies).
INTRAVENOUS THERAPY: **99-101.**
— constant infusion syringe: 292.
— hypoglycaemia: 149.
— intestinal obstruction: 196, 197.
— metabolic disease: 226.
— respiratory distress: 138.
— techniques: **271.**
Intraventricular haemorrhage: (131), 182.
Intubation (see under appropriate adjective).
Irritability
— cerebral: 178, 184.
— drug withdrawal: 15, 222.


**J**
JAUNDICE: **156-161.**
— bilirubin estimation: 156.
— causes: 159-161.
   — acholuric jaundice: 160.
   — breast milk: 160.
   — Crigler-Najjar disease: (161).
   — dehydration: 161.
   — drugs: 160, 305, 306.
   — Dubin-Johnson syndrome: (161).
   — fructose intolerance: 227.
   — galactosaemia: 226.
   — haemolytic disease: 154, 159.
   — hypothyroidism: 160.
   — infections: 159, 163.
   — maternal medication with sulphonamides: 16.
   — metabolic disease: 160.
   — physiological: 157.
   — polycythaemia: 228.
   — pyruvate kinase deficiency: 160.
   — Vitamin K: 16, 19, 306.
— concern to mother: 79.
— indications for exchange transfusion: 152.
— kernikterus: 156, 186.
— persistent, in haemolytic disease: 155, 158.
— prognosis: 185.

— prolonged: 155, 158.
— treatment: 158-159.
Jitteriness: 176.
— cerebral hyperexcitability: 178.
— congenital thyrotoxicosis: 10.
— distinction from fits: 176.
— drug withdrawal: 222.
— maternal phenothiazines: 19.
— not a symptom of hypoglycaemia: 150.


**K**
Karyotype (see Chromosomes).
Keratitis
— infective causes: 164.
Kernikterus (see also Jaundice): 156, 186.
— due to water-soluble Vitamin K: 19.
— indication for exchange transfusion, not for giving up hope: 186.
— Moro reflex: 177.
— prevention: 157-159.
— relationship to hyperbilirubinaemia: 156.
KIDNEY
— agenesis: 9.
— cystic: 199.
— damage (colistin): 305.
— enlargement in abdominal distension: 199.
— enlargement in Beckwith's syndrome: 30.
— enlargement in infective illness: 165.
— hydronephrosis: 199.
— nephritis: (165).
— nephrosis, congenital: (67, 165).
— renal vein thrombosis: 199, 200.
Kleihauer test: (65).
Klumpke's palsy: 48.


**L**
Labelling the newborn: 75.
Lactase deficiency: 203.
Lactate, blood
— normal standards: 330.
— in respiratory distress: 132.
Lanugo (see Hair).
Large-for-dates babies
— babies of diabetic mothers: 9.
— identification: 89.
Laryngeal oedema: 9, 145.
Lethargy: 240.
— cerebral depression: 178.
— feeding difficulties: 80.
— hyponatraemia: 18.
— maternal medication with reserpine: 17.
— metabolic disease: 225.
Leukaemia: 220.

349

Leukocytes
— in infective illness: 166.
— normal standards: 333.
Leukopenia
— babies of mothers with disseminated lupus erythematosus: 12.
Listeriosis: 159, 168.
— maternal: 21.
— meconium staining of amniotic fluid: 29.
Liver — enlargement:
— Beckwith's syndrome: 30.
— chorionepithelioma: 12.
— galactosaemia: 226.
— haemolytic disease: 152.
— heart failure: 213.
— infective causes: 164.
— leukaemia: 220.
— subcapsular haematoma: 206.
— inborn metabolic errors and haemorrhage: 208.
— normal size: 83.
— rupture: 48, 218.
Lobar emphysema (see Congenital lobar emphysema).
Low-birthweight baby (see also under Preterm, Fetal growth retardation, Small-for-dates baby).
LOW-BIRTHWEIGHT BABIES
— classification: 89.
— continuing care: **233-235.**
— problems: 90.
— talking to parents: 43.
— transfer to Special Care Nursery: 45.
Lumbar puncture: 182, 279.
LUNGS (see also Pulmonary, Respiratory distress).
— accessory lobe as cause of respiratory distress: 117.
— congenital cysts as cause of respiratory distress: 118, 121.
— congenital lobar emphysema: 122.
— cystic adenomatoid malformation as cause of ascites: (67).
— heart failure: 213.
— massive pulmonary haemorrhage: 117, 120.
— pneumonia: 119.
— pulmonary surfactant: 119.
— transient tachypnoea: 120.

**M**

Magnesium, blood
— hypomagnesaemia: 189.
— normal standards: 330.

Malaria
— maternal: 23.
— neonatal: 164.
— treatment: 171.
MALFORMATIONS
— anencephaly: 179.
— Arnold-Chiari: 55, 179.
— Beckwith's syndrome: 30.
— cardiac: 214.
— choanal atresia: 53.
— cleft palate and cleft lip: 42, 59.
— congenital dermal sinus: 180.
— diaphragmatic hernia: 50.
— diastematomyelia: 180.
— Down's syndrome: 4, 42, 223.
— duodenal atresia: 194.
— exomphalos: 54.
— gastroschisis: 54.
— gastro-intestinal: 192.
— genitalia: 60-64.
— Hirschsprung's disease: 192-196, 198.
— hooded prepuce: 64.
— hydranencephaly: 180.
— hydrocephalus: 179.
— hypospadias: 42, 64.
— imperforate anus: 60.
— malrotation of gut: 194.
— maternal drugs: 14.
— microcephaly: 164, 180.
— multiple: 223.
— myelomeningocele: 54.
— needing URGENT treatment: **49-58.**
— neurological: 54, **179-180.**
— oesophageal atresia: 49.
— omphalocele: 54.
— Pierre Robin syndrome: 51.
— pulmonary: 121-122.
— pyloric stenosis: 193.
— skeletal: 258-260.
— small gut atresia: 194.
— talipes equinovarus: 57.
— talking to parents of malformed babies: 41.
— transfer to Special Care Nursery: 45.
— vertebral: 259.
Malignant disease
— congenital: 11, 220-221.
— maternal: 11.
Malpresentation: (9).
Malrotation of gut: 194, 196.
Marrow aplasia: 208, 215.
Masculinization: 60.
Massive pulmonary haemorrhage: 117, 120.
MATERNAL DISEASE: **6-26.**

351

— *Pseudomonas aeruginosa:* 111, 120, 163, 168.
— respiratory syncytial virus: (163).
— rubella virus: 25, 163, 164, 165, 243.
— *Salmonellae:* 21, (165).
— *Shigellae:* 21, (165).
— *Staphylococcus pyogenes:* 165, 167, 169.
— streptococcus, group B β haemolytic: 162.
— *Toxoplasma gondii:* 23, 163, 164, 165, 172, 215.
— *Treponema pallidum:* 23, 159, 163, 164, 165, 172.
— TRIC agent: 26, 171.
— vaccinia virus: 25, 164, 165.
— varicella-zoster virus: 24, 164, 165.
— variola virus: 25, 164, 165.
— *Vibrio fetus:* 22, 168.
Milia: 78, 251.
Milk, choice of
— cardiac failure: 216.
— diarrhoea: 201.
— low-birthweight baby: 96, 98.
Moebius's syndrome: 175.
Mongol (see Down's syndrome).
'Mongolian blue spots': 249.
Moniliasis (see Candidiasis).
Monosaccharide intolerance: 203.
Moro reflex: **177.**
— kernikterus: 186.
— unpleasant experience: 81.
Morphological standards: **321-327.**
MOTHERS (see also Maternal)
— breast feeding: 76.
— consent for blood transfusion: 277.
— introduction to: 113.
— keeping mothers informed: 46, 153, 234, 277.
— observations of infants' behaviour: 173, 240.
— observations of physical signs: 198.
— participation in care: 235.
— rooming-in: 76.
— talking about ill or deformed baby: **41-44.**
— worries: **78-80.**
Motor function: 176.
Mouth-to-mouth respiration: 35, 36, 38, 136.
Movement: 176.
— lateralising signs: 178.
Mucoviscidosis (see Cystic fibrosis).
Multiple pregnancy (see Twins).
Mumps
— maternal: 24.
Muscles (see also Muscle tone, Hypertonia and Hypotonia)

— absence of abdominal muscles: 199.
— lateralising signs: 178.
— myoclonus—drug withdrawal: 15.
Myasthenia gravis: 13, 17, (187).
Mycoplasma infection: 25, 164, 165, 169.
Myelomeningocele: **54-57.**
Myocarditis: 214.
Myoclonus (see Muscle).
Myopathy: 4, 187.

**N**
Naevi: 249.
Napkin rash: 252.
Narcotic addicts, infants of: 222.
Nasal discharge
— choanal atresia: 53.
— drug withdrawal: 222.
— osteomyelitis of maxilla: 245.
Nasolachrymal duct—blocked: 244.
Nasotracheal intubation: 134, 139, 291.
Neck-righting reflex: 92.
Necrotizing enterocolitis: 167, 194, **202.**
Nephrotic syndrome: (67, 165)
Neuroblastoma: (67), 199, 220, 221.
NEUROLOGICAL DISORDERS: **179-191.**
— abnormal behaviour: 181.
— anencephaly: 179.
— brachial plexus palsy: 48.
— cerebral depression: 178.
— cerebral hyperexcitability: 178.
— fits: **188-191.**
— hydranencephaly: 180.
— hydrocephalus: 179.
— hypotonia: **186-187.**
— intracranial haemorrhage: 182.
— investigations: **181-184.**
— kernikterus: 186.
— management: 181-184.
— microcephaly: 180.
— myelomeningocele: 54.
— peripheral nerve palsies: 48.
— prognosis: 185, 191.
— spinal cord transection: 181.
— spinal malformations: 180.
Neurological examination: **173-178.**
— assessment of gestational age: **91-92.**
— not a routine: 173.
— repeated in low-birthweight babies: 233.
Nitrogen washout: (123), 131.
Note keeping (see Record keeping).
Notes—blank pages: iv, 2, 28, 74, 86, 88, 230, 232, 262, 286, 296, 308, 310, 318, 320, 336.
Nursery (see Special Care Nursery, Intensive Care Nursery).

Nystagmus: 175, 176.
Oedema (see also Hydrops fetalis): **255.**
— heart failure: 213.
— laryngeal: 9, 145.
— late respiratory distress: 238.
Oesophageal atresia: **49-50.**
— diagnosis: 7.
— management: 50.
— single umbilical artery: 31.
— symptoms
— birth asphyxia: 37.
— drooling mucus: 9, 49.
— maternal polyhydramnios: 7.
— respiratory distress: 117.
Oligohydramnios: 9.
Omphalocele: 30, 54.
Ophthalmia (see Conjunctivitis).
Ophthalmology (see Eyes).
Ophthalmoscopy
— indications for: 241.
— limited value in neurological examination: 175.
— technique: 241.
Opisthotonus (see also Hypertonus)
— kernikterus: 186.
— maternal phenothiazines: 19.
Organicacidaemias: 118, 187, 226.
Osmolality, plasma
— angiography: 213.
— dehydration fever: 163.
— diarrhoea: 201.
— Gastrografin enemata: 197.
— normal standards: 331.
— rapid changes: 306.
Osteochondrodystrophy: 258.
Osteogenesis imperfecta: 48, 259.
Osteomyelitis
— maxilla: 169.
— treatment: 169.
Osteopetrosis: 259.
Ovarian cysts: (199).
Overfeeding
— diarrhoea: 204.
— WARNING: 98.
OXYGEN THERAPY, general principles: **107-109.**
— apnoeic attacks WARNING: 109, 143.
— control of: 108, 126.
— indications for: 107.
— not the birthright of the low-birthweight baby!: 125.
— respiratory distress: 124-126.
— retrolental fibroplasia WARNING: 107, 109, 242.

— toxicity to lungs: 107, 125.
— transport of ill babies: 115.

**P**
Pallor
— haemorrhage: 209.
— infective illness: 165.
Palsy (see under appropriate adjective).
Paralytic ileus (see Ileus).
Parents (see Mothers, Fathers).
Paroxysmal tachycardia: 214.
Patent ductus arteriosus: 214.
Pemphigus: 250.
Periodic respiration: 142.
Periostitis: 164.
Peritonitis: 193.
Pertussis
— immunisation not recommended after neonatal neurological abnormalities: (186).
Petechiae (see Purpura).
pH (see Acid-base status).
Phallus (see Genitalia).
Phenobarbitone therapy
— fits: 190.
— jaundice: 159.
Phenylketonuria: (84, 225).
Phosphate, plasma
— normal standards: 331.
Phototherapy: 159.
Physiotherapy
— during ventilator therapy: 137.
Pierre Robin Syndrome: 37, **51-53.**
Pigmentation, abnormal
— café-au-lait and white spots: 249.
— congenital adrenal hyperplasia: 63.
— incontinentia pigmenti: 251.
— 'mongolian' blue spots: 249.
— pigmented naevus: 249.
Pinnae (see Ears).
PLACENTA: (67), **69-71.**
Placental transfusion: 30.
Plasma (see Biochemical standards).
Pleural effusion: (117).
*Pneumocystis carinii*: 117, (163).
Pneumomediastinum (see Pneumothorax).
PNEUMONIA: **119-120.**
— in Pierre Robin syndrome: 53.
— differential diagnosis of paroyxsmal tachycardia: 214.
— infective causes: 164.
— respiratory distress: 117, **119-220.**
PNEUMOTHORAX: **140-141.**
— as cause of respiratory distress: 117.

355

— supplements: 234, 235.
Vitamin B1
— in metabolic disease: 226.
Vitamin B12
— in metabolic disease: 226.
Vitamin D
— ? causing hypercalcaemia: 19.
— routine administration: 234.
Vitamin E
— deficiency: 234.
— not given routinely: 236.
Vitamin K
— causing jaundice: 19, 306.
— deficiency: 207, 209.
— routine administration: 76.
Volvulus: 192, 194, 196.
VOMITING: **192-197.**
— congenital adrenal hyperplasia: 64, 192.
— drug withdrawal: 15, 222.
— galactosaemia: 226.
— heart failure: 213.
— infections: 163.
— metabolic disease: 226.
— regurgitation of feeds: 80.
— transfer to Special Care Nursery: 45.

**W**
Weighing: 77, 233.
Weight (see also Birthweight).
Weight gain

— discharge from hospital: 235.
— excessive: 213, 233.
— pre-term babies: 233.
Weight loss
— congenital thyrotoxicosis: 10.
— infective diarrhoea: 201.
— in pre-term infants: 233.
— in the baby who 'goes off': 240.
— parenteral infections: 163.
Werdnig-Hoffman disease: (187).
Wharton's jelly: 30.
Wilson-Mikity syndrome: 117, 238.

**X**
Xanthochromia: 183.
Xiphisternum — prominent: 79.
X-rays (see Radiology).

**Z**
Zygosity: 69.

**Final acknowledgements**
We are greatly indebted to our secretaries, Miss M. Middleton, Miss M. Hayter, Mrs. C. Souter, Mrs. M. Bayno and Mrs. L. Milner, for all the trouble they have taken and talent they have shown in typing the manuscript. We are also very appreciative of the patience, interest and skill of the printers.

# Name Index